LH-RH and its Analogues
Fertility and Antifertility Aspects

New Developments in Biosciences 1

W DE G
Walter de Gruyter
Berlin · New York 1985

LH-RH and its Analogues
Fertility and Antifertility Aspects

Editor
Manfred Schmidt-Gollwitzer †

Co-Editor
Rosemarie Schley

W
DE
G
Walter de Gruyter
Berlin · New York 1985

Editor
Prof. Dr. med. Manfred Schmidt-Gollwitzer †

Co-Editor
Rosemarie Schley
c/o Schering AG
Müllerstr. 170–178
D-1000 Berlin 65

This book contains 174 illustrations and 54 tables

Library of Congress Cataloging in Publication Data

Main entry under title:

LH-RH and its analogues.

(New developments in biosciences ; 1)
Proceedings of an international workshop held in 1983 and sponsored by Schering AG, Berlin.
1. Luteinizing hormone releasing hormone–Analogs–Physiological effect–Congresses. 2. Fertility, Effect of drugs on–Congresses. I. Schmidt-Gollwitzer, Manfred, 1942-1984. II. Schley, Rosemarie, 1938- III. Schering A.G. IV. Title: LH-RH and its analogues. V. Series. [DNLM: 1. Fertility–drug effects–congresses. 2. LH-FSH Releasing Hormone–analogs & derivatives–congresses. 3. LH-FSH Releasing Hormone–physiology–congresses. W3 NE865 v.l / WK 515 L6912 1983]
QP572.L85L45 1985 · 599'.016 85-6729
ISBN 0-89925-031-9 (U.S.)

CIP-Kurztitelaufnahme der Deutschen Bibliothek

LH-RH and its analogues : fertility and antifertility aspects / ed. Manfred Schmidt-Gollwitzer. Co-ed. Rosemarie Schley. – Berlin ; New York : de Gruyter, 1985.
(New developments in biosciences ; 1)
ISBN 3-11-010055-X

NE: Schmidt-Gollwitzer, Manfred [Hrsg.]; GT

3 11 010055 X Walter de Gruyter · Berlin · New York
0-89925-031-9 Walter de Gruyter, Inc., New York

Opening remarks

On behalf of Schering AG I would like to cordially welcome you to our Berlin headquarters. We have been looking forward to this meeting and trust that we shall be able to contribute to the scientific success of this International Workshop on LH-RH agonists and antagonists.

Since the isolation, structural analysis, and synthesis of the hypothalamic LH-/FSH-releasing hormone in 1971, the progress made in this particular field of research has been remarkable. Synthetic analogues have been developed and extensively studied in basic biological and preclinical experiments as well as in clinical trials covering a broad range of possible diagnostic and therapeutic applications. The scientific literature has already achieved an impressive volume and it appears that the number of conferences and expert meetings on this subject is also becoming conspiciously high.

One may therefore ask whether such a meeting like the one which we are about to start is really needed. I think the answer is a clear-cut "yes". Nowadays scientific data are generated at a breathtaking speed on an international level and need to be evaluated and re-evaluated at close intervals and the accumulated knowledge must be sifted and edited by the relevant experts. If this were left undone, then one couldn't help but underline a statement made by the great Russian poet Tolstoj who once said "What is called science today consists of a haphazard heap of information, united by nothing". Personally I much prefer to adopt Herbert Spencer's opinion that "science is organized knowledge". It is in this sense that I welcome our workshop and think that it is needed.

Concluding my address I would like to draw your attention to a more technical feature of this workshop, i. e. the mode of publication of its transactions. As some of you may know, Schering used to publish quite a number of reports and outstanding scientific symposia and workshops in a series of books headlined "Advances in the Biosciences".

The first volume of this series appeared in 1967 with the transactions of an International Symposium on "Advances in Endocrinology" which was held in honor of a pharmacologist of world-wide fame, Professor Karl Junkmann, former head of Schering's main laboratories in Berlin.

The "Biosciences" were very well accepted by the scientific community and very soon they became an internationally much wanted source of information. The last volume was issued in 1975, and since then we have been continuously asked – for not to say pressed – to resume the publication of the results of important symposia and workshops in this way. We are now prepared to follow these requests and, making use of the opportunity as offered by the present workshop, shall publish its transactions as another volume within this series. I hope you will be pleased by this decision.

Once again, ladies and gentlemen, welcome to Berlin. The workshop is now open and I would like to call on Professor Zander for his opening remarks.

Berlin, October 1983 G. Laudahn

Opening remarks

Having been honoured with the task of presenting some opening remarks to this workshop, I gave the subject of opening remarks some thought and came to the conclusion that it is difficult or even impossible to find any good definition for them. I will therefore confine myself to one or two general aspects of the subject:

1. With regard to the time taken up, they should be as short as possible. This can be demonstrated by two examples.
   The first example comes from Berlin. Adolph v. Menzel was a great painter who lived here during the last century. It is said that he was asked on a very official occasion to make an opening address. He accepted and when he came slowly to the podium everybody in the audience respectfully waited for what he had to say. – All he said was – "Möge" – which could be freely translated as "Let us hope . . ." – and left the podium.
   The second example comes from an old friend and famous endocrinologist. Years ago, after about an hour of opening remarks for a symposium, as his last opening remark he finally quoted Goethe, with two words "mehr Licht", meaning "more light", adding that Goethe is reported to have said these words just before he died.
2. A second aspect of opening addresses is that the person who is asked to make them can basically say anything he wants. This is wonderful. He can talk about the weather, about the nice people who have sponsored and organized the meeting or about the pleasant surroundings. And he can also talk about the important things he has done in life, taking care that his personal contributions to science are not forgotten.
3. A final aspect is that the speaker is allowed to say things everybody in the auditory already knows. In our case for example, that research on the chemical structure, physiology and pharmacology of LH-RH and its analogues belongs to the great achievements in the endocrinology of reproduction of the last ten years. A further example, directed more at the future is that we are looking forward to learning new facts during this workshop on the chemistry, pharmacology and clinical use of LH-RH analogues.

In summarizing my thoughts regarding opening remarks, I came to the conclusion that a combination of the one word of Adolph von Menzel and the two words of Goethe may be an acceptable solution to the problem, namely: "Möge . . ." or let us hope that we all enjoy this workshop and "mehr Licht" or "more light" . . . which does not need any explanation.

Munich, October 1983 J. Zander

Contents

Physiological basis for clinical use of LH-RH and its analogues

H. M. Fraser

Introduction

Luteinizing hormone releasing hormone (LH-RH) is the most important signal from the brain controlling the synthesis and release of luteinizing hormone (LH) and follicle stimulating hormone (FSH) from the pituitary gland and hence ovarian and testicular function. The structural characterisation of LH-RH as a decapeptide, pyro Glu-His-Trp-Ser-Tyr-Gly-Leu-Arg-Pro-Gly NH_2 [1, 2] rapidly led to the synthesis of the molecule. The development of antagonistic and agonistic analogues of LH-RH and production of antibodies to neutralize its action has helped us understand its physiological role (fig. 1). This manipulation of LH-RH has led to improved methods of both stimulating and inhibiting fertility as well as providing new therapy for diseases involving the pituitary gonadal axis (fig. 1).

The nature of the LH-RH signal

It has been known since the early 1970s that LH is released in a pulsatile manner in a large number of species investigated induding man [3–7]. Since LH-RH is secreted by neurones it was assumed that LH-RH discharge was of a pulsatile nature forming a one-to-one relationship with pulses of LH. Effects of immunoneutralization of LH-RH in the rat and sheep gave strong support to this concept [8–11]. Intravenous injection of antibodies to LH-RH causes an immediate cessation of pulsatile release of LH indicating that the pulses are totally dependent on a stimulus from hypothalamic LH-RH immediately preceding them (fig. 2). Because of the technical difficulties of simultaneous measurement of LH-RH in hypophysial portal blood and LH in peripheral blood this relationship has been difficult to establish. Recently, this problem has been overcome and the relationship established in unanesthetized sheep [12, 13] (fig. 3).

It is generally accepted that LH-RH is the single releasing hormone responsible for LH and FSH release, although claims for isolation of a separate FSH-RH continue [14]. Injection of antibodies to LH-RH show how the rapid cessation of LH release contrasts with the considerably less marked effect on FSH [8, 11, 15]. This cannot be

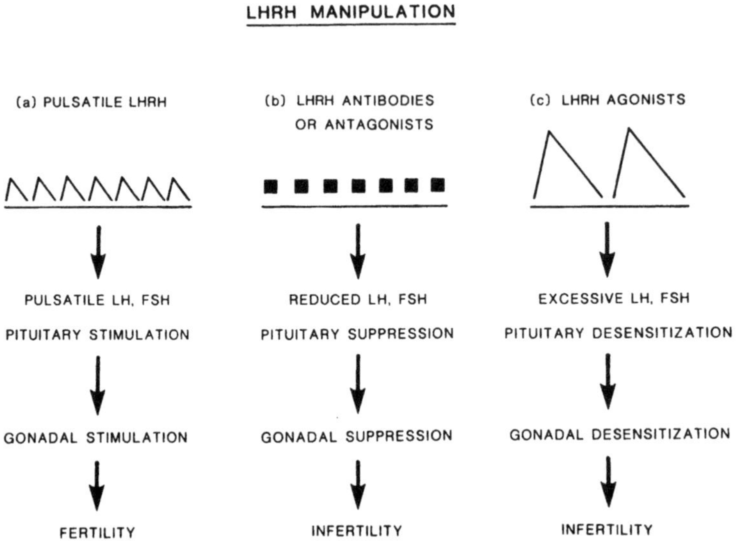

Fig. 1 Scheme illustrating how (a) pituitary-gonadal function is stimulated by regular pulses of LHRH from the hypothalamus or when LHRH is administered in this manner to treat hypogonadotrophic hypogonadism. Conversely (b) LHRH action is prevented by neutralization by antibodies or by blocking the LHRH receptor by chemical antagonists. This results in suppression of gonadotrophin release and, if maintained, to infertility. LHRH agonists (c) given by daily administration or continuous infusion, initially cause pituitary and gonadal stimulation but when the natural hormonal patterns are overridden in this way pituitary-gonadal desensitization occurs.

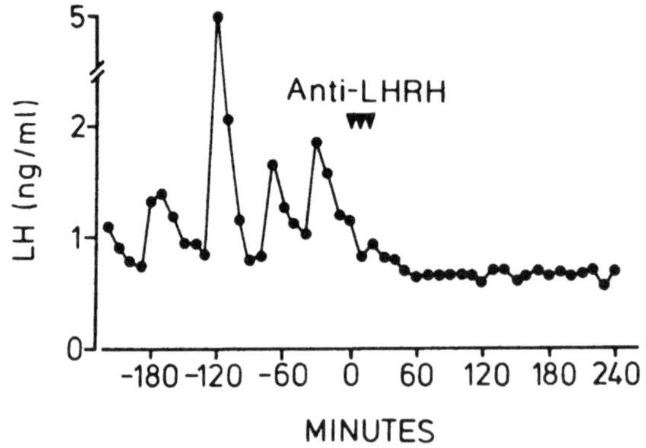

Fig. 2 Effect of intravenous injection of antibodies to LHRH on pulsatile release of LH in the ewe. (From [11].)

fully explained by differences in the half-lives of the 2 hormones and probably reflects differences in control of release at the pituitary level, FSH being subject to greater selective negative control by gonadal steroids or inhibin. Perhaps the most convincing evidence we have for LH-RH controlling both pituitary hormones is the

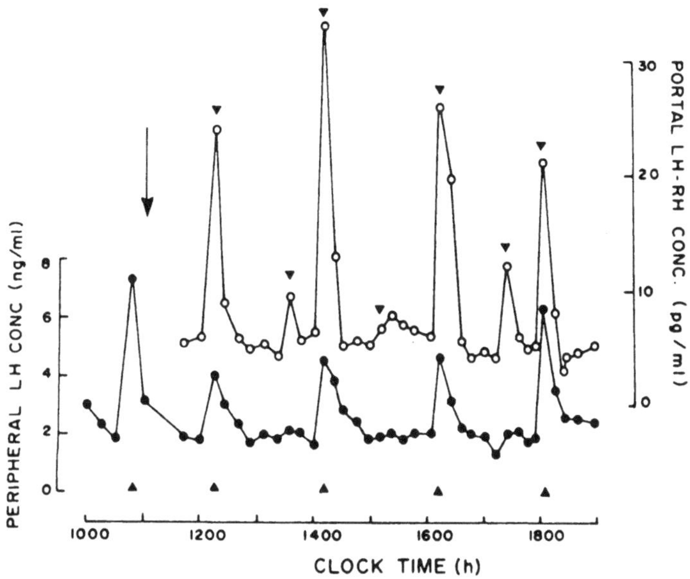

Fig. 3 Concentration of LHRH (0) in hypothalamo-hypophysial portal blood and LH (●) in peripheral blood of an ovariectomized ewe. The arrow (↓) indicates the time the portal vessels were cut. Note close relationship between LHRH pulses (▼) and LH pulses (▲). (From [12].)

fact that repeated pulsatile administration of the decapeptide in humans with LH-RH deficiency (see below) or in experimental animals with low output of endogenous LH-RH, full pituitary and gonadal function can be expressed.

Role of LH-RH during the menstrual cycle

Follicular phase

While measurement of changes in LH-RH pulse frequency at different stages of the menstrual cycle in primates has yet to be achieved, we can imply from measurement of serum LH pulses in the monkey and human during the follicular phase that LH-RH is discharged at a rate of one pulse every 60–90 min [16, 17]. Neutralization of LH-RH by active or passive immunization blocks LH pulses and leads to a reduction in oestradiol secretion from the developing follicle in rats [18, 19], hamsters [20], sheep and monkeys [15, 21].

Despite knowledge of the rate of LH pulses, the early use of LH-RH to stimulate follicular growth in amenorrheoic patients with defective LH-RH secretion did not take this physiological mode into account, perhaps because of the previous use of "unphysiological" gonadotrophin preparations for this purpose. Thus, when LH-RH was administered 3 times daily the number of ovulatory cycles which were induced was unsatisfactory [22].

One of the major influences in the recognition of the need for mimicking the physiological mode of LH-RH release came from studies on replacement of LH-RH in rhesus monkeys in whom LH-RH secretion was blocked by lesions in the medal basal hypothalamus [23–25]. Successful re-initiation of ovulatory cycles was optimally achieved by replacing uniform LH-RH pulses at a rate of every 60–90 min [26]. Longer intervals or infusions were unsuccessful [26, 27]. During recent years application of this approach to treat amenorrheoic women by delivering LH-RH by means of programmed pumps has become widespread and is highly effective in inducing fertile ovulatory cycles [28, 29].

The LH-RH agonists, originally developed to treat hypogonadotrophic hypogonadism by means of long-lived pituitary stimulation were theoretically defunct for this purpose. Indeed, early studies in women receiving repeated injections demonstrated decreased pituitary responsiveness [30]. While use of agonists to stimulate fertility has been virtually abandoned such observations led to the observation that repeated agonist administration to cycling women during the follicular phase prevented ovulation [31]. Studies on experimental animals receiving chronic high dose administration of LH-RH or its agonists had previously demonstrated an impairment of a number of reproductive functions [32–34] and these studies led to observations of suppression of ovulation in monkeys after daily agonist administration during the follicular phase [35]. Continued agonist administration maintained the suppressive effect on ovulation in women and monkeys [36–41] leading to a new approach to contraception devoid of the metabolic effects of steroids [42, 43].

The mechanism of the antifertility effects of the agonists are believed to involve 1. pituitary desensitization and 2. attenuation of the ability of oestrogen to induce an LH surge [35, 44, 45] down regulation of the follicle by abnormal exposure to gonadotrophin [46, 47] and 3. a direct ovarian effect of the agonist [48]. There may be species differences in these mechanisms. For example, daily agonist injections in rats stops oestrous cycles, but in contrast to the primate, the ovaries consist of a preponderance of luteal tissue [49, 50]. Also while LH-RH receptors of high affinity are present on the rat ovary to mediate the direct effects of LH-RH on steroidogenesis, binding sites of low affinity are present in the human ovary [51, 52] making similar direct action of LH-RH agonists from doses administered for contraception unlikely.

One problem in using continuous daily LH-RH agonist to prevent ovulation has been the individual variations in response with regard to serum concentrations of oestradiol, and hence follicular growth. Thus some monkeys and women respond with low oestrogen production while others have marked fluctuations in oestradiol suggesting waves of follicular development in the absence of ovulation [36–41]. We do not know whether these differences are related to differences in pattern of gonadotrophin output and whether these follicles are being driven by the gonadotrophins induced by the agonist or by more normal pulses of endogenous gonadotrophins occurring betwen agonist administrations. It also needs to be established if over- riding endogenous gonadotrophin secretion further by several agonist administrations during the day, or by constant infusion, is more effective in suppressing ovarian function. If we are to use LH-RH agonist regimens more effectively to suppress ovarian function more work must be done to elucidate these mechanisms. Problems in controlling follicular development during continuous daily agonist treatment have led to dissatisfaction in some quarters concerning the acceptability of this regime for contraception. There is concern that complete suppression of follicular development with low oestrogen production would lead to menopausal symptoms, while fluctuations in follicular development would cause unacceptable irregular bleeding and risks of "unopposed" oestrogen. This has lead to investigation of more complex treatment regimens such as intermittent high dose exposure during critical stages of follicular development [53, 54] or agonist treatment followed by progestagen supplementation to control bleeding [55]. Thus, while suppression of ovulation by LH-RH agonist can undoubtedly act as a contraceptive we still have to decide on the optimal approach in utilising this property.

The development of potent LH-RH antagonists for clinical use will provide a unique opportunity of studying the effects of selective gonadotrophin deprivation at different stages of follicular development in women. Application for contraception and therapeutic suppression of ovarian steroidogenesis may require higher doses than LH-RH agonists, but because the mechanism of action involves a relatively simple receptor blockade at the pituitary, responses may be more uniform.

Role of LH-RH during the mid-cycle LH surge

As the follicle developes, the rising concentrations of oestradiol in the blood reaches a critical concentration which triggers the LH surge. This may be brought about by an increased secretion of LH-RH together with an increase in pituitary responsiveness. While the latter effect is well established, difficulties in measuring hypopysial portal blood concentrations of LH-RH have helped to raise controversy over its role during the period of the LH surge in the primate (fig. 4)

In the rat, measurement of LH-RH in the hypophysial portal blood has revealed a clear rise in LH-RH co-incident with the LH surge [56, 57]. The dependence of the pre-ovulatory LH surge on the presence of LH-RH during this period in the rat, hamster and sheep is revealed by the ability of injection of LH-RH antibodies or LH-RH antagonists, only a few hours prior to the expected time of the LH surge, to block it and prevent ovulation [15, 20, 59, 61].

Measurement of LH-RH in the hypophysial portal blood or primates during an LH surge has obvious problems. While early data indicated an increased LH-RH concentration [62] other experiments detracted from the importance of LH-RH in inducing an LH surge, suggesting the oestrogen-induced increased pituitary respon-

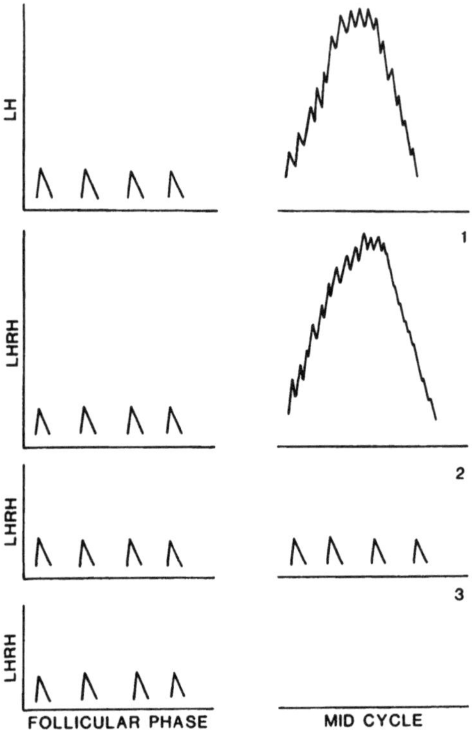

Fig. 4 Schematic diagram to illustrate the alternative patterns of LHRH release for driving LH pulses during the follicular phase of the cycle and during the mid-cycle LH surge. In the follicular phase, a simple one-to-one relationship exists. During the LH surge an LHRH surge may also occur as in the rat (1), but in primates and LHRH surge can be achieved by uniform pulses of LHRH (2) or may be without LHRH (3) provided there has been previous LHRH priming and the correct quota of oestradiol.

siveness was all that was required. For example, LH-RH antibodies were unable to block the LH surge in macaque monkeys despite the fact that they were active in blocking follicular development when injected during the early follicular phase and could suppress gonadotrophin levels in ovariectomised animals [15, 63]. Studies by Knobil's group in monkeys in whom endogenous LH-RH secretion was blocked by lesions in the medial basal hypothalamus showed that an unvarying input of exogenous LH-RH could induce an LH surge suggesting that LH-RH had only a "permissive" role in this regard [23–26]. Furthermore, stopping LH-RH injections 24h prior to oestrogen injection still resulted in an LH surge which led these authors to call oestrogen "a GnRH" [64]. This was supported by studies on rhesus monkeys in which the pituitary stalk was disconected and a silastic barrier inserted between the hypothalamus and pituitary but a positive feedback could still be demonstrated if oestrogen were administered immediately afterwards [65]. These results suggest that in the primate, in contrast to rodents and sheep, there is a "fail-safe" mechanism for inducing an LH surge which can operate for at least a day by the action of oestrogen on a pituitary gland previously exposed to appropriate LH-RH priming.

This conclusion has recently been challenged by Norman et al. [66] on the basis that all endogenous LH-RH had not been eliminated in these models.

What of the physiological situation? Following on the principal of a one-to-one relationship between LH pulses and LH-RH pulses, then the high pulse frequency towards the time of the LH surge in monkeys and in women [16, 17, 67] would clearly implicate LH-RH pulses as the driving force prior to and during the LH surge. Two recent experiments support an active hypothalamic component during the LH surge. Using push-pull cannulae LH-RH has recently been shown to increase during the ostrogen-induced LH surge in ovariectomized monkeys [68]. Also, injection of a potent LH-RH antagonist prevented the LH surge in ovariectomized monkeys [69], a feat which has been difficult to demonstrate with previously tested weaker antagonists.

As far as the clinical application of this information is concerned, it seems that for the induction of an LH surge in ovulation in hypogonadal patients, an unvarying pulsatile LH-RH stimulation will suffice [28, 29]. Conversely, while the new antagonists might be used to block the LH surge, this late interuption of follicular development may not be a viable contraceptive approach because of the "unopposed" oestrogen which would ensue. Antagonist administration would be preferable at an early stage of follicular growth.

While the evidence that pulses of LH-RH during gonadotrophin secretion induces follicular development is very convincing, it should also be noted that under certain conditions constant low dose infusions of LH-RH can also induce successfull development and ovulation [70].

LH-RH and luteal function

The role of LH-RH, or the gonadotrophins, in control of the corpus luteum in the primate and in women is incompletely understood and the variety of approaches used to investigate its dependence on the gonadotrophins have produced some conflicting results. One complicating factor is due to the likelihood that the LH produced by the mid-cycle surge alone can maintain luteal function for several days [71, 72]. Pituitary LH pulses (hence LH-RH pulses) occur at a considerably reduced frequency during the luteal phase [16], presumably as a result of negative feedback action of progesterone on the hypothalamus. This would suggest 2 phases of gonadotrophin support, an initial "free running" period after the LH surge, followed by continued independence or maintainance by infrequent LH pulses.

Evidence for independent luteal function is provided by recent observations in rhesus monkeys either hypophysectomised [73] one day after ovulation or treated with

LH-RH antagonist throughout the luteal phase [74]. Both approaches resulted in normal luteal function.

In contrast, administration of antiserum to hCG in an attempt to neutralize LH in monkeys on days 15–18 of the cycle caused a shortening of cycle length [75]. In agreement with the concept of LH dependence of the corpus luteum, in a few isolated incidens in which hypogonadotrophic women have had ovulation induced by LH-RH only to be followed by failure of the delivery pump during the luteal phase, the corpus luteum has ceased to function [28]. This situation has recently been tested experimentally in rhesus monkeys with lesions in the medial basal hypothalamus [76]. Once ovulatory cycles were restored by pulsatile administration of LH-RH, the effects of discontinuing LH-RH were observed. When the infusion was stopped during the early luteal phase there was a gradual premature decline in plasma progesterone levels and menses occurred 5–8 days later. When LH-RH infusion was continued until the mid luteal phase then stopped, plasma progesterone concentrations fell markedly to non detectable levels within the first day. These results suggest that the corpus luteum is dependent on LH-RH and hence LH but is more susceptible to LH withdrawal by the mid-luteal phase, by which time the stimulatory effects of the LH surge have subsided.

It is well established that high doses of LH-RH or its agonists can have a deleterious effect on the corpus luteum in monkeys and in women. It is of interest that single injections are ineffective during the early luteal phase but are luteolytic when injected after the mid-luteal phase [77, 78]. One mechanism for this inhibitory effect may be a reduction in releasable LH after the initial stimulation.

While the above results are difficult to reconcile with the studies suggesting independent luteal function, it does seem that during pulsatile LH-RH treatment for induction of fertility that LH-RH pulses should be maintained during the luteal phase or replaced by hCG to produce long-acting support for the corpus luteum. While a luteolytic agent has been a popular target for contraceptive developers, the effects of LH-RH agonists during the normal cycle are, alas, overriden by hCG [79, 80], suggesting the approach would be unsuccessful if conception occurred.

The recent availability of highly potent LH-RH antagonists will provide a much needed additional approach for studying the LH-RH and gonadotrophin dependency of the corpus luteum during different stages of the luteal phase as well as providing a further line of attack against the corpus luteum of early pregnancy.

LH-RH in the male

Measurement of secretion patterns of LH-RH in the male has received little attention, but from studies on passive immunization against LH-RH we can assume that a similar relationship between LH-RH and LH pulses exists as in the female [8, 10]. Chronic neutralization of LH-RH by active immunization has been studied in detail in a variety of experimental animals from rats to primates. It leads to reduction in pituitary content of LH and FSH and reduced numbers of LH-RH receptors; reduced serum levels of LH, FSH and testosterone; decreased LH binding to Leydig cells and a drastic suppression of their steroidogenic capacity involution of seminal vesicles and prostate; suppression of spermatogenesis; and a reduction in agression and mating behaviour [81–84].

Conversely, in rams during the inactive phase of the breeding season when testicular function is suppressed due to low gonadotrophin (LH-RH) stimulation, then pulsatile administration can reactivate LH and FSH release and increase testosterone secretion [85]. Furthermore, in men with LH-RH deficiency, pulses of LH-RH delivered at 60–90 min intervals causes an increase in serum testosterone, formation of secondary sexual characteristics, restoration of testicular function and potential fertility [86].

For contraception in men it is desirable to suppress FSH to prevent spermatogenesis but leave LH stimulation testosterone production via the Leydig cell intact in order to conserve potency etc. From what we know about the effects of active immunization against LH-RH, and from studies in rats with LH-RH antagonists it is likely that suppression of LH-RH activity in this way would fail to dissociate between these effects [94]. Chronic administration of LH-RH agonists either by injections or by constant infusion or long-acting preparations also have inhibitory effects on the male reproductive system [87, 88] although there is a range of susceptibility according to species [89, 90] and with age. The mechanism of these effects is thought to involve pituitary desensitization followed by down regulation of Leydig cell function leading to suppression of spermatogenesis [91]. It is also established in the rat that LH-RH agonists, even in nanogram doses, have significant effects on testicular steroidogenesis, causing stimulation during the first day of exposure, thereafter becoming inhibitory [92]. Insufficient studies have been performed on the primate or human testis to determine if similar changes occur but it does appear that while the Leydig cells of the rat posses high affinity receptors for LH-RH through which these effects can be mediated [93], such receptors have not been demonstrated on the human Leydig cell [52]. Preliminary studies on the inhibitory effects of chronic administration of LH-RH agonists in men indicated that sperm numbers could be markedly reduced, but since this was accompanied by suppressed testosterone it also led to decreased libido and impotence [87]. The prospects for male contraception via LH-RH manipulation serum seem to be dependent on the acceptability and efficacy of testosterone replacement to maintain libido and potency. We also do not know the answer to the fundamental question of how far sperm numbers need to be suppressed for infertility [95].

References

[1] Matsuo, H., Y. Bata, R. M. G. Nair et al.: Biochem. Biophys. Res. Cummun. **43** (1971) 1334–1339.
[2] Guillemin, R.: Contraception 5 (1972) 1–19.
[3] Gay, V. L., V. A. Sheth; Endocrinology **90** (1982) 158–162.
[4] Yen, S. S. C., C. C. Tsai, F. Naftolin et al.: J. Clin Endocr. Metab. **34** (1972) 671–676.
[5] Stanten, R. J., C. W. Bardin: J. Clin Invest. **52** (1973) 2617–2628.
[6] Lincoln, G. A.: Nature **252** (1974) 232–233.
[7] Lincoln, G. A.: J. Endocr. **69** (1976) 213–226.
[8] Lincoln, G. A.., H. M. Fraser: Biol. Reprod. **21** (1979) 1239–1245.
[9] Snabes, M. C., R. P. Kelch: Neuroendocrinology **29** (1979) 34–41.
[10] Ellis, G. B., C. Desjardins, H. M. Fraser: Neuroendocrinology **37** (1983) 177–183.
[11] Fraser, H. M., A. S. McNeilly: J. Reprod. Fert. **69** (1983) 569–577.
[12] Clarke, I. J., J. T. Cummins: Endocrinology **111** (1982) 1737–1739
[13] Levine, J. E., K. Y. F. Pau, V. D. Ramirez, et al.: Endocrinology, **111** (1982) 1149–1455.
[14] McCann, S. M.: Present status of LH-RH: its physiology and pharmacology. In: Role of peptides and proteins in control of reproduction, pp. 3–26. (Eds. S. M. McCann, D. S. Dhindsa). Elsevier Biomedical, New York 1983.
[15] Fraser, H. M., A. S. McNeilly, R. M. Popkin: Passive immunization against LH-RH: elucidation of the role of LH-RH in controlling LH and FSH secretion and LH-RH receptors. In: Immunological Aspects of Reproduction in Mammals (Ed. B. Crighton). Butterworths, 1984.
[16] Backstrom, C. T., A. S. McNeilly, R. M. Leask, et al.: Clinical Endocrinology **17** (1982) 29–42.
[17] Marut, E. L., R. F. Williams, B. D. Cowan et al.: Endocrinology, **109** (1981) 2270–2272.
[18] Fraser, H. M., A. Gunn: Nature, **244** (1973) 160–161.
[19] Popkin, R., H. M. Fraser: Molec. Cell. Endocr. (1983).
[20] de la Cruz, A., A. Arimura, K. G. de la Cruz et al.: Endocrinology, **98** (1976) 490–497.
[21] McNeilly, A. S., H. M. Fraser, D. T. Baird; J. Endocr. (1984).
[22] Nillius, S. J.: Gonadotropin-releasing hormone for induction of ovulation in women. In: Human Ovulation, pp. 385–404. (Ed. E. S. E. Hafez). Elsevier North-Holland Biomedical Press, 1979.
[23] Knobil, E.: Rec. Prog. Horm. Res. **36** (1980) 53–88.
[24] Wildt, L., A. Hausler, G. Marshall et al.: Endocrinology **109** (1981) 376–385.
[25] Knobil, E., T. M. Plant, L. Widt et al.: Science, N. Y., **207** (1980) 1371–1373.
[26] Pohl, C. R., D. W. Richardson, J. S. Hutchison et al.: Endocrinology **112** (1983) 2076–2080.
[27] Belchetz, P. E., T. M. Plant, Y. Nakai et al.: Science, N. Y. **202** (1978) 631–633.
[28] Leydendecker, G., L. Wildt: J. Reprod. Fert. **69** (1983) 397–409.
[29] Skarin, G., S. J. Nillius, L. Wide: Fertil Steril **40** (1983) 454–460.
[30] Dericks-Tan, J. S. E., E. Hammer, H. D. Taubert: J. Clin Endocrinol. Metab. **45** 597–600.
[31] Nillius, S. J., C. Bergquist, L. Wide: Contraception **17** (1978) 537–545.
[32] Johnson, E. S., R. L. Gendrich, W. F. Withe; Fertil. Steril. **27** (1976) 853–860.
[33] Corbin, A., C. W. Beatie: Endocr. Res. Commun. **2** (1975) 445–458.
[34] Banik, U. K., M. Givner: J. Reprod. Fert. **44** (1975) 87–94.
[35] Fraser, H. M., N. C. Laird, D. M. Blakeley: Endocrinology **106** (1980) 452–457.
[36] Fraser, H. M.: Endocrinology, **112** (1983) 245–253.
[37] Vickery, B. H.: Female contraceptive potential of "super" agonists of LH-RH as assessed in infrahuman primates. In: LH-RH peptides as male and female contraceptives, pp. 338–354. (Ed. G. Zatuchni). Lippincoltt, USA 1982.
[38] Bergquist, C., S. J. Nillius, L. Wide: Lancet **II** (1979) 215–217.

[39] Bergquist, C., S. J. Nillius, L. Wide: Fertil Steril **38** (1982) 190–193.
[40] Schmidt-Gollwitzer, M., W. Hardt, K. Schmidt-Gollwitzer et al.: Contraception **23** (1981) 187–195.
[41] Schmidt-Gollwitzer, M., W. Hardt, K. Schmidt-Gollwitzer et al.: The contraceptive use of buserelin, a potent LH-RH agonist: Clinical and Hormonal Findings. In: LH-RH Peptides as Male and Female Contraceptives, pp. 199–215. (Ed. G. Zatuchni). Lippincott, USA 1982.
[42] Sandow, J., R. M. Clayton, H. Kuhl: Pharmacology of LH-RH and its analogues. In: Endocrinology of human infertility: new aspects, pp. 221–246. (Ed. P. Crossignani). Academic Press, London 1981.
[43] Sandow, J.: Clinical Endocrinology **18** (1983) 571–592.
[44] Fraser, H. M.: J. Endocr. **91** (1981) 525–530.
[45] Bergquist, C., S. J. Nillies, L. Wide: Clinical Endocrinology **16** (1982) 147–151.
[46] Friedrich, F., P. Kemeter, H. Salzer et al.: Acta Endocrinol. **78** (1975) 332–342.
[47] Cusan L., C. Auclair, A. Belanger et al.: Endocrinology **104** (1979) 1369–1376.
[48] Hsueh, A. J., P. B. C. Jones: Endocrine Reviews **2** (1981) 437–461.
[49] Sandow, J.: Gonadotropic and antigonadotropic actions of LH-RH analogues. In: Neuroendocrine Perspectives, vol. 1, pp. 339–395. (Eds. E. E. Muller, R. M. MacLeod). Elsevier Biomedical Press, Amsterdam 1982.
[50] Popkin, R. M., H. M. Fraser, R. G. Gosden: J. Reprod. Fert. **69** (1983) 245–252.
[51] Popkin, R., T. A. Bramley, A. Currie et al.: Biochem. Biophys. Res. Commun. **14** (1983) 750–756.
[52] Popkin, R., T. A. Bramley, A. Currie et al.: This volume (1984).
[53] Sheenan, K. L., R. F. Casper, S. S. C. Yen: Science **215** (1982) 170–172.
[54] Werlin, L. B., G. D. Hodgen: J. Clin. Endocr. Metab. **56** (1983) 844–848.
[55] Hardt, W., K. Schmidt-Gollwitzer, J. Nevinny-Stickel et al.: Geburtshilfe und Frauenheilkunde **42** (1982) 874–877.
[56] Sarkar, D. K., S. A. Chiappa, G. Fink et al.: Nature **264** (1976) 461–463.
[57] Levine, J. E., V. D. Ramirez: Endocrinology **111** (1982) 1449–1445.
[58] Koch, Y., P. Chobsieng, U. Zor et al.: Biochem. Biophys. Res. Commun. **55** (1973) 623–629.
[59] Fraser, H. M., A. S. McNeilly: Biol. Reprod. **27** (1982) 548–555.
[60] Schally, A. V., A. Arimura, D. H. Coy: Vit. Horm **38** (1980) 257–323.
[61] Bex, F. J., A. Corbin: Antifertility effects of LH-RH and its agonists. In: Reproductive Processes and Contraception, pp. 109–141. (Ed. K. W. McKerns). Plenum Press, New York–London 1981.
[62] Neil, J. D., J. M. Patton, R. A. Dailey et al.: Endocrinology **101** (1977) 430–434.
[63] McCormack, J. T., T. M. Plant, D. L. Hess et al.: Endocrinology **100** (1977) 663–667.
[64] Wildt, L., A. Hausler, J. S. Hutchinson et al.: Endocrinology **108** (1981) 2011–2013.
[65] Ferin, M., H. Rosenblatt, P. W. Carmel et al.: Endocrinology **104** (1979) 50–52.
[66] Norman, R. L., P. Gliessmann, S. A. Lindstrom et al.: Endocrinology **111** (1982) 1874–1882.
[67] Djahanbakhch, O., P. Warner, A. S. McNeilly et al.: submitted.
[68] Levine, J. E., H. G. Spies: Abstract 37. Meeting of Society for the Study of Reproduction, (1983).
[69] Asch, R. H., J. P. Balmaceda, M. R. Borghi et al.:J. Clin. Endocr. Metab. **57** (1983) 367–372.
[70] McLeod, B. J., W. Haresign, G. E. Lamming, J. Reprod. Fert. **68** (1983) 489–495.
[71] Varde Wiele, R. L., J. Bogmil, I. Dyrenfurth et al.: Recent. Prog. Horm. Res. **26** (1979) 63–104.
[72] Asch, R. H., M. Abou-Samra, G. D. Braunstein et al.: J. Clin Endocr. Metab. **55** (1982) 154–161.
[73] Balmaceda, J. P., M. R. Borghi, D. H. Coy et al.: J. Clin. endocr. Metab. **57** (1983) 866–868.
[74] Moudgal, N. R., G. J. MacDonald, R. O. Greep: J. Clin. Endocrinol. Metab. **35** (1972) 113–115.
[75] Hutchinson, J. S., A. J. Zeleznik: Abstract 94. Meeting of Society for the Study of Reproduction, (1983).

[76] Casper, R. F., S. S. C. Yen: Science **205** (1979) 408–410.
[77] Lemay, A., F. Labrie, A. Belanger et al.: Fertil. Steril. **32** (1979) 646–51.
[78] Casper, R. F., S. S. C. Yen; Science **205** (1979) 408–410.
[79] Casper, R. F., K. L. Sheehan, S. S. C. Yen: Contraception **21** (1980) 471–478.
[80] Bergquist, C., S. J. Nillius, L. Wide; (1980) Contraception **22** (1980) 341–348.
[81] Fraser, H. M., R. M. Popkin, A. S. McNeilly et al.: Mol. Cell. Endocrinol. **28** (1982) 321–331.
[82] Fraser, H. M., R. M. Sharpe, G. A. Lincoln et al.: LH-RH antibodies: Their use in the study of hypothalamic LH-RH and testicular LH-RH-like material and possible contraceptive applications. In: Progress Towards a Male Contraceptive. (Eds. S. L. Jeffcoate, M. Sandler). John Wiley & Sons. Ltd. 1982.
[83] Chappel, S. C., W. E. Ellinwood, C. Huckins et al.: Biol. Reprod. **22** (1980) 333–342.
[84] Lincoln, G. A., H. M. Fraser, T. J. Fletcher: J. Reprod. Fert. **66** (1982) 703–708.
[85] Lincoln, G. A., R. V. Short: Recent Prog. Horm. Res. **36** (1980) 1–52.
[86] Hoffman, A. R., W. F. Crowley: N. Engl. J. Med. **307** (1982) 1237–1241.
[87] Linde, R., G. C. Doelle, N. Alexander et al.: N. Engl. J. Med. **305** (1981) 663–667.
[88] Bint Akhtar, F., G. R. Marshall, E. J. Wickings et al.: J. Clin Endocr. Metab. **56** (1983) 534–540.
[89] Sandow, J.: Inhibition of pituitary and testicular function by LHR analogues. In: Progress Towards a Male Contraceptive pp. 19–40. (Ed. S. L. Jeffcoate, M. Sandler). John Wiley & Sons, Chichester 1982.
[90] Wickings, E. J., P. Zaidi, E. Nieschlag: J. Androl **2** (1981) 72–79.
[91] Labrie, F., A. Belanger, L. Cusan et al.: J. Androl, **1** (1980 209–228.
[92] Sharpe, R. M., D. G. Doogan, I. Cooper: Molec. Cell. Endocrinol. **32** (1983) 57–71.
[93] Sharpe, R. M., H. M. Fraser: Biochem. Biophys. Res. Commun. **95** (1980) 256–262.
[94] Rivier, C., J. Rivier, N. Vale: Endocrinology **108** (1981) 1998–2001.
[95] Nieschlag, E., M. H. Clazi: Perspectives and prospectives in male fertility control. In: Progress Towards a Male Contraceptive, pp. 245–250. (Ed. S. L. Jeffcoate, M. Sandler). John Wiley & Sons, Chichester 1982.

Hypothalamic control of gonadotropin secretion and ovarian function

L. Wildt, G. Leyendecker

Introduction

The concept that the neural control of gonadotropin secretion is mediated by gonadotropin releasing hormone (GnRH) discharged from the hypothalamus into the pituitary portal circulation and that ovarian hormones, in turn, regulate the secretion of gonadotropic hormones via negative and positive feedback loops has evolved from the pioneering work performed by Harris and Hohlweg and Junkmann more than four decades ago. Since then, studies in experimental animals and women have provided further insights into the functioning of the neuroendocrine control system that governs the ovarian cycle. In the course of these studies, salient differences became apparent between the mechanisms that direct the estrous cycle of laboratory rodents and those which govern the menstrual cycle of higher primates [1]. While in the rat neural mechanisms that link chronobiological signals and steroid levels to GnRH release play a critical role in the control of gonadotropin secretion and the timing of ovulation, such mechanisms seem not to be essential in primates, and hypothalamic GnRH secretion appears to be but a permissive component of the control system governing gonadotropin secretion and ovarian function during the menstrual cycle [2, 3, 4]. Experimental evidence derived from studies on the physiology and pathology of the human ovarian cycle and from therapeutic use of GnRH for induction of ovulation in hypothalamic failure suggests that this concept, which has been developed by Ernst Knobil and his colleagues in the rhesus monkey, may apply likewise to the human female [5, 6, 7]. The following chapter represents a brief summary of findings pertinent in this regard.

Hypothalamic control of gonadotropin secretion

The secretion of gonadotropic hormones from the pituitary gland is a rhythmic, pulsatile phenomenon. This was first recognized in the ovariectomized rhesus monkey and subsequently in other species, including man [8, 9, 10, 11]. Frequency of these pulses ranges from one pulse every 20 minutes in the rat to one pulse every 60–90 minutes in the agonadal human female. Because of its characteristic frequency of one pulse per hour in the monkey, this secretory pattern has been termed "circhoral" [8].

Pulsatile release of gonadotropins appears to be the consequence of pulses of GnRH discharged into the pituitary portal circulation. This view is supported by the direct observation of pulses of GnRH in the pituitary portal effluent of monkeys and sheep [12, 13] and human pituitary blood [14], and by the demonstration that antisera against GnRH block pulsatile gonadotropin release [15]. The intermittent secretion of GnRH appears to be the consequence of a synchronous discharge of GnRH-containing neurons, activated by some neuronal pulsegenerator or oscillator [3, 16]. This was suggested by the observation [2], that neuroactive drugs interrupt pulsatile LH secretion and has been substantiated by the results of recordings of multiunit-acitivity in the area of the arcuate nucleus, which have shown striking correlation between electrical activity and the inititation of LH pulses [3].

Complete isolation of the mediobasal hypothalamus (MBH) from the remainder of the brain does not interfere with pulsatile gonadotropin secretion in the rhesus monkey; the circhoral oscillator, which directs pulsatile GnRH release in this species, must therefore reside in this area of the central nervous system [17]. Within the MBH, the arcuate nucleus appears to contain the neuronal elements directing pulsatile GnRH release and to mediate hypothalamic control of gonadotropin secretion, since bilateral destruction of this nucleus by radiofrequency lesions completely abolished gonadotropin secretion [18].

The physiologic significance of pulsatile gonadotropin release did not become apparent until attempts were made to restore gonadotropin secretion in ovariectomized monkeys with hypothalamic lesions by the administration of exogenous GnRH. While continuous administration of the decapeptide was able to induce an initial increase in circulating LH and FSH levels, it failed invariably to sustain this increment. This was achieved, however, when continuous infusion was replaced by intermittent administration of GnRH with the physiologic frequency of one pulse per hour. This, and the additional observation that a shift from pulsatile to continuous mode of infusion promptly inhibited previously reestablished gonadotropin secretion, has led to the conclusion that the function of the hypothalamic control system that directs gonadotropin secretion is obligatorily intermittent and that the pattern, and not the amount, of GnRH delivered to the pituitary is of critical importance for the maintenance of gonadotropin secretion [3, 16, 19].

Frequency of hypothalamic GnRH secretion appears to play a much more important role than amplitude in this regard [20]. Increasing the frequency of pulsatile GnRH infusion from one to two or three pulses per hour led to a decline of circulating gonadotropin levels, while 5 pulses per hour completely abolished gonadotropin secretion in a manner similar to that observed during constant infusion. Decreasing the frequency of GnRH pulses from one pulse per hour to one pulse every three hours, on the other hand, was followed by a decline of LH levels and a increase of FSH concentrations, resulting in a dramatic change of the FSH/LH ratio [20].

The decline of plasma gonadotropins observed at high frequency stimulation may be related to the effect of desensitization or down-regulation, while the change of the FSH/LH ratio observed during slow frequency stimulation can be explained by an increase of the pituitary response to GnRH and by the different disappearance times of FSH and LH from the circulation. The increase in size of the LH bolus is more than matched by the time available for its disappearance. This is not the case for FSH, and this glycoprotein accumulates in the circulation. Minor changes in frequency of hypophysiotropic stimulation, therefore, not only alter the concentrations of LH and FSH, but also have major effects on their relative proportions. In contrast, major changes in amplitude of GnRH pulses have shown to posses but minor regulatory potential in the ovariectomized monkey [20].

Pulsatile gonadotropin secretion during the menstrual cycle

Amplitude and frequency of pulsatile gonadotropin secretion change in the course of the menstrual cycle. This is particularly apparent during the human menstrual cycle, where distinct pulses of LH can be detected. Earlier studies have established that the follicular phase of the cycle is characterized by high frequency, low amplitude pulses while during the luteal phase low frequency, high amplitude pulses prevail [9, 10]. The temporal aspects of this changing pattern of pulsatile gonadotropin secretion have been examined recently in women at 2–4 day intervals during different phases of the menstrual cycle or daily around the time of the midcycle surge [21, 22, 23]. Some results of these studies are shown on figure 1. Frequency of LH pulses declined progressively during the luteal phase, reaching a nadir immediately before onset of menstruation. Pulse amplitude appeared to increase during this time. Within the first days following onset of menstruation, pulse frequency increased dramatically and reached a stable plateau after 4 to 6 days. This was associated with a decrease in pulse amplitude. No further increase of LH pulse frequency was observed during the midcycle surge, but a dramatic increase of pulse amplitude occurred at this time.

Frequency of pulsatile LH secretion has shown to be reduced by progesterone, while estradiol was without effect in this regard [24, 25]. The reduction of LH pulse frequency observed during the luteal phase of the cycle may be attributed therefore to the inhibitory action of progesterone on the hypothalamic pulse generator directing gonadotropin secretion, while the increase of pulse frequency during the early follicular phase reflects withdrawal of this inhibition. The changes in frequency of pulsatile LH secretion during the entire menstrual cycle may thus be viewed as being the consequence of the changing titers of progesterone produced by the corpus luteum [23]. This view is supported by the observation that estradiol levels do not change significantly at the time around menstruation, when the most dramatic changes in

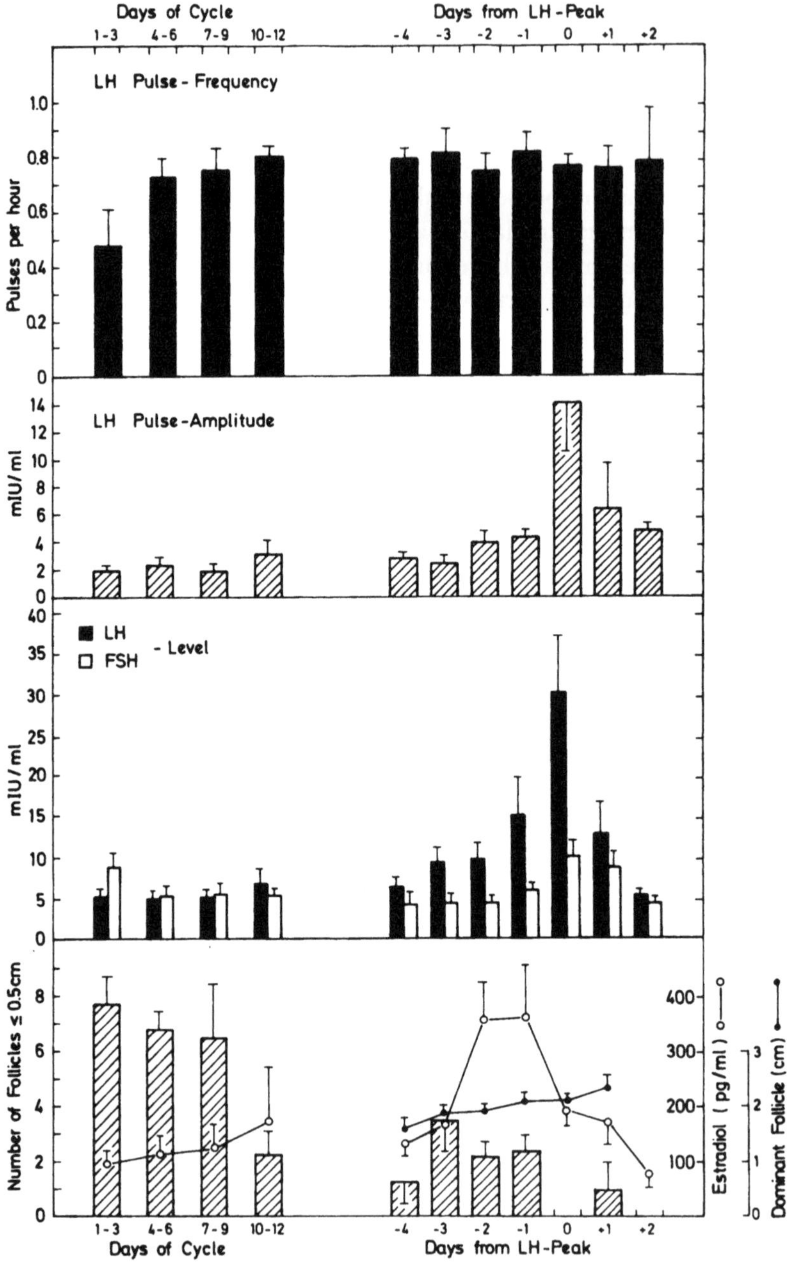

Fig. 1 Frequency and amplitude of pulsatile LH secretion, mean LH and FSH serum levels, estradiol concentrations, number of follicles ≤ 5 mm in diameter (hatched bars) and diameter of the dominant follicle during the follicular phase of the human menstrual cycle. Blood samples were obtained at 15 minute intervals over 8 hour periods 2–4 days apart or daily around the midcycle surge. Data are normalized to the onset of menstruation (left side) or the day of the LH surge (right side) and represent mean + SEM of 3–14 observations.

pulse frequency occur. The effects of progesterone in this context appear to be exerted in a more time – than concentration – dependent manner, since the lowest pulse frequency was observed immediately before menstruation when progesterone has already surpassed peak levels in the circulation.

It has been proposed that the reduction of pulse frequency of gonadotropin secretion occasioned by progesterone is responsible for the increase of FSH serum levels observed at the end of the luteal phase and reinitiation of follicular development that occurs at this time [26]. The observations, however, that normal menstrual cycles can be induced by the pulsatile administration of GnRH at an unvarying frequency and that the pattern of FSH secretion at the end of the luteal phase of those cycles as well as follicular development during the subsequent follicular phase are not different from those observed during the normal menstrual cycle argue against this hypothesis [4, 7, 27]. The physiological significance of the changes in frequency of pulsatile gonadotropin secretion during the menstrual cycle, if any remains, is still to be elucidated.

The changes in amplitude of LH pulses observed during the follicular phase of the cycle can be accounted for by the negative and positive feedback actions of estradiol on gonadotropin secretion. During the luteal phase, however, LH pulse amplitude was found to be higher than during the early or midfollicular phase of the cycle. If this is the consequence of an antiestrogenic effect of progesterone, a reduction of pulse frequency or a combination of both of these factors is not known.

Control of gonadotropin secretion by ovarian steroids

The overall pattern of gonadotropin secretion during the entire menstrual cycle, – low, tonic secretion during the follicular and luteal phase, interrupted by a massive discharge at midcycle – has shown to be primarily determined by time and concentration dependet inhibitory and stimulatory actions of ovarian estradiol [1, 2, 28]. Progesterone, secreted from the dominant follicle immediately before ovulation, appears to enhance the stimulatory action of estradiol [7, 28], while the elevated levels of this steroid produced by the corpus luteum completely block this action of estrogen [2].

Estradiol and progesterone could modulate gonadotropin secretion by actin at the hypothalamus, the pituitary gland or at both of these sites. Considerable effort has been devoted to the elucidation of the site(s) at which estradiol exerts its inhibitory and stimulatory actions on gonadotropin secretion. Compelling evidence in favor of a pituitary site of action has been provided by Knobil and his colleagues [3, 29]. In experiments using ovariectomized monkeys with hypothalamic lesions, gonadotropin secretion was reestablished by the intermittent administration of GnRH. An increment in circulating estradiol was then produced that first inhibited gonadotropin secretion. This inhibition, however, was only transient and was followed by a massive discharge of LH and FSH which was indistinguishable from that observed in response to estradiol administration in monkeys with intact central nervous systems. Since this occurred in the presence of an unvarying pulsatile GnRH replacement regimen, it was concluded that estradiol exerts its feedback actions at the level of the pituitary gland and that changes in hypothalamic GnRH secretion are not necessary in this regard [3, 29].

The additional observation that normal ovulatory menstrual cycles could be induced in animals with hypothalamic lesions, but intact ovaries, by applying, the same unvarying pulsatile GnRH replacement regimen, has led to the conclusion, that hypothalamic GnRH secretion plays an obligatory, but only permissive role in the control system that governs the menstrual cycle of the rhesus monkey, and that gonadotropin secretion during the cycle is controlled by ovarian estrogen acting directly at the pituitary gland [3, 4].

Estradiol could exert its stimulatory effects on gonadotropin secretion either by sensitizing the pituitary to an unvarying, pulsatile GnRH stimulus or by activating some other secretory mechanism. The second of these possibilties is supported by the results of experiments, in which estradiol was injected in castrated lesioned monkeys at various timer after discontinuation of GnRH infusion. Discharges of LH and FSH could be induced when the steroid was injected up to 48 hours after termination of GnRH infusion, but not thereafter [30]. These observations are consonant whith the report by Ferin and colleagues that estrogen can induce gonadotropin discharges when administered shortly after pituitary stalk section [31] and suggest, that the steroid itself can act as a releasing hormone, when the pituitary is adequately prepared by GnRH. These findings also explain the earlier observation, that inhibition of endogenous GnRH secretion by neuroactive drugs as well as its neutralization by the acute administration of antiserum against the decapeptide were unable to block the positive feedback actions of estradiol [2, 15].

In contrast to the pituitary site of action of estradiol, the progesterone blockade of estradiol induced' gonadotropin discharges must be exerted at the central nervous system, since increments in circulating progesterone levels that block estrogen induced' gonadotropin discharges in intact monkeys failed to do so in animals with hypothalamic lesions on GnRH replacement [32]. Further experiments suggest that the blocking action of progesterone is not effected by an interruption of GnRH release, but appears to be caused by the release of an inhibitory agent from the hypothalamus [33]. The facilitatory action of progesterone, on the other hand, seems to be exerted at the pituitary gland since estrogen induced' gonadotropin discharges were advanced in time during progesterone treatment of lesioned monkeys on GnRH replacement [32].

Pulsatile gonadotropin secretion in amenorrhoic women

Similar to monkeys with hypothalamic lesions that abolish endogenous GnRH production and pulsatile gonadotropin secretion, a variety of circumstances that compromise normal ovarian function in women are characterized by the absence or by the severe reduction of pulsatile gonadotropin release. Since the common final defect in those patients appears to be a reduction of hypothalamic GnRH secretion, their condition is referred to as "hypothalamic amenorrhea", a term coined by Klinefelter and associates more than forty years ago for characterization of patients suffering from amenorrhea of suprapituitary origin.

That absence or reduction of GnRH secretion is cause of hypothalamic amenorrhea is strongly suggested by the demonstration, that normal menstruation cycles resulting in ovulation, corpus luteum formation and pregnancy could be induced in such patients by the chronic intermittend administration of an unvarying amount of GnRH [6, 7, 27, 34, 35]. The results of these studies have led to the conclusion that the concept of the permissive action of hypothalamic GnRH in the control of gonadotropin secretion during the menstrual cycle, that has been prosposed by Knobil for the rhesus monkey, applies likewise to the human female. In addition, they have opened new ways for the treatment of patients suffering from infertility as a consequence of hypothalamic amenorrhea.

Based on studies in amenorrhoic patients [5], prepuberal subjects [35] and prepuberal monkeys [36], the view has been advanced that hypothalamic amenorrhea is part of a pathophysiological continuum of ovarian insufficiency resulting from hypothalamic dysfunction and represents the more severe degrees on a sliding scale of impairment of hypothalamic GnRH secretion [5, 7, 27]. It was furthermore proposed that the extent of this impairment in patients presenting with amenorrhea can be assessed by the response to gestagen, clomiphene and GnRH administration. This concept has been substantiated by examining the 24 hour pattern of pulsatile gonadotropin secretion and follicular development in women with hypothalamic amenorrhea graded according to these criteria [23]. The results of this study are shown in figure 2.

In the most severe form of hypothalamic amenorrhea, gonadotropin secretion was found to be compromised to an extent similar to that observed in lesioned monkeys and no evidence for pulsatile secretion was found. In most patients, however, pulsatile gonadotropin secretion could be observed and frequency and amplitude of LH pulses increased with decreasing grades and severity of the disorder. In the more severe grades, this increase in pulsatile LH secretion became only apparent during sleep. In less severe grades, it extended over the whole 24 hour day and reached, with respect to frequency, values comparable to that observed during the early follicular phase of the cycle. The increase in pulsatile LH secretion was reflected by an increasing number of ovarian follicles determined by ultrasonography. Amplitude of the LH

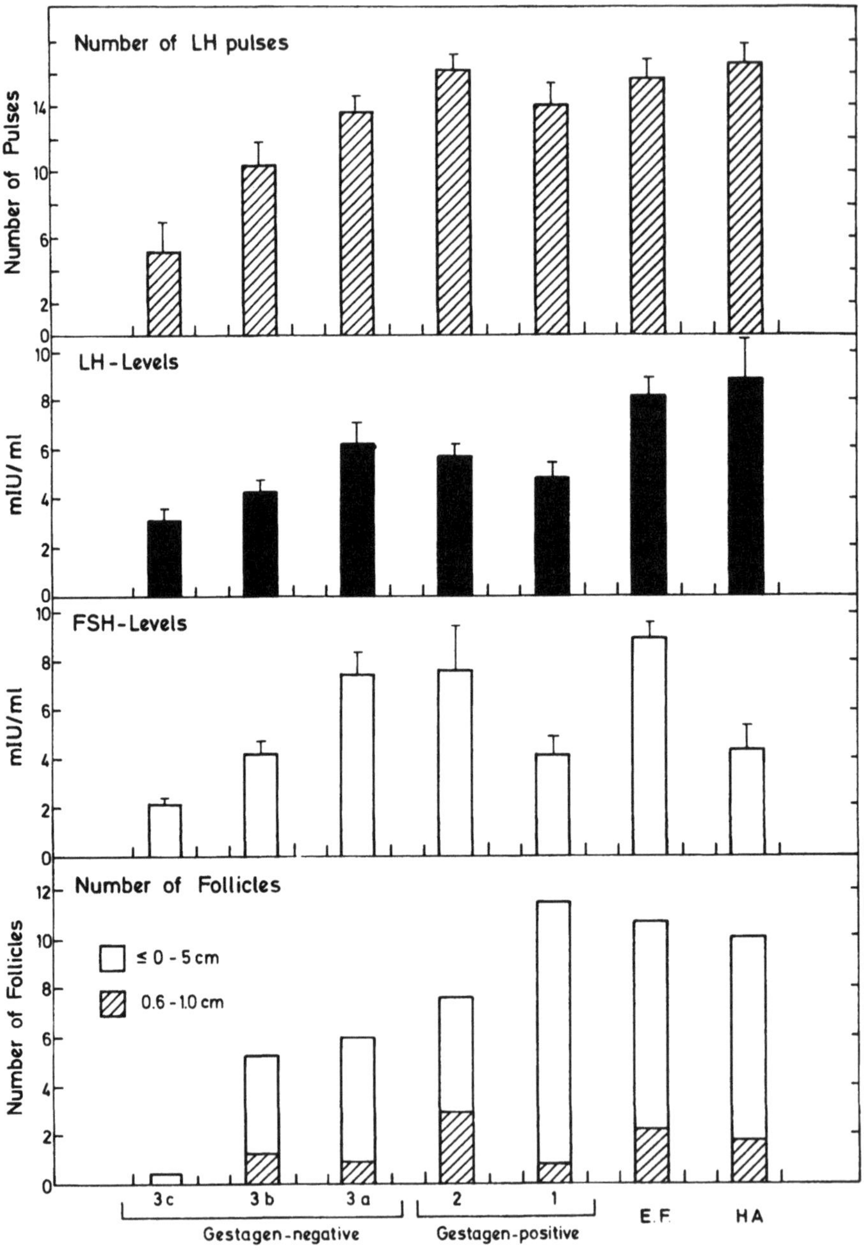

Fig. 2 Number of LH pulses over 24 hours, mean LH and FSH serum levels and number of follicles as determined by ultrasonography in patients with hypothalamic (n=24) or hyperandrogenemic (HA, n=6) amenorrhea. The numbers on the bottom line refer to grade of hypothalamic amenorrhea (1 clomiphene-positive, 2 clomiphene-negative. 3c no response, 3b prepuberal and 3a adult response to 100 μ GnRH iv.). Blood samples were obtained at 15 minute intervals over 24 hours. Values of the early follicular phase (EF) are given for comparison. Data represent mean + SEM. From Wildt et al., with permission [23].

pulses, however, always remained lower than in women during the early follicular phase of the cycle, and this was reflected by subnormal mean LH levels.

This pattern of gonadotropin secretion in patients with hypothalamic amenorrhea is similar to that observed during the course of normal puberty [35]. Primary hypothalamic amenorrhea may therefore be viewed as a consequence of an arrest at some early stages of pubertal development; secondary hypothalamic amenorrhea may be perceived as regression into puberty [5, 7, 23, 27]. These observations support the view of hypothalamic amenorrhea as a part of a pathophysiological continuum and demonstrate that the extent of the impairment of hypothalamic GnRH secretion, as reflected by a reduced frequency of pulsatile LH release, can be reliably assessed by simple functional tests.

It is tempting to speculate that the reduction of LH pulse frequency and amplitude observed in patients with hypothalamic amenorrhea reflect a corresponding reduction of frequency and amplitude of hypothalamic GnRH secretion. That amplitude of GnRH pulses in subjects with intact ovaries, in contrast to ovariectomized monkeys, may indeed have regulatory potential is suggested by the results of experiments, in which women suffering from identical grades of hypothalamic amenorrhea were infused with different doses of GnRH at a constant frequency, resulting in different amplitudes of GnRH pulses. A critical amplitude had to be surpassed for the induction of ovulatory cycles and with increasing amplitudes, higher levels of LH, FSH estradiol and luteal progesterone were achieved. These observations strongly suggests that the amplitude of the GnRH pulse can determine the magnitude of the pituitary and ovarian response by changing the setpoint of the feedback system operating between the ovary and the anterior pituitary gland [7, 27]. In addition, they lend further support to the view, that corpus luteum insufficiency and anovulatory cycles are part of a pathophysiological continuum of hypothalamic failure and that amenorrhea simply reflects a more severe grade of impairement of hypothalamic GnRH secretion [5, 7, 27].

The nature of the inhibitory inputs restraining the activity of the hypothalamic pulse generator in hypothalamic amenorrhea are unknown. It has been demonstrated that administration of the opiate antagonist naloxone to patients suffering from hypothalamic amenorrhea reinitiates and sustains pulsatile LH release [23, 27]. It has also been shown that naloxone administration is followed by an increase of LH pulse frequency when administered during the luteal phase of the cycle [38]. These observations suggest, that inhibitory inputs impinging on the neuronal oscillator that directs pulsatile LH release can be mediated by endogenous opiates. Whether this occurs in hypothalamic amenorrhea remains to be shown.

While hypothalamic amenorrhea is characterized by a reduced frequency and amplitude of pulsatile LH secretion, the reverse obtains in some patients suffering from hyperandrogenemic amenorrhea. In those patients, gonadotropin secretion throughout the 24 hour day is characterized by LH pulses occurring at a "supraphysiologic" frequency and amplitude [23, 29]. In contrast, FSH levels are markedly suppressed, and it is tempting to speculate, that this is the consequence of a supraphysiologic frequency of hypothalamic GnRH secretion. If this increase in frequency and amplitude of LH secretion is cause of hyperandrogenemia, or merely the consequence of a disturbance in other components of the control system that governs gonadotropin secretion, is unclear at present. Once established, however, this pattern of gonadotropin secretion could sustain and further aggravate pituitary and ovarian dysfunction.

Conclusions

The data presented in this chapter have led to the construction of a model of the neuroendocrine control system that directs the primate ovarian cycle, which differs in some major aspects from that proposed for the laboratory rodent [1, 3, 7]. In the rat, the induction of the preovulatory surge of gonadotropins is dependent upon the discharge of a large bolus of (GnRH into the pituitary portal circulation that results from an action of estrogen at the central nervous system and is linked to circadian rhythms [1]. In primates, including the human female, hypothalamic GnRH secretion plays but a permissive role in this regard and gonadotropin secretion during the menstrual cycle, including the midcycle surge, is controlled by estradiol acting directly at the pituitary gland. The ovary, therefore, and not the brain, is timing ovulation and determines the course of the primate ovarian cycle, which can evolve in the presence of an unvarying, pulsatile signal delivered from the hypothalamus. This model, which is much simpler than that proposed for the rat, has provided the basis for a new understanding of the pathophysiology of some forms of human reproductive failure, which came to be viewed as being the consequence of a reduced activity of the hypothalamic pulse generator that directs GnRH secretion. This has led to new therapeutic regimens for the succesful treatment of some of these disorders.

References

[1] Goodman, R. L., E. Knobil: Neuroendocrinology **32** (1981) 57–63.
[2] Knobil E.,: Recent Progr. Horm. Res. **30** (1974) 1–46.
[3] Knobil, E.: Recent Progr. Horm. Res. **36** (1980) 53–88.
[4] Knobil, E., T. M. Plant, L. Wildt et al.: Science **207** (1980) 1371–1373.
[5] Leyendecker, G.: Eur. J. Obstet. Gynecol. Reprod. Biol. **9** (1979) 175–186.
[6] Leyendecker, G., T. Struve, E. J. Plotz: Arch. Gynäkol. **229** (1980) 177–190.
[7] Leyendecker, G., L. Wild: In "Neuroendocrine Aspects of Reproduction" (Ed. R. L. Norman), pp. 295–323. Academic Press, New York 1983.

[8] Dierschke, D. J., A. N. Bhattacharya, L. E. Atkinson et al.: Endocrinology **87** (1970) 850–853.
[9] Yen, S. S. C., C. C. Tsai, F. Naftolin et al.: J. Clin. Endocrinol. Metab. **34** (1972) 671–675.
[10] Santen, R. J., C. W. Bardin: J. Clin. Invest. **52** (1973) 2617–2628.
[11] Gay, V. L., N. A. Sheth: Endocrinology **90** (1972) 158–162.
[12] Carmel, P. W., S. Araki, M. Ferin: Endocrinology **99** (1976) 243–248.
[13] Clarke, I. J., J. T. Cummins: Endocrinology **111** (1982) 1737–1739.
[14] Antunes, J. L., P. W. Carmel, E. M. Housepian et al.: J. Neurosurg. **49** (1978) 382–386.
[15] McCormack, J. T., T. M. Plant, D. L. Hess et al.: Endocrinology **100** (1977) 663–667.
[16] Knobil, E.: Biol. Reprod. **24** (1980) 44–49.
[17] Krey, L. C., W. R. Butler, E. Knobil: Endocrinology **96** (1975) 1073–1087.
[18] Plant, T. M., L. C. Krey, J. Moossy et al.: Endocrinology **102** (1978) 52–62.
[19] Belchetz, P. E., T. M. Plant, Y. Nakai et al.: Science **202** (1978) 631–633.
[20] Wildt, L., A. Häusler, G. Marshall et al.: Endocrinology **109** (1981) 376–385.
[21] Wildt, L., K. A. Brensing, G. Leyendecker: Acta Endocrinol. **99**, Suppl. 246 (1982) 82–33.
[22] Wildt, L., I. Hebold, G. Leyendecker: Acta Endocrinol. **105**, Suppl. 264 (1983) 148.
[23] Wildt, L., H. Schwilden, G. Wesner et al.: In "Brain and Pituitary Peptides II" (Eds G. Leyendecker, H. Stock, L. Wildt), pp. 28–57. Karger, Basel 1983.
[24] Goodman, R. L., F. J. Karsch: Endocrinology **107** (1980) 1286-1290.
[25] Soules, M. R., R. A. Steiner, D. K. Clifton et al.: J. Clin. Endocrinol. Metab. **58** (1984) 378–383.
[26] Hanker, J. P., E. Nieschlag, H. P. G. Schneider: Acta Endocrinol. **96**, Suppl. 240 (1981) 75–76.
[27] Leyendecker, G., L. Wildt: J. Reprod. Fertil. **69** (1983) 397–409.
[28] Leyendecker, G., L. Wildt, H. Gips et al.: Arch. Gynäkol. **221** (1976) 29–45.
[29] Nakai, Y., T. M. Plant, D. L. Hess et al.: Endocrinology **102** (1978) 1008–1014.
[30] Wildt, L., A. Häusler, J. S. Hutchinson et al.: Endocrinology **108** (1981) 2011–2013.
[31] Ferin, M., H. Rosenblatt, P. W. Carmel et al.: Endocrinology **108** (1979) 50–52.
[32] Wildt, L., J. S. Hutchinson, G. Marshall et al.: Endocrinology **109** (1981) 1293–1294.
[33] Pohl, C. R., D. W. Richardson, G. Marshall et al.: Endocrinology **110** (1982) 1454–1455.
[34] Leyendecker, G., L. Wildt, M. Hansmann: J. Clin. Endocrinol. Metab. **51** (1980) 1214–1216.
[35] Boyar, R. M., J. Finkelstein, H. Roffwarg et al.: New Engl. J. Med. **287** (1972) 582–586.
[36] Wildt, L., G. Marshall, E. Knobil: Science **207** (1980) 1373–1375.
[37] Quigley, M. E., K. L. Sheehan, R. F. Casper et al.: J. Clin. Endocrinol. Metab. **50** (1980) 949–954.
[38] Ropert, J. F., M. E. Quigley, S. S. C. Yen: J. Clin. Endocrinol. Metab. **52** (1981) 583–585.
[39] Yen, S. S. C.: Clin. Endocrinol. **12** (1980) 177–208.

Induction of ovulation in amenorrhea infertile women with pulsatile administration of gonadotropin releasing hormone

D. Berg, H. Mickan, H.-K. Rjosk, E. Kuss, J. Zander

Introduction

In the past few years several investigators have demonstrated the efficacy of pulsatile administration of gonadotropin releasing hormone (GnRH) for induction for ovulation in patients with primary or secondary amenorrhea [1–3]. Based on the successful treatment schedule reported by Leyendecker et al. [4] we began in November 1980 treating patients with presumed hypothalamic anovulatory infertility with GnRH administered intravenously in a pulsatile form. It is our purpose to determine the clinical value of this new mode of ovulation induction in terms of effectiveness and safety.

Methods

Selection of patients

A group of 42 patients, aged 22–36 years, was selected for treatment. 6 patients had a primary amenorrhea and 36 a secondary amenorrhea for periods longer than six months. The patients were subdivided into two main groups according to their response to a progesterone challenge. Group I consisted of 17 patients with no bleeding in response to progesterone withdrawal, whereas group II consisted of 25 patients who bled in response to progesterone withdrawal.

All patients included in this study presented a normal tubal factor, as verified by hysterosalpingography or laparoscopy, normal or low serum FSH levels, and no clinical evidence of hyperandrogenemia. In every case, the husband had a normal spermiogram, or only occasionally a slight asthenozoospermia. Two patients with hyperprolactinemia were also included in this study because of intolerance to dopamine agonists.

GnRH infusion

A portable infusion pump (Zyklomat, Ferring GmbH, Kiel) was used to deliver intermittently 5 μg or 20 μg GnRH in 50 μl solution every 90 min through an intravenous catheter inserted in a forearm vein. Following withdrawal bleeding, GnRH was administered for periods of 8 to 52 days. Two days after the rise of basal body temperature, the Zyklomat pump was removed and 3 injections of 2.500 IU hCG were administered every second day. In two cases, in which interpretation of the basal body temperature and of the cervical score was uncertain, the GnRH infusion was continued until a menstrual bleeding or pregnancy occurred.

Hormonal assay methods

The clinical surveillance of our patients by means of basal body temperature records and cervical score was supplemented by daily determination of FSH, LH, oestrone-glucuronide and pregnanediol-glucuronide in early morning urine samples. This proceeding seems to be convenient for the clinical routine surveillance, since daily blood sampling or collection of 24-hour urine would have been very cumbersome from a practical point of view. Furthermore a good correlation exists between gonadotropin and ovarian steroid concentration in serum, 24-hour urine and early morning urine [5–7].

FSH, LH and testosterone were measured directly, without pretreatment of the serum and urine samples, using commercially available radioimmunoassay kits. Antisera for the radioimmunological determination of oestrone-glucuronide and pregnanediol-3-glucuronide were the kind gift of Dr. Samarajeewa (Courtauld Institute of Biochemistry, The Middlesex Hospital Medical School, London). ^{125}Iodine labelled derivatives of the steroid-glucuronides were used as tracers. These were synthesized and purified in our laboratory according to a method developed for the preparation of iodine labelled catecholoestrogens [8]. Steroidglucuronides were also measured directly in the urine samples.

The endocrine profile of 8 control cycles of normally mestruating women is shown in figure 1.

Results and discussion

The 42 patients were subjected to a total of 77 treatment cycles. The results of the therapy in patients with positive and negative response to progesterone challenge are summarized in table 1. 64 treatment cycles were ovulatory, representing an ovulation rate of 83%. 23 patients conceived. 22 singleton and 2 twin pregnancies were

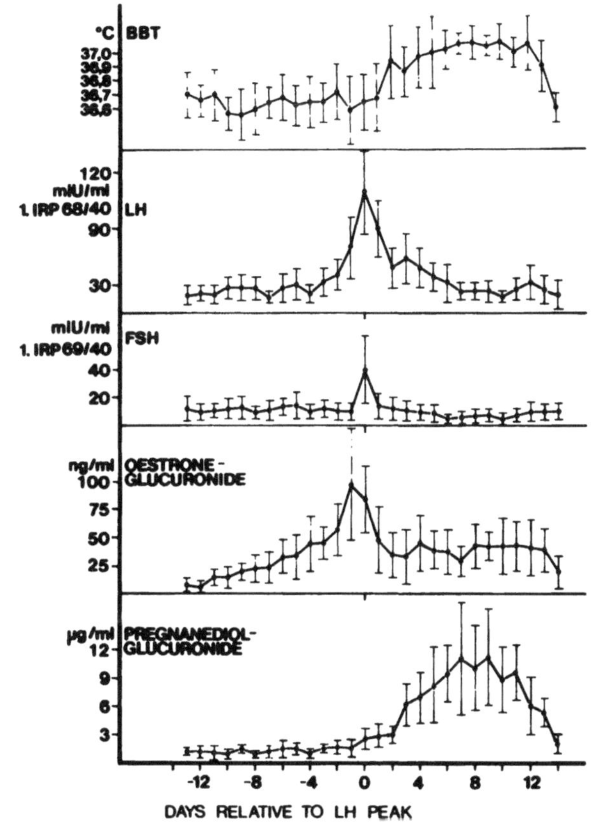

Fig. 1 BBT and urinary excretion of LH, FSH, oestrone-glucuronide and pregnanediol-glucuronide (morning urine) in spontaneous ovulatory cycles (n = 8, mean ± SD).

confirmed by ultrasonography. This represents a pregnancy rate of 31.2% when referred to the total of treatment cycles and of 54.8% when referred to the total of patients treated. Ovulation and pregnancy rates were similar in both groups.

17 pregnancies developed normally out of which 9 patients have already delivered healthy mature children. One patient had a premature birth of twins in the 32nd week of gestation, and 7 pregnancies developed so far without problems. There were 7 abortions between the 6th and 15th week of gestation.

Both patients with hyperprolactinemic amenorrhea conceived during the first treatment cycle. In spite of their raised prolactin concentration (1000–2500 µE/ml) ovulation occurred after 12 to 14 days of treatment. It may be concluded that the intermittent administration of GnRH normalized gonadotropin secretion, thereby inducing physiological ovarian function, even in the presence of increased prolactin levels [9].

Table 1 Summary of clinical results with GnRH in patients with primary or secondary amenorrhea and infertility

	Group I	Group II	Group I + II
Total no. of patients	17	25	42
Total no. treatment courses	30	47	77
Ovulation			
Patients	15	22	37 (88.0%)
Courses	25	39	64 (83.1%)
GnRH-treatment length days (mean ± SD)	18.1 ± 3.2	14.9 ± 4.4	16 ± 4.7
Pregnancy achieved			
Patients	9	14	23 (54.8%)
Courses	9	15	24 (31.2%)
Births	4	6	10
Abortions	2	5	7
Still pregnant	3	4	7

Group I: no bleeding in response to progesterone challenge
Group II: bleeding in response to progesterone challenge

Serious side effects which might have resulted from the pulsatile GnRH administration were unusual. In only two instances the infusion of GnRH had to be interrupted. One patient developed severe thrombophlebitis with fever caused by the i.v. catheter; in the other patient a technical defect of the Zyklomat pump remained unnoticed.

Minor complications, such as minimal bleeding or inflammatory reaction at the catheter site were more frequently observed. In these patients the catheter had to be resited.

None of the treated patient presented any clinical signs of ovarian hyperstimulation. This observation was reinforced by the concentration pattern of LH, oestrone-glucuronide and pregnanediol-glucuronide throughout the treatment cycles (fig. 2). The degree of ovarian stimulation, however, seems to depend on the dosis of GnRH administered. 4 patients with positive response to progesterone challenge received, in two subsequent treatment cycles, first 20 μg GnRH and then 5 μg per pulse. All cycles were ovulatory. Neither the pelvic examination nor the cervical score offered any clinical evidence for an increased stimulatory effect when 20 μg GnRH per pulse were administered. However, the oestrone-glucuronide concentrations in early morning urine were in this case clearly higher (fig. 3). The fact that the two twin pregnancies observed in our study occurred in the group II patients treated with 20 μg GnRH might also suggest a tendency to hyperstimulation under such conditions of treatment.

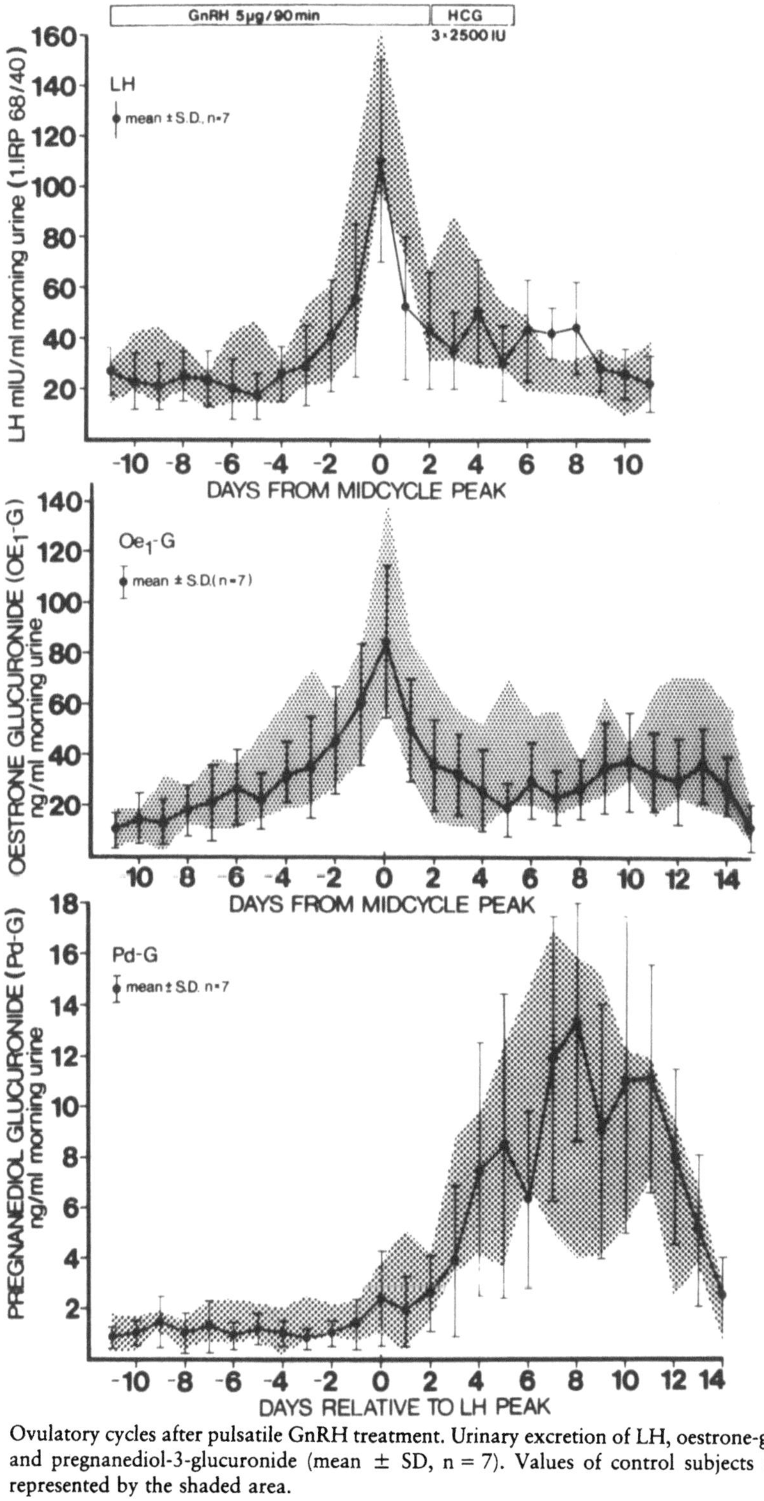

Fig. 2 Ovulatory cycles after pulsatile GnRH treatment. Urinary excretion of LH, oestrone-glucuronide and pregnanediol-3-glucuronide (mean ± SD, n = 7). Values of control subjects (n = 8) are represented by the shaded area.

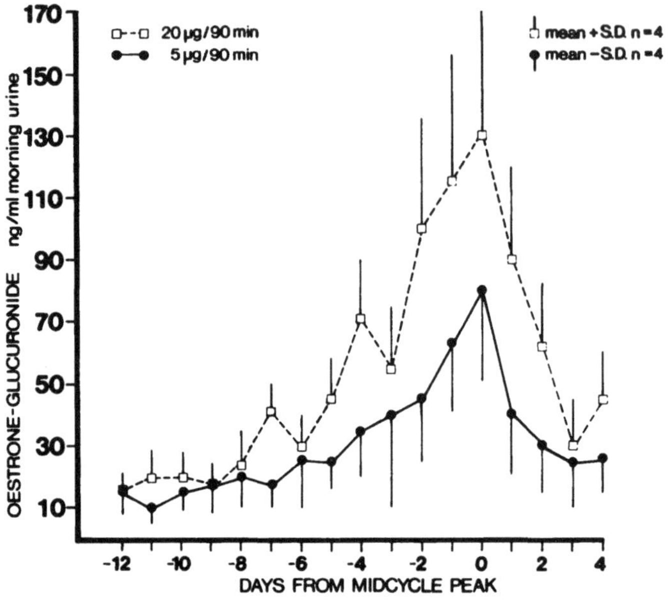

Fig. 3 Urinary excretion of oestrone-glucuronide in 4 patients with positive response to progesterone challenge using different dosis of GnRH.

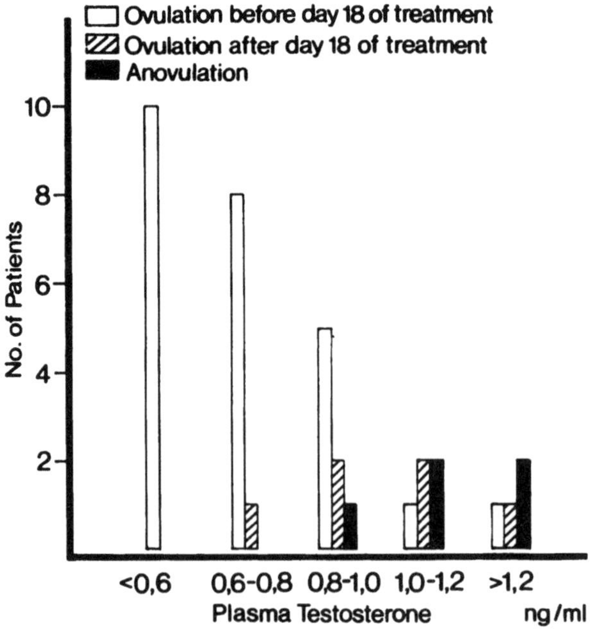

Fig. 4 Ovulation rate and time of ovulation as a function of plasma testosterone concentration.

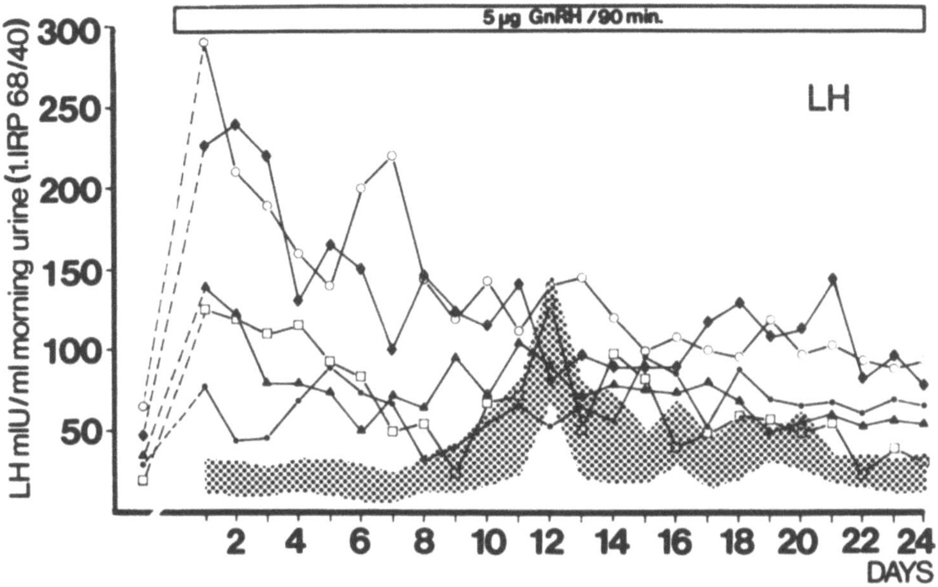

Fig. 5 Anovulation during pulsatile GnRH treatment in 5 patients with positive response to progesterone challenge. Urinary excretion of LH.

Five of 42 patients, all with secondary amenorrhea, remained anovulatory throughout all 8 treatment cycles performed. The mean duration of GnRH infusion was 29 days. In another group of 6 patients, ovulation occurred always after at least 18 days of treatment. None of these patients showed any typical symptoms of hyperandrogenemia, nor did the ovaries present any polycystic alterations by ultrasound. Occasionally slightly increased levels of serum LH were observed before treatment. Nevertheless, the elevated levels of androgens observed before and during treatment (fig. 4) appeared to be the factor responsible for the secondary amenorrhea, even though there were no clinical signs of hyperandrogenemia. Thus, even though the number of patients considered is relatively low, it may be concluded that there undoubtedly is a tendency of delayed ovulation, or even anovulation with increasing serum androgen levels (5–12 determinations/patient were performed).

The LH concentrations of those patients who did not ovulate during the treatment present further evidence for a hyperandrogenemic ovarian insufficiency [10]. Under normal or slightly increased pretreatment levels of LH, there was a pronounced increase immediately after beginning of the therapy, which tended to normalize in the course of time (fig. 5). Similar conclusions arise from the oestrone-glucuronide profile of these patients. Four out of five patients had clearly elevated concentrations of oestrone-glucuronide at the beginning of the treatment. These high levels decreased throughout the therapy (fig. 6).

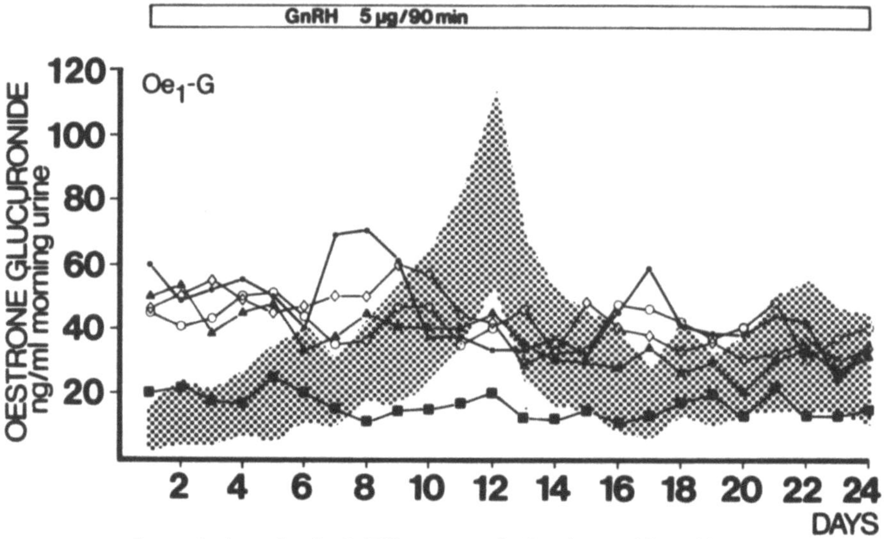

Fig. 6 Anovulation during pulsatile GnRH treatment in 5 patients with positive response to progesterone challenge. Urinary excretion of oestrone-glucuronide.

A certain therapeutical effect was observed also from the clinical point of view. Four out of these 5 patients had an anovulatory bleeding after 27 to 52 days of treatment. To what extent a sufficiently long GnRH treatment is capable of normalizing the ovarian function in these cases remains as yet unclear [11].

Summarizing, from the data presented in this study, it may be concluded that the pulsatile administration of GnRH is an efficient and convenient method for the induction of follicle maturation and ovulation in the clinical routine practice. It certainly represents a convincing therapeutical advance in the treatment of infertility in hypothalamic amenorrhea.

References

[1] Leyendecker, G., T. Struve, E. J. Plotz: Arch. Gynecol. **229** (1980) 177–190.

[2] Schoemaker, J., A. H. M. Simons, G. J. C. van Osnabrugge et al.: J. Clin. Endocrinol. Metab. **52** (1981) 882–885.

[3] Berg, D., H. Mickan, S. Michael, et al.: Arch. Gynecol. **233** (1983) 205–210.

[4] Leyendecker, G., L. Wildt, M. Hansmann: J. Clin. Endocrinol. Metab. **51** (1980) 1214–1216.

[5] Adlercreutz, H., J. Brown, W. Collins et al.: J. Steroid. Biochem. **17** (1982) 695–702.

[6] Collins, W. P., P. O. Collins, M. J. Kilpatrick et al.: Acta. Endocrinol. (Copenh) **90** (1979) 336–348.

[7] Denari, J. H., Z. Farinati, P. R. F. Casas et al.: Obstet. Gynecol. **58** (1981) 5–9.

[8] Berg, D., R. Sonsalla, E. Kuss: Acta Endocrinol. (Copenh) **103** (1983) 282–288.

[9] Berg, D., H.-K. Rjosk, F. Jänicke et al.: Geburtsh. u. Frauenheilk. **43**, in press.

[10] Schwartz, U., L. Moltz, J. Hammerstein: Gynäkologie **14** (1981) 119–130.

[11] Weber, J. M., H. J. T. Coelingh Bennink, G. P. J. Alsbach et al.: Acta. Endocrinol. (Copenh) **103**, Suppl. 256, (1983) 77.

Effects of different substituents in the A-ring of estradiol on its potency in sensitizing pituicytes to gonadotropin releasing hormone

G. Emons, R. Knuppen, P. Ball, K. J. Catt

Introduction

For the elucidation of the cellular mechanisms regulating gonadotrophin release, the knowledge of those structural features of the estrogen molecule that are essential for its bioactivity is most important. As a first step to detect the relations between structure and biological activity of estrogens, we designed a series of studies where the relative potencies of estradiol and selected A-ring modified estrogens were compared. As experimental arrangement we chose the estrogen effect on spontaneous and gonadotrophin releasing hormone (GnRH) stimulated LH release by cultured pituitary cells. This model offers some major advantages: a) estrogen target cells (*i. e.* the gonadotrophs) can be directly confronted with defined concentrations of the test substance. Errors caused by differences in resorption from the injection site, peripheral metabolism etc. which usually complicate *in vivo* studies are avoided; b) changes in the concentration of the test substance either due to chemical decomposition or metabolism can be monitored and be taken into account. c) interferences by other factors such as changes in hypothalamic GnRH pulse amplitude and/or frequency which might be also modulated by estrogens are excluded.

Recently we demonstrated that the effect of estrogens on pituitary sensitivity to GnRH is biphasic [1]. Thus the testing of estrogens over a broad range of concentrations yields bell-shaped dose response curves for LH release with characteristic maximal effective doses (ED max.) for each substance tested. These ED max. can be easily defined mathematically and hence provide a clear parameter for the relative potency of the estrogen tested. In that study, we were also able to demonstrate that the introduction of an additional hydroxy- or methyl-group in position 2 or 4 of the phenolic A-ring of the estradiol molecule leads to characteristic changes in its bioactivity [1]. In this paper we now report on the effects of systematic modifications of the A-ring of the estradiol molecule by substituents of different size and negative polarization.

Materials and methods

Steroids

Estradiol was commercially available, 2- and 4-hydroxyestradiol, 2- and 4-aminoestradiol, 2- and 4-nitroestradiol were prepared from estradiol according to Stubenrauch and Knuppen [2]. The monomethyl ethers of 2- and 4-hydroxyestradiol were synthesized as previously described [3]. 2- and 4-methylestradiol were prepared from estrone as described in an earlier paper [1]. The purity of these 2- and 4-substituted estrogens was greater than 99.9% as shown by mass spectrometry, using the technique of selected ion monitoring; contamination with estradiol was less than 50 ppm. 2- and 4-fluoroestradiol were generously provided by Dr. D. Pfeiffer, Dr. G. R. Merriam, and Dr. N. J. MacLusky.

Pituitary cell preparation and culture

Adult female Sprague-Dawley (200–300 g) or Wistar (200–250 g) rats of random stages of the estrous cycle (obtained from Charles River Laboratories, Chicago, or Winkelmann, Borchen-Kirchborchen, Western Germany) were used for the preparation of primary cultures of pituitary cells as described previously [1]. Briefly, pituitaries were cut into pieces, treated with Trypsin, DNAse I, Soybean Trypsin Inhibitor, and EDTA before they were dispersed by trituration. The cells were suspended in Medium 199, containing L-glutamine, 0.14% sodum bicarbonate, 100 U/ml penicillin, 100 μg/ml streptomycin sulfate and 10% horse serum, pretreated with dextran coated charcoal. Cell viability assessed by Trypan blue exclusion was consistently >85%. The cell suspension was then diluted with the above medium to a concentration of 2×10^5 viable cells/ml, and 1 ml aliquots were added to 22 × 10 mm wells and maintained at 37 °C in a water-saturated atmosphere of 5% CO_2 in air. Cells were allowed to attach to the wells for at least 40 h before experiments were begun.

Experimental protocol

Pituitary cells prepared as described above were incubated in quadruplicate for 48 h in the presence of 10^{-11} to 10^{-6} M or 10^{-13} - 10^{-6} M concentrations of the estrogens to be studied. All estrogens were stored at the respective predilution at O °C in ethanol containing 1% ascorbic acid. Shortly before use, 20 μl aliquots of the respective estrogen solution were added to 10 ml of prewarmed (30 °C) medium. Control cultures were incubated with medium to which ethanol containing 1% of ascorbic acid had been added (20 μl/10ml of medium). The media were changed every 12 h until 48 h, when media were changed again and collected after 4 h for assay of basal

LH-release. The cells were then incubated for a further 4 h period with 5×10^{-10} M GnRH in fresh medium without ethanol, ascorbic acid, or steroids, and the medium was saved for assay of the GnRH stimulated LH-release. Cell loss during media changes was carefully monitored (approx. 20% over the whole experiment). It showed no relation to the estrogen tested nor to the different concentrations, but was identical in all cultures, including the controls. All experiments were repeated at least once. Estradiol was run as reference in every experiment.

Radioimmunoassay and statistical analysis

The LH content of incubation media was measured by RIA as described previously [4] and expressed in terms of the RP-1 standard preparation. Maximal effective doses (ED max.) were calculated using a Kruskall-Wallis test for effect of treatment, followed by a Nemenyi test for comparisons between individual groups (for details see [1]).

Results

Incubation of pituitary cells with increasing doses of most of the estrogens tested led at low steroid concentrations to a dose dependent increase of the LH-response to a submaximal GnRH-stimulus (5×15^{-10} M). This positive effect was lost at higher steroid concentrations. Thus, we obtained bell-shaped dose response curves with comparable maxima but significant differences in the estrogen concentrations at which maximal LH-release was observed. These maximal effective doses (ED max.) are given in table 1. With 4-nitroestradiol probably only the first half to the curve

Table 1 Maximal effective concentrations (ED max.) of estradiol and selected A-ring modified estrogens

Substance tested	ED max. [M]
estradiol (E_2)	10^{-11}
4-hydroxyestradiol (4-OHE_2)	10^{-11}
4-fluoroestradiol (4-FE_2)	10^{-11}
2-fluoroestradiol (2-FE_2)	10^{-10}
2-methylestradiol (2-CH_3E_2)	10^{-9}
2-methyl 4-hydroxyestradiol (2-$CH_3$4-OHE_2)	10^{-9}
4-hydroxyestradiol 4-methyl ether (4-$OHE_2$4-Me)	10^{-9}
2-hydroxyestradiol (2-OHE_2)	10^{-8}
2-aminoestradiol (2-NH_2E_2)	10^{-8}
4-aminoestradiol (4-NH_2E_2)	10^{-8}
4-nitroestradiol (4-NO_2E_2)	10^{-8}
2-hydroxyestradiol 2-methyl ether (2-$OHE_2$2-Me)	10^{-7}
4-methylestradiol	n. d.
2-nitroestradiol	n. d.

was covered by the range of concentrations tested, with 2-nitroestradiol and 4-methylestradiol no significant effect was observed with the doses used. The basal LH-release by the pituicytes seems to have been affected in a similar way, but the effects are less pronounced or sometimes missing (figs. 1–4) and were thus not used to calculate relative potencies.

Discussion

The data reported here demonstrate that besides the naturally occurring estrogens E_2, 2-OHE_2, 4-OHE_2, 2-OHE_2 2-Me and 4-OHE_2 4-Me also a number of synthetic estrogens can sensitize the pituitary to GnRH: 2- and 4-FE_2, 2-CH_3E_2, 2-CH_3 4-OHE_2, 2- and 4-NH_2E_2, and 4-NO_2E_2. 2-NO_2E_2 and 4-CH_3E_2 seem to have no sensitizing effect – at least at the concentrations tested. For the other estrogens studied, clear ED max. could be calculated, which allow a comparison of their relative potencies. The finding that the catecholestrogen 4-OHE_2 is significantly more potent than the isomeric 2-OHE_2 is in agreement with numerous *in vivo* studies (for review confer[1]). The demonstration that 4-OHE_2 is equipotent with E_2 in this

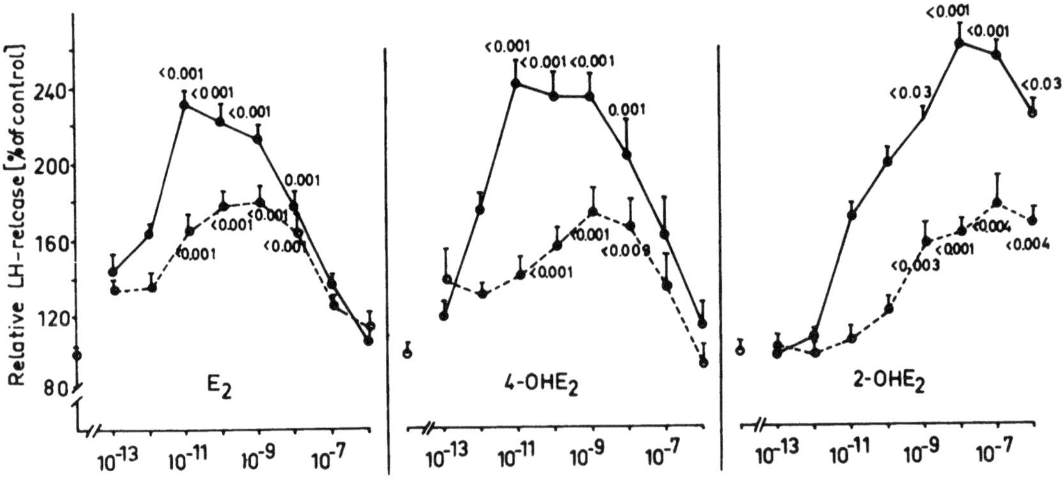

Fig. 1 Effects of increasing concentrations of E_2, 4-OHE_2, and 2-OHE_2 upon LH release (O- - -O- - -O) and the LH response to 5×10^{-10} M GnRH (O- - -O- - -O). The data from 5 independent experiments run in quadruplicate were pooled for each steroid concentration. LH values (mean + SE) are expressed in terms of percent increase as compared to control cultures (no steroid = 100%). In this and subsequent Figures, absolute LH values for controls varied between 0.8–1.5 µg RP-1 per 2×10^5 cells/4h for GnRH stimulated LH release and 50–120 ng per 2×10^5 cells/4h for basal LH release. Numbers above the curves indicate P-values for comparison of differences from controls for GnRH stimulated LH release, and numbers below the curves are those for basal LH release.

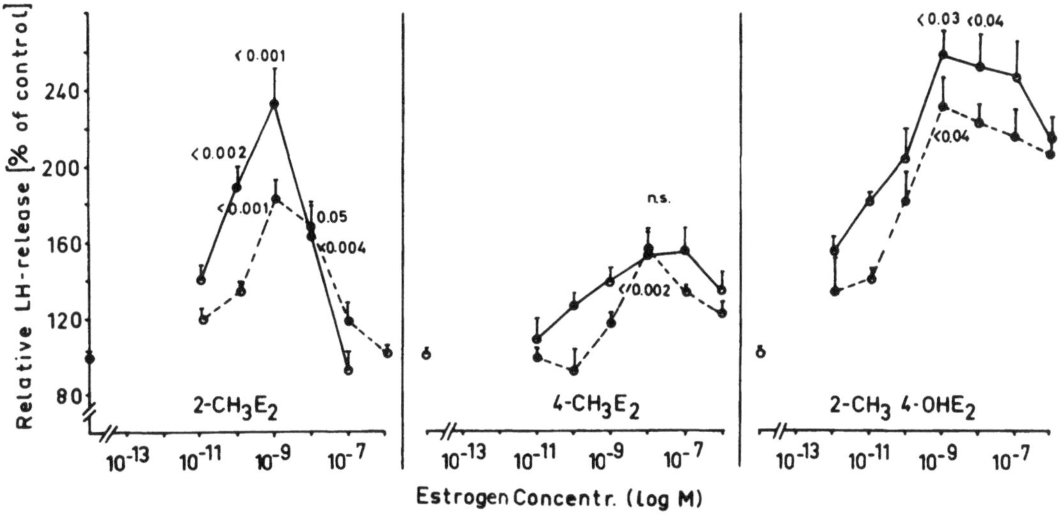

Fig. 2 Effects of increasing concentrations of methylestrogenes on basal and GnRH stimulated LH release. The data from 2 independent experiments run in quadruplicate were pooled for each steroid concentration. For further details see figure 1.

model corroborates our recent finding that these two estrogens are equipotent in their effects on LH-release in the ovariectomized ewe, when comparable blood levels of E_2 and 4-OHE_2 are achieved. Thus, former theories that 4-OHE_2 is less potent than E_2 which were mainly based on the comparison of the doses of either steroid administered systemically, have to be revised, especially as it is now well known [6, 7] that the peripheral clearance of 4-OHE_2 is faster than that of E_2.

The data obtained on the methyl-substituted estrogens confirm earlier findings of our group [8] on the effects of minipump infusions of 2-CH_3E_2, 4-CH_3E_2, and 2-$CH_3$4-OHE_2 on uterine growth and LH-release in long term ovariectomized rats. In that study, 2-CH_3E_2 and 2-$CH_3$4-OHE_2 increased uterine weight and had the well known negative and positive effects on serum LH levels, whereas 4-CH_3E_2 was inactive. Our present results on the effects of 2- and 4-FE_2 are in good agreement with the data of Krey et al. [9] on the effects of these substances on LH release, induction of sexual behavior and translocation of estrogen receptors *in vivo*, where the fluoroestrogens acted as potent estrogens.

To the best of our knowledge this is the first report that 2- and 4-NH_2E_2 and 4-NO_2E_2 have effects on LH-release. The same holds for 2-OHE_2 2-Me and 4-OHE_2 4-Me. These catecholestrogen monomethyl ethers had hitherto been regarded as inactive metabolites of the parent 2-OHE_2 or 4-OHE_2, respectively.

The interpretation of the data accumulated in table 1 and figure 5 with regard to the structure-activity-interrelationship is very complex. It is true that in this model at least factors other than the interaction of the test substance with the pituicyte are

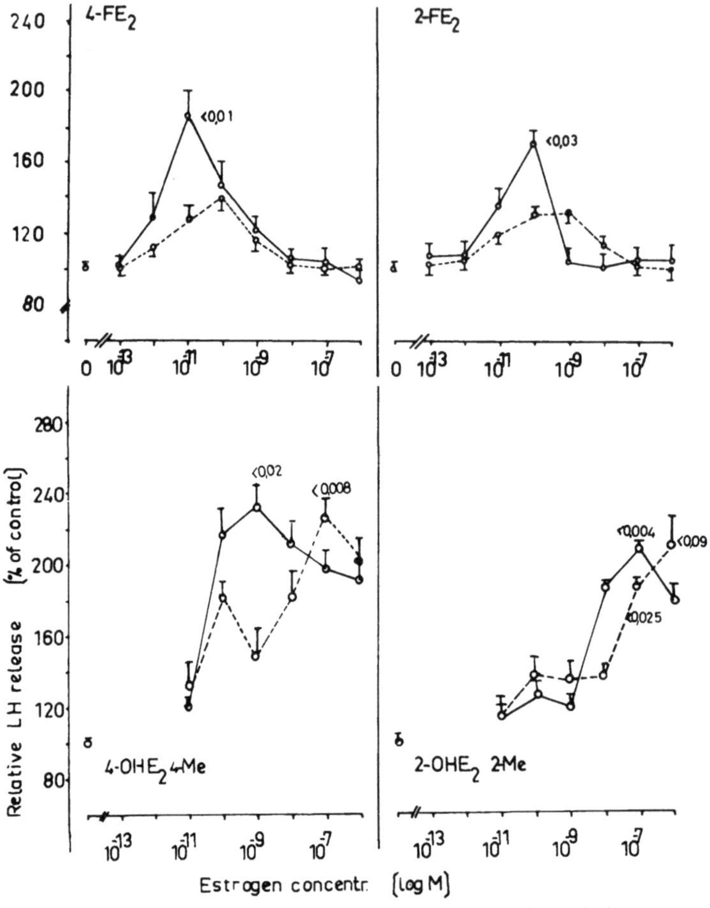

Fig. 3 Effects of increasing concentrations of fluoroestrogenes and catecholestrogen monomethyl ethers on basal and GnRH stimulated LH release. The data from 2 independent experiments were pooled for each steroid concentration. For further details see figure 1.

excluded. But there still remains the question of differences in the metabolism by the pituicytes themselves and of chemical stability. In our previous study [1] we had demonstrated that at least the very labile catecholestrogens 2- and 4-OHE_2 are stable under our culture conditions. It might be inferred that the same holds for the comparatively stable methyl-, fluoro-, and nitro-derivatives. For 2- and 4-NH_2E_2 this issue remains to be studied. As to the possible metabolism of the estrogens tested by the pituicytes, there is still much work to be done:

Thus the interpretations given now are bound to be preliminary and speculative:

1. The introduction of a small and strongly electronegative substituent in position 4 of the E_2 molecule does not decrease the estrogenic potency (ED max.: E_2 = 4-OHE_2

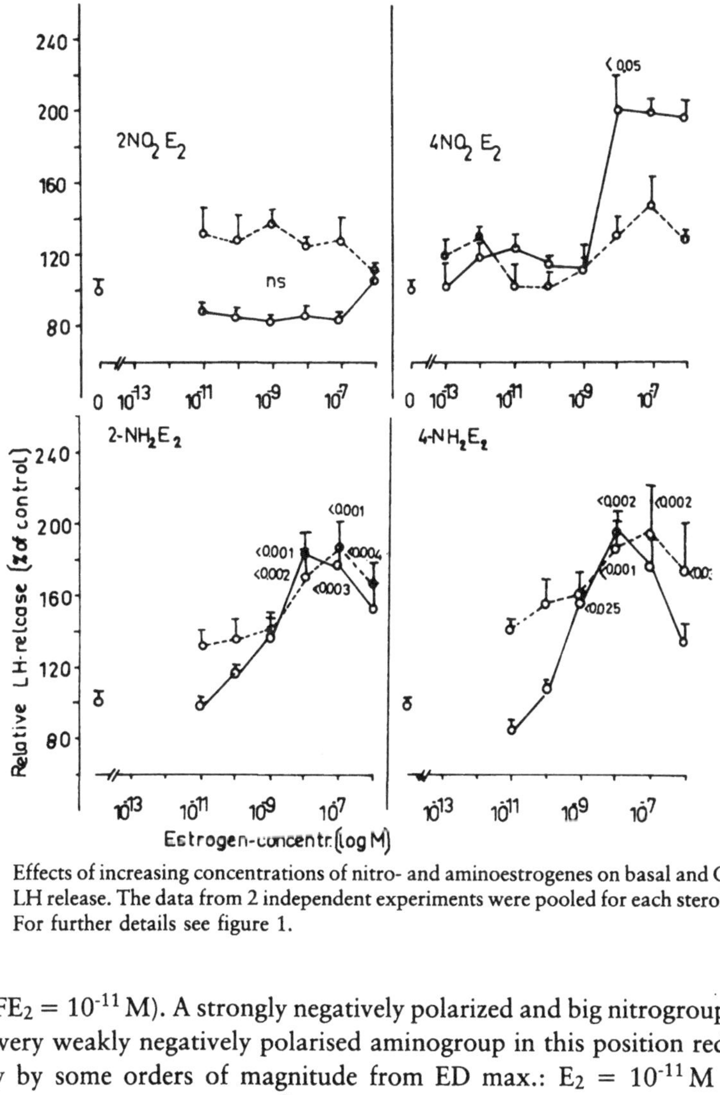

Fig. 4 Effects of increasing concentrations of nitro- and aminoestrogenes on basal and GnRH stimulated LH release. The data from 2 independent experiments were pooled for each steroid concentration. For further details see figure 1.

= 4-FE_2 = 10^{-11} M). A strongly negatively polarized and big nitrogroup in position 4 or a very weakly negatively polarised aminogroup in this position reduces estrogenicity by some orders of magnitude from ED max.: E_2 = 10^{-11} M to ED max.: 4-NO_2E_2 and 4-NH_2E_2 = 10^{-8} M.

2. The same substituents in position 2 have quite different effects: 2-FE_2 is slightly (Ed max. = 10^{-10}M) and 2-OHE_2 is significantly (Ed max. = 10^{-8}M) weaker than E_2. 2-NO_2E_2 is completely devoid of estrogenic activity. Interestingly the very weakly negatively polarised aminogroup in position 2 has the same effect as in position 4 (ED max.: 2-NH_2E_2 = 4-NH_2E_2 = 10^{-8}M).

3. With a non-polar methylgroup the effects are different: In position 2 of the E_2 or 4-OHE_2-molecule it decreases estrogenic potency from ED max. = 10^{-11}M (E_2) to

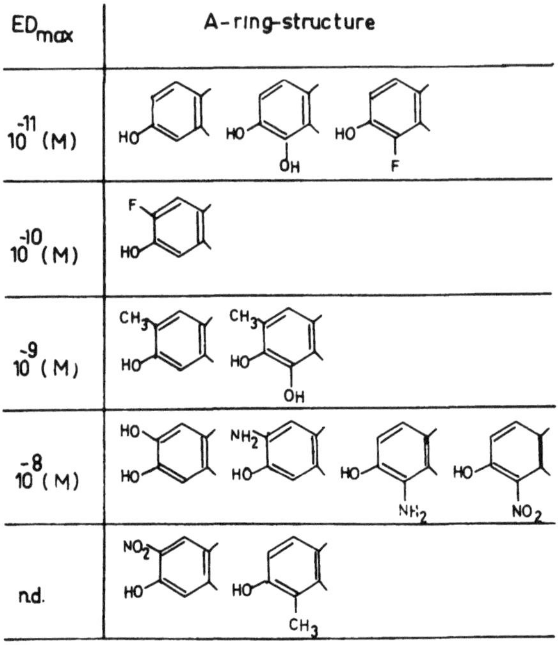

Fig. 5 A-ring structure and maximal effective dose (ED max.) of estradiol and selected A-ring modified estrogens.

10^{-9}M (2-CH_3E_2 and 2-CH_3 4-OHE_2), in position 4 it abolishes estrogenicity (4-CH_3E_2).

4. This finding suggests that the change in estrogenic potency caused by the substitutions is not only a function of the size of the substituent but also of its polarity, mesomeric and inductive properties. Though the nitro- and methylgroups are comparable in size, their effects are quite opposite: 2-NO_2E_2 inactive, 2-CH_3E_2 still active, 4-NO_2E_2 still active, and 4-CH_3E_2 inactive.

5. The monomethylethers of catecholestrogens (2-$OHE_2$2-Me and 4-OHE_2 4-Me) do not fit into this pattern. But here, cleavage of the methyl ether by the pituicytes yielding the parent 2-OHE_2 and 4-OHE_2 is most probable and might account for the biological activity of these compounds.

Thus, all substances tested that have a strong polar group in position 4 are more potent than their respective 2-isomer. The most potent ones of the 4-substituted estrogens are the natural 4-OHE_2 and the synthetic 4-FE_2 which is comparable with 4-OHE_2 as to electronegativity and size of the substituent. Both these substances are equipotent with E_2. Those substances that have a weaker (4-NH_2E_2) or bigger (4-NO_2E_2) negatively polarised substituent in position 4 are less potent. The one carrying a non-polar substituent (4-CH_3E_2) is inactive. The substances with substitution in position 2 are all still active, though to a lesser extent, except for 2-NO_2E_2 which is inactive. One highly speculative, though intriguing theory might reconcile these findings: E_2 has to be converted to 4-OHE_2 before is becomes active. Substances that cannot be 4-hydroxylated are still active as long as they have also an electronegative substituent in position 4. The one with a methyl group in that position is inactive, the one with a nitrogroup in position 2, which probably hampers 4-hydroxylation by electronic effects on the aromatic system is also devoid of estrogenicity. For the other estrogens tested with substituents in position 2 there is still the theoretical possibility of being 4-hydroxylated though it should be assumed that substituents in position 2 generally decrease estrogenic potency. However, as exciting as this working hypothesis may be, it has to be checked by quite a lot of sober experiments.

Acknowledgements

The authors wish to express their gratitude to Drs. D. Pfeiffer, G. R. Merriam, and N. J. MacLusky (NICHD, Bethesda and Yale University School of Medicine, New Haven) for the gift of 2- and 4-FE_2 and to the NIAMDD for the support with radioimmunoassay reagents. This study was supported by a travel grant for G. Emons by the Deutsche Forschungsgemeinschaft.

References

[1] Emons, G., R. Knuppen, P. Ball et al.: Endocrinology, in press.
[2] Stubenrauch, G., R. Knuppen: Steroids **28** (1976) 733–741.
[3] Emons, G., B. Klinger, O. Haupt, et al.: Horm. Metab. Res. **14** (1982) 376–379.
[4[Solano, A. R., M. L. Dufau, K. J. Catt: Endocrinology **105** (1979) 372.
[5] Brack, C., R. Chatelain, G. Emons et al.: Acta Endocrinol **Suppl 256**, 235.
[6] Pfeiffer, D. G., N. J. MacLusky, G. Emons et al.: J. Steroid Biochem 17 (1982) LXXIV.
[7] Ball., P., G. Emons, H. Kayser. et al.: Endocrinology, in press.
[8] Ball, P., G. Emons, O. Haupt et al.: Acta Endocrinol. **102**, 150–152.
[9] Krey, L. C., N. J. MacLusky, D. G. Pfeiffer et al.: In "Catecholestrogens", (Eds. G. R. Merriam, M. B. Lipsett), pp. 249–263. Raven Press, New York 1983.

Present status of LH-RH analog chemistry

D. H. Coy, M. V. Nekola, S. J. Hocart

Introduction

In peptide analog work, as with other areas of medicinal chemistry, the usual primary objectives of analog design can perhaps be summarized as follows:

a) Increased biological activity
b) Prolonged activity
c) Selectivity
d) Antagonist discovery and design
e) Selective antagonist development

The success of LH-RH research in areas a), b) and d) is quite apparent and has really provided a framework upon which expectations concerning structure-activity studies on many other peptides have been based. Analog research on somatostatin, the opiate peptides, and several other peptides with wide bioactivity spectra, such as the neuro-GI peptides, is currently providing answers to questions raised in areas c) and e).

LH-RH analogs with increased agonist activity

Research in this area, although highly successful at an early stage, has shown no further important advances since 1976, perhaps because existing analogs were so active that additional increases were not really necessary either from a research or commercial point of view. Given the length of time since this particular LH-RH analog work was completed, the development of the superagonists has been frequently reviewed (see for instance ref. [1]) and will only be discussed briefly in this report.

Basically, modifications to just two residues of the LH-RH decapeptide chain (tab. 1) were responsible for increasing in vivo gonadotropin releasing activities up to 50-fold relative to LH-RH. The first of these was the incorporation of an ethylamide group in place of glycine at the C-terminus [2] and the second, replacement of glycine in position 6 by alkyl D-amino acids [3]. D-amino acids with very bulky side-chains, such as D-Phe and D-Trp [4] and D-Ser(tBu) [5], were even more effective in in-

Table 1 Sequences of the major LH-RH superagonist analogs undergoing commercial development

					LH-RH					
1	2	3	4	5	6	7	8	9	10	
pGlu –	His –	Trp –	Ser –	Tyr –	Gly –	Leu –	Arg –	Pro –	Gly –	NH_2
a)					D-Leu				$NHCH_2CH_3$	
b)					D-Trp					
c)					D-Trp				$NHCH_2CH_3$	
d)					D-Ser(tBu)				$NHCH_2CH_3$	
e)					D-Ser(tBu)				$NHNHCO_2NH_2$	
f)					D-B-Nal					

creasing activity. Combinations of D-Ala and D-Leu in position 6 together with a C-terminal ethylamide group were also very effective in increasing potency [6, 7]. Combinations of D-Phe and D-Trp with the ethylamide modification gave no increases in *in vivo* activity over the normal D-Phe-6 and D-Trp6 analogs [4].

Quite a number of the LH-RH superagonists are now undergoing clinical evaluations and commercial development. The principal ones are shown in table 1 and are compared structurally to LH-RH itself. Analog (a) is being developed by Abbott, (b) by Tulane University, (d) by Hoechst, (e) by ICI, and (f) by Syntex.

Based on the complex antagonist sequences which have evolved, further improved superagonist analogs are entirely feasable, should this prove to be desirable in the future.

LH-RH antagonist analogs

Since the concept represented such a novel approach to birth control, the development of competitive antagonists of LH-RH was given high priority in structure-activity work with the hormone. This was despite considerable initial scepticism that potent competitive antagonists of structures as complicated as a decapeptide could ever be synthesized. Perhaps one of the principal benefits from LH-RH chemistry has been the demonstration that peptide competitive inhibitors are entirely feasable with binding affinities orders of magnitude higher than the natural parent peptides. Antagonists of other peptides are now being discovered on an almost routine basis.

Unlike superagonist analog studies which have remained essentially static for a number of years, the antagonist analog area continues to be very productive and has made steady progress for at least 10 years towards ever increasing potencies. It must be emphasized that structural modifications responsible for superagonist activity were also responsible for increasing antagonist activities to readily detectable levels in the early analogs. Among the first examples of this then novel approach to antagonist design were [desHis-2, D-Ala-6]-LH-RH [3], in which the D-Ala-6 superagonist substitution greatly increased the binding affinity of the very weakly active desHis-2 analog, and [desHis-2, desGly-10]-LH-RH ethylamide [8] in which the Fujino ethylamide modification plays the same role. This latter analog was the first to counteract the effects of an LH-RH injection *in vivo* in the rat [8].

The evolution of the LH-RH inhibitors from these two early peptides to the present, highly potent and long-acting materials has also been reviewed [1, 9]. We wish only to point out several landmark discoveries which were primarily responsible for improving *in vivo* LH-RH antagonism. These must include the use of D-aromatic rather than alkyl amino acids in position 6 which, as with the agonists, considerably boosted antagonist activities [10]. The use of D-Phe in position 2 [11] rather than simple elimination of His represented a significant improvement as did the replacement of pGlu-1 by D-pGlu [12] and, even better, Ac-D-Phe [13]. D-p-Cl-Phe [14] rather than D-Phe in position 2 and Ac-D-p-Cl-Phe in place of Ac-D-Phe in position 1 [15] alone and in combination were responsible for 10 to 20-fold increases in antiovulatory activities in the rat. In combination, all of these changes resulted in conversion of the first analogs with barely detectable antiovulatory activity after single injections of 1–2 mg to more recent analogs which block ovulation at a dose of just a few ug. The antiovulatory assay system itself, in which analogs are injected at 12 noon on proestrus in 4-day cycling rats and their effectiveness measured by counting ova on the following day has also, in its speed and reliability, contributed enormously to this field.

Given the great number of effective LH-RH antagonists reported, it is, however, difficult to come up with strict generalizations, we have attempted to summarize the most important effective modifications and these are shown in table 2.

Table 2 LH-RH substitutions contributing to high antagonist activity

Ac-A-B-C-Ser-Tyr-E-Leu-F-Pro-G-amide	
A:	D-4-halophenylalanines, D-B-naphthylalanine
B:	D-4-Cl-Phe, certain other D-4-halo-Phe's, D-B-Nal
C:	D-Trp, certain other D-amino acids resembling Trp
E:	D-Arg, D-Lys, certain other basic amino acids
F:	Arg or Lys
G:	Gly or, better, D-Ala

Current antagonist analog designs

One undesirable characteristic of the most potent LH-RH antagonists was their poor solubility in aqueous solvent systems which was brought about by the high proportion of lipophilic amino acid substitutions. In recent work, we began to examine ways to circumvent this by introducing highly charged, hydrophilic amino acids such

Table 3 Antiovulatory activities of position 6 analogs of Ac-[D-p-Cl-Phe-1,2,D-Trp-3,X-6,D-Ala-10]-LH-RH in the rat

Amino acid (X)	Dose (μg)	% Inhibition of Ovulation
D-Arg	3.0	100
D-Lys	3.0	50
D-4-aminomethyl-Phe	7.5	100
	3.0	67
D-diaminobutyric acid	3.0	0
D-homo-Arg	15.0	100
	3.0	0

Table 4 Antiovulatory activities of position 4 analogs of Ac-[D-p-Cl-Phe-1,2,D-Trp-3,X-4,D-Arg-6,D-Ala-10]-LH-RH in the rat

Amino acid (X)	Dose (μg)	% Inhibition of Ovulation
D-Arg	3.0	100
Lys	7.5	15
D,L-4-aminomethyl-Phe	7.5	0
Diaminobutyric acid	7.5	0

as Lys and Arg into positions which would have minimal adverse effects on biological activity. The most obvious position with which to accomplish this was the sixth, usually occupied by D-aromatic amino acids. We were suprised to find that D-Lys-6 analogs were just as active and had much improved solubility characteristics. [16]. D-Arg-6 analogs actually showed a two-fold improvement over corresponding D-Phe-6 analogs.

The present generation of antagonists virtually all contain D-Arg in position 6. Many studies have been made to discover more effective position 6 replacements, however, no great improvement in biological activity has been reported so far. We have tried (tab. 3) a number of basic replacements with varying side-chain lengths and also a D-p-aminomethyl-Phe-6 substitution [17] which combines both aromaticity and high basicity. These combined properties did not improve antiovulatory activity. Basic amino acid substitutions in position 4 (tab. 4), position 7, position 3, position 2, and position 1 all resulted in great losses of activity. In a related study of Arg in position 8, it was unexpectedly found [17] that other basic amino acids such as Lys retained full activity. However, none of the position 8 analogs, which included manipulations of side-chain length and other characteristics (tab. 5), had improved activities.

A detailed study was made of position 1 in relation to the D-Arg-6 replacement [18]. The most important conclusion to be drawn from this was that very hydrophobic

Table 5 Antiovulatory activities of position 8 analogs of Ac-[D-p-Cl-Phe-1,2,D-Trp-6,X-8,D-Ala-10]-LH-RH in the rat

Amino acid (X)	Dose (μg)	% Inhibition of Ovulation
Arg	3.0	100
Lys	3.0	100
D,L-4-aminomethyl-Phe	7.5	80
Diaminobutyric acid	3.0	10
4-amino-Phe	7.5	20
His	7.5	15
Gln	15.0	0

Table 6 Blockade of ovulation on estrus when [Ac-D-B-Nal-1,D-p-Cl-Phe-2,D-Trp-3,D-Arg-6,D-Ala-10]-LH-RH was injected on diestrus I

Amount Injected (μg)	# Ovulating/ # Injected	% Inhibition of Ovulation
0	5/5	0
10	5/7	29
100	0/7	100

Table 7 Stability of a solution of [Ac-D-B-Nal-1,D-p-Cl-Phe-2,D-Trp-3,D-Arg-6,D-Ala-10]-LH-RH after being stored at room temperature in 40% propylene glycol in saline

Day Injected (2.5 μg/0.5 ml/rat	# Ovulating/ # Injected	% Ovulation Blockade
0	0/6	100
4	0/6	100
11	0/5	100
48	0/3	100
62	0/4	100
89	0/4	100
131	0/4	100

amino acids gave significant improvements in activity. Thus, [D-B-Nal-1,D-p-Cl-Phe-2,D-Trp-3,D-Arg-6,D-Ala-10]-LH-RH and the corresponding D-p-Br-Phe-1 analog are presently among the most active analogs to have been reported. One reason for their potent antiovulatory effects may be their extremely prolonged activity (up to 48 h) after injection [18]. In fact, blockade of ovulation can be achieved when the Ac-D-B-Nal-1 analog is injected days before the proestrous gonadotropin surge (tab. 6). Research by Dr. K. J. Catt and co-workers on the binding of this type of analog to intact cells clearly reveals high affinity binding and also greatly lowered receptor-ligand dissociation rates relative to, for instance, the superagonists (personal communication). Another impressive physical property of the D-B-Nal-1 analog is its excellent stability in dilute solution. Solutions in 40% propylene glycol/saline can routinely be stored at room temperature for at least 6 months without discernible loss of biological activity (tab. 7).

The increased tolerance for large, lipophilic amino acids at the N-terminus of D-Arg-6 analogs is further illustrated by the high activity of Ac-[D-B-Nal-1,2,D-Trp-3,D-Arg-6,D-Ala-10]-LH-RH. This analog has full activity at a dose of 3 ug (0% at 1 ug) [18] and is, therefore, almost as active as the corresponding D-p-Cl-Phe-2 analog. In the D-Phe-6 series, D-B-Nal in position 2 results in far greater loss of activity.

Conclusions

Although little new chemistry has been performed on LH-RH agonist analogs, steady progress has been made in the development of competitive antagonists with increasing antiovulatory activity and much prolonged time course of action. Despite the large numbers of analogs that have been made and the already intensive studies on each residue of the peptide chain, opportunities for new structure-activity studies and the discovery of more active analogs still remain numerous.

Acknowledgement

This research was supported by NIH Contract NICHD HD-2-2809.

References

[1] Schally, A. V., A. Arimura, D. H. Coy: Vitamins and Hormones, pp. 257–323. Academic Press, New York 1980.
[2] Fujino, M., A. Kobayashi, M. Obayashi et al.: Biochem. Biophys. Res. Commun. **49** (1972) 863–869.
[3] Monahan, M. M. S. Amoss, H. A. Anderson et al.: Biochemistry 12 (1973) 4616–4620.
[4] Coy, D. H., J. A. Vilchez-Martinez, E. J. Coy et al.: J. Med. Chem. **19** (1976) 423–425.
[5] Konig, W., J. Sandow, R. Geiger: Peptides: Chemistry, Structure, and Biology, pp. 883–885. Ann Arbor Science Publishers, Ann Arbor, MI, 1975.
[6] Fujino, M. I. Yamakazi, S. Kobayashi et al.: Biochem. Biophys. Res. Commun. 57 (1974) 1248–1256.
[7] Coy, D. H., E. J. Coy, A. V. Schally et al.: Biochem. Biophys. Res. Commun. 57 (1974) 335–340.
[8] Coy, D. H., J. A. Vilchez-Martinez, E. J. Coy et al.: J. Clin. Endocrinol. Metab. 37 (1973) 331–333.
[9] Coy, D. H., M V. Nekola, J. Erchegyi et al.: LH-RH Reptides as Female and Male Contraceptives, pp. 37–45, Harper and Row, NY, 1981.
[10] de la Cruz, A., D. H. Coy, J. A. Vilchez-Martinez et al.: Science **191** (1976) 195–197.

[11] Beattie, C. W., A. Corbin, T. J. Foell et al.: Contraception **13** (1976) 341–353.
[12] Rivier, J, W. Vale: Life Sciences **23** (1978) 869–873.
[13] Channabasavaiah, K., J. M. Stewart: Biochem. Biophys. Res. Commun. **86** (1979) 1266–1274.
[14] Coy, D. H., I. Mezo, E. Pedroza et al.: Peptides: Structure and Biological Function, pp. 775–779. Pierce, Rockford, IL, 1979.
[15] Erchegyi, J., D. H. Coy, M. V. Nekola: Biochem. Biophys. Res. Commun. **100** (1981) 915–920.
[16] Coy, D. H., A. Horvath, M. V. Nekola: Endocrinology **110** (1982) 1445–1447.
[17] Hocart, S. J., D. H. Coy, D. H. Coy, Peptides: Proc. 8th American Peptide Sym. Pierce, Rockford, IL, 1983, in press.
[18] Coy, D. H., M. V. Nekola: Hormonal Control of the Hypothalamo-Pituitary-Gonadal Axis. Plenum Press, NY, 1983, in press.

Pharmacology of GnRH analogues

C. Rivier, J. Rivier, W. Vale

Introduction

The long-term effects of both GnRH agonists and antagonists on reproductive functions are well established. As the mechanisms through which both types of analogs inhibit reproductive parameters become better understood, these peptides are being considered as therapeutic agents that do not only regulate fertility, but also in pathological conditions where a marked lowering of steroid secretion is desired.

While some years ago, the potency of the GnRH antagonists then available did not permit their use in meaningful long-term experiments, we presently have antagonists which are powerful enough to be used over extended periods of time. Since, in the long range, both agonists and antagonists will inhibit reproductive functions, the question arises as to which class of analogs would be best suited to control fertility.

We describe here the effects of the prolonged exposure to both types of analogs on reproductive functions in the rat, discuss what we know of their respective mechanisms of action and compare their effects in the rat.

Male rat

In the adult male rat, a first injection of GnRH agonists causes marked elevations in plasma LH and FSH levels [1]. Subsequent daily administrations of the analogs for 7 days are followed by blunted, though significant, increases in LH, but not FSH, release. As a consequence, the LH : FSH ratios are significantly augmented over control values [2].

Baseline levels of testosterone (T), which are slightly elevated on day 2, are significantly depressed from day 4 through day 7 [2]. As in the case of the gonadotropins, stimulated T levels are significantly higher on day 1 than any other day, and though each daily administration of the agonists significantly stimulates testosterone secretion, a blunting of the response is rapidly observed [2].

Plasma Progesterone (Po) levels, which are not significantly elevated 2 hrs after the first injection of the agonists, show a ten-fold increase 2 hrs after the second administration of the peptide and stay elevated for over 5 hrs. A-induced increases of Po are diminshed on days 3 and 4 and do not occur on days 5 through 7. Baseline Po levels remain unchanged [2].

These changes in steroid secretion can be linked to studies from several groups that have documented a defect in the steroidogenic pathways of gonadotropin-desensitized Leydig cells leading to decreased androgen production and accumulation of earlier intermediates [3–6]. Such enzymatic defects may account for the increased levels of circulating Po observed in agonist-treated rats, as well as for the lower levels of testosterone. We have also investigated a possible effect of the agonists on the steroidogenic pathways leading to the secretion of testosterone. Steroid production by the Leydig cells of nonpretreated rats incubated with LH was measured in the absence of presence of agonists [7]. We found no direct inhibitory effect of $10-^{9}$ M agonist on spontaneous or LH-stimulated steroidogenesis by these cells. On the contrary, T secretion tended to be slightly elevated in the presence of the agonist [7]. These data indicate that during short-term incubations, GnRH agonists does not appear to exert a direct effect on steroidogenic pathways.

Since, apart from the testis, the adrenal is also known to produce Po, we conducted experiments designed to investigate the respective contributions of both organs to the agonist induced Po secretion. We first examined the steroid production by isolated Leydig cells of control and agonist treated rats incubated with increasing doses of LH over a 3-h incubation period [7]. We observed that Po secretion, which was absent in control tests, was increased in a dose-related fashion by LH in Leydig cells of rats killed 24 h after a single injection of the agonist, but was blunted when the rats had been treated for 2 and 5 days. 17-Hydroxyprogesterone secretion showed a similar pattern. Production of androstenedione was slightly stimulated by the highest dose of LH only in tests of rats having been treated for 5 days, while T secretion showed a progressive blunting as the length of SA administration *in vivo* increased. Baseline levels of T (i.e., in the absence of LH) were also decreased in Leydig cells of rats having received the agonist. These results, which are in keeping with the enzymatic blocks observed in gonadotropin or LH-RH agonist-treated rats indicate that the Leydig cells of nonpretreated rats secrete little, if any, Po, but that they will secrete this steroid in response to GnRH agonists [7].

These results indicate that the chronic treatment of adult male rats with GnRH agonists results in non-physiological secretions of LH, FSH, testosterone and progesterone, which mediate the anti-reproductive effects of these analogs. Histological examination of the testes of male rats having received daily injections of GnRH agonists for 7 days indicates disrupted spermatogenesis, and depopulation of the germinal epithelium [1]. The diameter of the tubules is significantly decreased. It should be emphasized, however, that although most tubules of agonist-treated rats appear empty, some tubules consitently show evidence of ongoing spermatogenesis.

During the long-term treatment of adult male rats with GnRH antagonists, the secretion of LH, FSH and testosterone is inhibited at all times [8]. The amounts of LH and FSH in the pituitary is also significantly lower in antagonist-treated animals. Consistent with the dramatic decrease in circulating T, the weights of testes and androgen-dependent organs is also greatly reduced [8].

The tubular diameter of rats treated with GnRH antagonists is markedly decreased, and the germinal epithelium shows no sign of mitosis. In no tubules did we observed germinal cells beyond spermatogonia and a few spermatocytes [8]. It should be emphasized that while the doses of GnRH antagonists necessary to disrupt reproductive functions are much larger than those of agonists, the degree of inhibition of testicular weight and testosterone release is significantly higher [9].

These data indicate that both GnRH agonists and antagonists disrupt hormonal secretion and interfere with spermatogenesis. Measurement of actual fertility of male rats treated over long-time periods with either class of analogs has indicated, however, marked differences. When adult male rats were injected with the agonist [$DTrp^6$, Pro^9, NEt]-GnRH] (3 μg/kg), daily for 6 months, a significant number of agonist-treated rats remained fertile [9] (fig. 1). Daily administration of the antagonist [Ac-Δ^3,Pro^1,pcl-$DPhe^2$,$DTrp^{3,6}$,Nβ$MeLeu^7$]-GnRH (3 mg/kg) on the other hand, resulted in the absence of sexual activity which can be restored by the concomitant injections of low doses or androgen in the absence of recovery of spermatogenesis [10].

The comparison of the effects of GnRH agonists and antagonists in the male rats, thus indicates a number of differences in the long-term effects of these peptides. As mentioned above, the degree of inhibition of reproductive function is significantly higher for the antagonists than it is for the agonists, even though at the present time

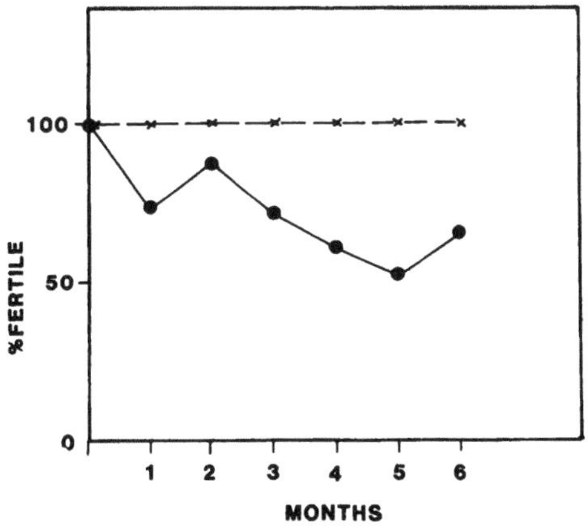

Fig. 1 Fertility of male rats injected daily with saline (x) or [$DTrp^6$, Pro^9, NEt]-GnRH (0). Each point represented the mean of 10 rats.

much larger doses of antagonists versus agonists are required. Furthermore, the antagonists cause a total arrest of spermatogenesis, while chronic exposure to the agonists is still accompanied by a certain degree of fertility.

Female rat

Puberty

The daily administration on GnRH agonists to immature female rats delays puberty (as assessed by the onset of vaginal opening) for the duration of the treatment [11]. As shown in table 1, 2.5 μg/kg of a GnRH agonist administered daily from day 24 through day 60 prevents vaginal opening in all treated animals [9]. Upon cessation of the treatment, vaginal opening is observed 3–8 days after the last injection, and the subsequent 3 estrous cycles appear normal.

The effect of GnRH antagonists on puberty is also illustrated in table 1. When the antagonist was administered from day 24 of age to female rats (1 mg/kg), vaginal opening was delayed by 10–14 days, but eventually occurred despite continuing administration of the analog. These data are also consitent with studies showing that passive immunization to endogenous GnRH only delayed puberty in female rats which did, however, achieve fertility.

Table 1 Effect of GnRH agonist or antagonist on the onset of puberty in the rat

Treatment	N	Day of the vaginal opening
Control	10	36.9 ± 0.84
2.5 μg/kg BW agonist	10	63.4 ± 1.52
Control	12	37.6 ± 0.83
1 mg/kg BW antagonist	12	43.5 ± 0.86

Agonist = DHis^{6}(imBzl),Pro^{9}-NEt]-GnRH
Antagonist = [Ac-DNAL(2)^{1},4FDPhe^{3},DArg^{6}]-GnRH

At the present time, we do not know whether GnRH agonist-treated animals would have eventually exhibited sexual maturation. The observation that some antagonist-treated female rats showed vaginal opening as early as 38 days of age (i.e., only 3 days later than most controls, while no agonist-treated animals reached puberty during the course of the treatment [9], would however suggest that the agonist was more effective than the antagonist to interfere with normal sexual maturation.

GnRH antagonists have been demonstrated to be more powerful to inhibit LH than FSH release. In collaborative studies, (Charlesworth *et al.* submitted), we have indeed repeatedly observed that even large doses of these antagonists would not lower plasma FSH levels by more than 50%. Since an increase in FSH, but not LH, secretion has been reported to represent the principal stimulus for puberty [12], it is possible that the "escape" seen in antagonist-treated rats may have been at least partially due to the inability of these analogs to totally inhibit FSH release. By contrast, the total absence of FSH stimulation in the presence of agonist [1], as well as the reported gonadal desensitization occurring with prolonged exposure to such analogs, may have been responsible for the higher effectiveness of agonist.

Estrus cycle

Daily administration of a GnRH agonist to regularly cycling female rats, starting on diestrus-II, interrupts cyclicity (and ovulation) for the duration of the treatment [11, 13]. Regular cycles were resumed 5–8 days after the last injection.

Studies on the antiovulatory effects of GnRH antagonists have shown that 0.5 μg of the most potent analogs can block ovulation when administered at noon on proestrus, while larger doses are necessary to be effective when injected on diestrus-II (C. Rivier, J. Rivier and W. Vale, unpublished). Daily administration of the antagonists completely block the estrus cycle, which resumes 6–9 days after cessation of the treatment [14].

As illustrated by these experiments, both GnRH agonists and antagonists can effectively interfere with normal cyclicity in the female rat, and this effect is totally reversible.

Pregnancy

It is well established that administration of GnRH agonists will interfere with gestation in the rat [13, 15–20]. We have observed that GnRH agonists (4 μg/kg) would terminate pregnancy when injected either from day 1 through 7, or 8 through 12 after mating, with the second regimen being slightly more effective [13]. GnRH agonists can also terminate pregnancy when administered after the LH-dependent time of gestation (day 12), an effect probably due to their extra-pituitary actions [21].

GnRH antagonists will also disrupt gestation, but their ability to do so varies with the stage of pregnancy [14, 22]. Much larger doses of the antagonist are required during the first week (10 mg/kg) than in the second week after mating (1 mg/kg). We have observed [9] that 10 times more antagonist was necessary to terminate pregnancy during days 1–7, than during days 8–12 [14]. By contrast, no effect of antagonist is observed after day 12 (C. Rivier and W. Vale, unpublished).

These data indicate that there are at least two differences between the antigestiational effects of GnRH agonists and antagonists in the female rat: the dose-dependent effectiveness (within each class of analogs) of the peptides to terminate pregnancy, and the temporal relationship between the abortifacient effects of both classes of peptides.

We have observed that exogenous administration of progesterone, PRL or hCG during the first week of pregnancy can reverse the deleterious effect of GnRH agonists, while during the second week only progesterone and hCG are effective [23] (tab. 2). These data suggested that during the first week after mating the antigestational properties of the agonists are at least partially mediated through inhibition of PRL secretion, a hormone which plays an essential luteotropic role in the rat. By contrast, since exogenous PRL is unable to prevent the abortifacient action of GnRH antagonists (tab. 3), it is probable that the effects of these analogs are not mediated through inhibition of PRL secretion. These data had led us to suggest that during the first week of gestation the differential ability of GnRH agonists and antagonists to modify PRL release were related to their relative efficacy to terminate pregnancy [23].

Results from replacement therapy during the second week of gestation indicate that the main mediator of both types of analogs' effects during that time is inhibition of LH release [23]. We have indeed reported that there is a striking parallelism between maximal antireproductive effects of GnRH antagonists and the time of LH-dependency of the corpus luteum [22], an observation which is in agreement with previously published studies on the effect of immunoneutralization of endogenous GnRH in pregnant rats [24] GnRH agonists, through their ability to cause pituitary desensitization, also induce abortion by depriving the corpus luteum of its tropic signal.

Finally, as previously mentioned, GnRH agonists (but not antagonists) can terminate pregnancy when administered during the third week after mating [21]. Since the

Table 2 Interaction between GnRH agonist, progesterone, PRL and hCG on the outcome of pregnancy in the rat

Treatment		No. pregnant at term	No. pups delivered/female
Vehicle	d1-7	6/6	9.8
Agonist	d1-7	0/6	0
Agonist + Po	d1-7	6/6	11.3
Agonist + hCG	d1-7	4/6	9.3
Agonist + PRL	d1-7	5/6	10.4
Vehicle	d8-12	6/6	9.9
Agonist	d8-12	0/6	0
Agonist + Po	d8-12	6/6	4.5 (dead)
Agonist + hCG	d8-12	6/6	9.0 (dead)
Agonist + PRL	d8-12	2/6	8.5 (dead)

Agonist = [DTrp^6,Pro^9,NEt]-GnRH
Doses: Agonist = 1.0 μg
Po = 4.0 μg
hHG = 0.5 1U
PRL = 0.3 mg

Table 3 Interaction between GnRH antagonist, progesterone, PRL and hCG on the outcome of pregnancy in the rat

Treatment		No. pregnant at term	No. pups delivered/female
Vehicle	d1-7	6/6	10.0
Antagonist	d1-7	3/6	10.0
Antagonist + Po	d1-7	6/6	10.8
Antagonist + hCG	d1-7	6/6	8.5
Antagonist + PRL	d1-7	3/6	16.0
Vehicle	d1-8	6/6	10.1
Antagonist	d1-8	0/6	0
Antagonist + Po	d1-8	6/6	8.7
Antagonist + hCG	d1-8	6/6	6.7
Antagonist + PRL	d1-8	0/6	0

Antagonist = [Ac-Δ-Pro^1, pCEl-$DPhe^2$,$DTrp^{3,6}$]-GnRH
Doses: Antagonist = 0.3 mg
Po = 4.0 mg
hCG = 0.5 1U
PRL = 0.3 mg

agonists are abortifacient in pregnant rats hypophysectomized at day 13 of gestation, they most probably act through an extrapituitary site of action, namely at the ovarian level, to inhibit luteal progesterone production [21]. On the other hand, while GnRH antagonists have also been reported to exert extrapituitary effects, we have been unable to demonstrate any antigestational action of these analogs during the third week of pregnancy [9]. Therefore, the effectiveness of GnRH agonists and the lack of effectiveness of GnRH antagonists during the last week of gestation can probably be attributed to the relative importance of the agonists' extra-pituitary effect in mediating these antireproductive effects. (Review in [25, 26].)

Conclusion

In conclusion, it is apparent that the long-term administration of both GnRH agonists and antagonists disrupts reproductive functions in the rat. While the mechanisms of action of the antagonists appear to primarily involve competitive blockade of pituitary GnRH receptors with a subsequent inhibition of gonadotropin (in particular LH) and steroid secretion, the effects of GnRH agonists are more complex, including desensitization to GnRH at the pituitary level (which is more marked for FSH than for LH), a loss of LH gonadal receptors, a decrease in PRL release, and direct (extrapituitary) gonadal actions. Furthermore, an important difference between the effects of GnRH agonists and antagonists resides in the fact that the administration of the antagonists is consistently accompanied by a marked decrease in plasma LH (and to a lesser degree, FSH) levels, while each daily injection of the agonists causes a measurable (though blunted) increase in LH (but usually not FSH) release.

The time-period during which GnRH analogs need to be present in the circulation to significantly alter reproductive parameters represents another element that differentiates their mode of action: GnRH antagonists need to occupy pituitary receptors on a continuous basis (and therefore be consistently present in the circulation) in order to be effective; on the other hand, since a large portion of the effects of GnRH agonists on reproduction appears to be mediated through pituitary and gonadal desensitization, periodic exposures to the peptide are sufficient to disrupt reproductive functions. This may explain at least in part why much larger doses of the antagonists than the agonists are required to be effective.

However, an important factor resides in the observation that the degree of inhibition of reproductive functions observed in the male rat with GnRH antagonists is significantly higher than it is for the agonists.

Over the past years, considerable progress has been made in the design of new GnRH antagonists, and future improvements in potencies may lead to peptides that will be active at much lower doses than those presently available. Because GnRH antagonists do not cause the periodic stimulation of gonadotropin and steroid release observed with GnRH agonists, they are believed to represent significant future tools in regulating reproductive functions.

Acknowledgements

This study was supported by NIH grants AM-20917, AA-03504, AM-26741, HD-13527; NIH contract NO 1-HD-0-2836; The Rockefeller Foundation; The Texas-Salk Institute Foundation; and The March of Dimes-Birth Defects Foundation. Research conducted in part by The Clayton Foundation for Research, California Division. Drs. C. Rivier and W. Vale are Clayton Foundation Investigators.

References

[1] Rivier C., J. Rivier, W. Vale: Endocrinology **105** (1979) 1191–1201.
[2] Rivier, C., W. Vale: Life Sci. **25** (1979) 1065–1074.
[3] Labrie, F., Godbont, A. Zelanger et al.: In "LH-RH Peptides as Female and Male Contraceptives", (Eds. G. I. Zatuchni, J. D. Shelton, J. J. Sciarra), pp. 246–260. Harper and Row, publishers, 1981.
[4] Catt, K. J., A. J. Baukal, T. F. Davies et al.: Endocrinology **104** (1979) 17–25.
[5] Harwood, J. P., R. N. Clayton, K. J. Catt: I. Properties and inhibition of luteal cell function. Endo. **107** (1980) 407–413.

[6] Reddy, P. V., S. Azhar, K. M. J. Menon: Endocrinology **107** (1980) 930–936.
[7] Rivier, C., J. Rivier, W. Vale: Intl. J. Fertility **25** (3) (1980) 145–150.
[8] Rivier, C., J. Rivier, W. Vale: Science **210** (1980) 93–95.
[9] Rivier, C., W. Vale, J. Rivier: J. of Med. Chem. (1983) in press.
[10] Rivier, C., J. Rivier, W. Vale: Endocrinology **108** (1981) 1998–2001.
[11] Vale, W., C. Rivier, M. Brown et al: In "Hypothalamic Peptide Hormones and Pituitary Regulation. Advances in Experimental Medicine and Biology", (Ed. J. C. Porter), pp. 123–156. (Proc. NIH Workshop, Bethesda, MD.) Plenum Press, New York 1977.
[12] Critchlow, W., M E. Bar-Sela: Neuroendocrinology **2** (1967) 101–162.
[13] Rivier, C., J. Rivier, W. Vale: Endocrinology **103** (1978) 2299–2305.
[14] Rivier, C., J. Rivier, W. Vale: Endocrinology **108** (4) (1981) 1425–1430.
[15] Humphrey, R. R., B. L. Windsor, D. C. Jones et al: Biol. Reprod. **19** (1978) 84–91.
[16] Humphrey, R. R., B. L. Windsor, J. R. Reel et al: Biol. Reprod. **16** (1977) 614–621.
[17] Corbin, A., C. W. Beattie, R. Rees et al: Fertility and Sterility **28** (1977) 471–476.
[18] Corbin, A., W. C. Beattie, R. Jones et al.: Int. J. Gynaecol. Obstet. **16** (1979) 359–372.
[19] Bex. F. J., A. Corbin: Endocrinology **105** (1979) 139–145.
[20] Rivier, C., J. Rivier, W. Vale: Contraception **19** (1979) 185–190.
[21] Bex, F. J., A. Corbin: Endocrinology **108** (1981) 273–280.
[22] Rivier, C., W. Vale: Biol. Reprod. **24** (1981) 1061–1067.
[23] Rivier, C., W. Vale: Endocrinology **110** (1982) 347–351.
[24] Nishi, N., A. Arimura, H. G. dela Cruz et al: Endocrinology **98** (1976) 1024.
[25] Hsueh, A. J. W., P. B. C. Jones: Endocrine Rev. **2** (1981) 437–461.
[26] Sharpe, R. M: J. Reprod. Fert. **64** (1982) 517–527.

Binding sites for LH-RH in the human – does LH-RH exert extrapituitary actions in man?

R. M. Popkin, T. A. Bramley, A. Currie, R. M. Sharpe, H. M. Fraser

Introduction

The presence of extrapituitary binding sites is now well documented particularly in the case of rat ovary [1, 2] and testicular Leydig cells [3, 4] where the binding sites appear to mediate direct actions of LH-RH and its analogues on steroidogenesis. Exogenous LH-RH and its agonists have been reported to exert both inhibitory [5, 6] and stimulatory actions on the gonads [7, 8]. It is likely that in the female the effects of LH-RH are dependent upon the stage of follicular development and/or period and extent of exposure to gonadotrophin. In the male, short-term exposure (<24 h) is stimulatory, while longer term exposure has inhibitory effects on steroidogenesis [9, 10, 11]. The physiological importance of a putative intragonadal LH-RH-like factor remains unsolved, though such factor(s) may play a role in the regulation of ovarian and testicular function [12]. However, the presence of high affinity extrapituitary LH-RH receptors clearly provides a potential site of action for exogenously administered LH-RH and its analogues. Particularly in the case of the rat where chronic administration of LH-RH is known to exert antifertility effects, the direct gonadal component of such actions is largely unsolved.

With the increased use of LH-RH and its analogues for both clinical and veterinary purposes [13, 14] the question of direct extrapituitary actions of LH-RH in species other than the rat is clearly important. Several reports have indicated that gonadal tissue from other species can respond to LH-RH, for example porcine granulosa cells [15] and rabbit ovarian tissue [16]. On the other hand the mouse appears immune to direct gonadal actions[17]. In addition sheep corpus luteal tissue failed to show specific binding of ^{125}I-LH-RH agonist in 3 separate experiments (R. M. Popkin, unpublished observations).

Due to difficulties involved in assessing direct gonadal actions of LH-RH in the human, we approached the question by examining the evidence for the presence of extrapituitary binding sites for LH-RH in human placental and gonadal tissue. The ability of human tissue to bind specifically ^{125}I-D(Ser) But [6] des Gly [10] LH-RH agonist was thus assessed and the binding characteristics compared to that of the rat.

Specific binding of ^{125}I-LH-RH agonist to rat ovarian tissue

Binding was measured using homogenates of whole rat ovarian tissue prepared from immature rats 48 h after administration of 50 IU pregnant mare's serum gonadotrophin (PMSG) to induce follicular development. 100 000 cpm ^{125}I-LH-RH agonist was used as the ligand, with non-specific binding being assessed in the presence of 10^{-5}M LH-RH agonist. After incubation on ice for 2 h separation of free hormone from receptor bound hormone was achieved by addition of 0.5 ml of 0.5% bovine immunoglobulin (IgG) followed by 1 ml of ice-cold 25% polyethylene glycol (PEG). After 30 minutes on ice, tubes were centrifuged at 3000 rpm for 10 minutes at 4 °C, the supernatant was discarded and the pellet counted.

Binding of the labelled ligand was displaced in the presence of various concentrations of unlabelled peptides. A typical displacement cure for LH-RH agonist, LH-RH and unrelated peptides is shown in figure 1. The characteristics of binding were identical to those found with rat anterior pituitary tissue, namely a high affinity site for LH-RH agonist with a 100–1000 lower affinity for LH-RH and minimal displacement by peptides unrelated to LH-RH. Similar binding characteristics have been reported for rat luteal tissue [1].

Specific binding of ^{125}I-LH-RH agonist to human corpus luteum homogenates

Human luteal tissue was obtained (with the informed consent of the patient) from patients undergoing laparotomy during the luteal phase of the cycle and post menopausal tissue from women undergoing hysterectomy.

After homogenization, tissue was incubated as described for rat ovarian tissue, with separation of free from bound hormone being achieved by centrifugation in the presence of PEG/IgG. The displacement curve obtained in 3 separate experiments using 3 different corpus luteum homogenates is shown in figure 2.

The characteristics of human luteal binding sites for LH-RH are similar to those of the rat pituitary and gonads as regards affinity for LH-RH (apparent Ka of 10^6M^{-1}) and specificity (only LH-RH and LH-RH agonist displacing binding). However, an important difference can be seen in the affinity for LH-RH agonist, the displacement curve being shifted to the right, giving an apparent Ka for LH-RH agonist which was 100–1000 fold lower than that estimated for rat tissue, and of similar order of magnitude to that of LH-RH (fig. 2). No specific binding of ^{125}I-LH-RH agonist was detectable with human post menopausal tissue.

Preliminary studies of LH-RH agonist binding to human corpora lutea recovered at different stages of the luteal phase showed that specific binding was present at all stages, with highest levels associated with the mid-luteal phase (Bramley, Popkin & Baird, in preparation).

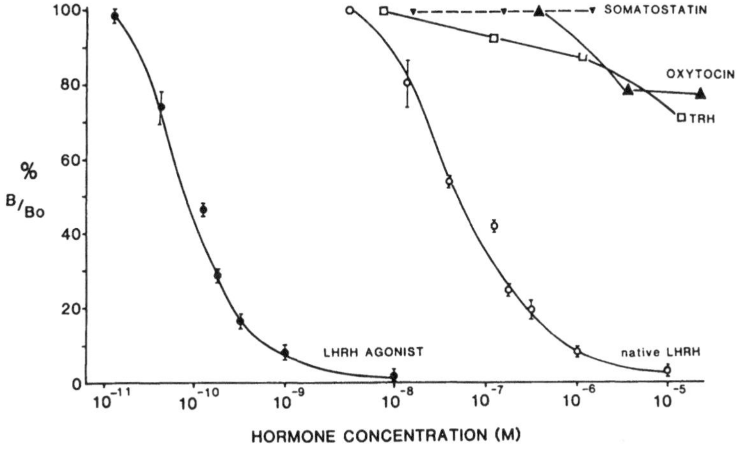

Fig. 1 Competition curves for binding of ^{125}I-LHRH agonist to rat ovarian homogenates in the presence of increasing concentrations of LHRH agonist (D-ser-t-Bu^6-*des*-GlyNH$_2$^{10} LHRH ethylamide), LHRH, oxytocin, somatostatin and TRH. The figure represents mean ± range of duplicate determinations at each point.

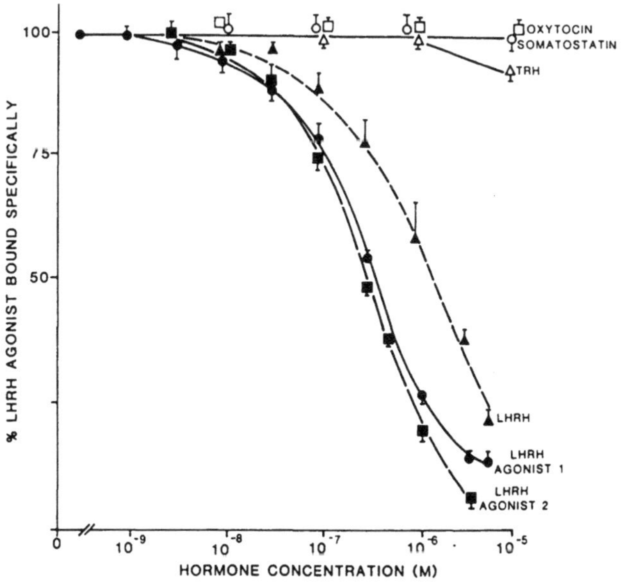

Fig. 2 Competition curves for binding of ^{125}I-LHRH agonist to human luteal tissue in the presence of increasing concentrations of unlabelled LHRH agonist$_1$, ((D-ser-t-Bu^6-*des*-GlyNH$_2$^{10}) LHRH ethylamide), LHRH agonist$_2$ (D-Nal (2)^6) LHRH, native LHRH, oxytocin, somatostatin and TRH. The figure represents the mean of 3 displacement curves obtained from 3 mid-luteal corpora lutea. The values of Bo for each corpus luteum were 9.500 cpm/75 ul, 4.900 cpm/50 ul, and 7.100 cpm/40 ul. Printed with permission[35].

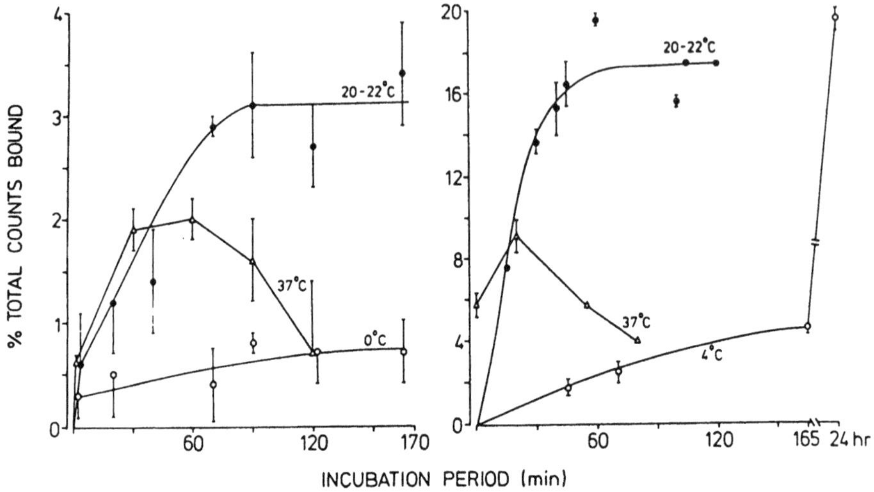

Fig. 3 Binding of ^{125}I-LHRH agonist to the 1.000 g fraction (left hand panel) and 10.000 g fraction (right hand panel) of term placenta at different temperatures. Each point represents the mean ± range of either duplicate or triplicate incubations and the results are representative of several experiments. Printed with permission[34].

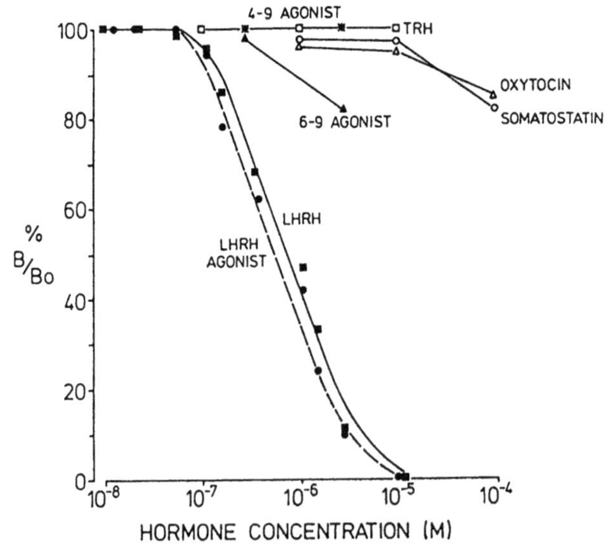

Fig. 4 Competition curves for binding of ^{125}I-LHRH agonist to human placental tissue in the presence of increasing concentrations of LHRH agonist ((D-ser-t-Bu^6-*des*-GlyNH$_2$^{10}) LHRH ethylamide), LHRH, 6–9 LHRH agonist, 4–9 LHRH agonist, somatostatin, oxytocin and TRH. Each point is the mean ± range of duplicate determinations. Printed with permission[34].

Specific binding of ^{125}I-LH-RH agonist to human placental tissue

Binding of ^{125}I-LH-RH agonist to both 1000 g and 10 000 g membrane preparations from human term placental tissue was time- and temperature-dependent (fig. 3). Incubations were routinely performed at 20 °C for 90 minutes, with separation of free from bound hormone by filtration through Whatman GF/C filters which had been presoaked in 2% BSA.

The displacement of binding by LH-RH and LH-RH agonist showed essentially the same characteristics as those shown for human luteal tissue (fig. 4). The apparent affinity of the placental binding site for LH-RH and LH-RH agonist was similar (6×10^7 M^{-1} and $4 \times 10^7 M^{-1}$ respectively).

Specific binding of ^{125}I-LH-RH agonist to isolated human Leydig cells

Testicular tissue was obtained by courtesy of Dr. T. B. Hargreave, from patients undergoing orchidectomy for prostatic carcinoma. The patients were aged 60–71 years and had not received prior hormone therapy. After removal of the testicular capsule, tissue was cut into cubes of approx. 0.5 g and the tissue then dispersed in a shaking water bath (170 cycles/min) by incubation for 15 minutes at 34 °C following the addition of 2 mls/g Krebs-Ringer bicarbonate solution containing collagenase (0.5 mg/ml), BSA (0.5 mg/ml), Trypsin inhibitor (0.5 mg/ml) and DNA ase (0.25 mg/ml). Cells were resuspended at a concentration of 10×10^6 nucleated cells/ml in M199 containing Hank's salts and BSA (1 mg/ml) and aliquots of 2×10^6 cells incubated with 300 000 cpm ^{125}I-LH-RH agonist and various concentrations of unlabelled peptides for 15 minutes at 21 °C. Cells were then placed on ice for 10 minutes, diluted five-fold with cold medium and the cells pelleted by centrifugation at 4 °C for 10 minutes at 1000 g. The proportion of Leydig cells was determined by staining of acetone-fixed cells for 3B-hydroxysteroid dehydrogenase and varied from 2–11% according to the cell preparation.

For 2 separate preparations of cells. LH-RH agonist, and to a lesser extent LH-RH, depressed binding in a dose dependent manner, whereas the other peptides tested were inactive at the same hormone concentrations (fig. 5).

Discussion

From the data presented in figures 1–3 it is clear that specific binding sites for LH-RH and LH-RH agonist are present in extra-pituitary sites in the human. Although the sites are specific, the affinity for LH-RH agonist is 100–1000 fold lower than that found in the rat. Neverthless the affinity for native LH-RH is comparable

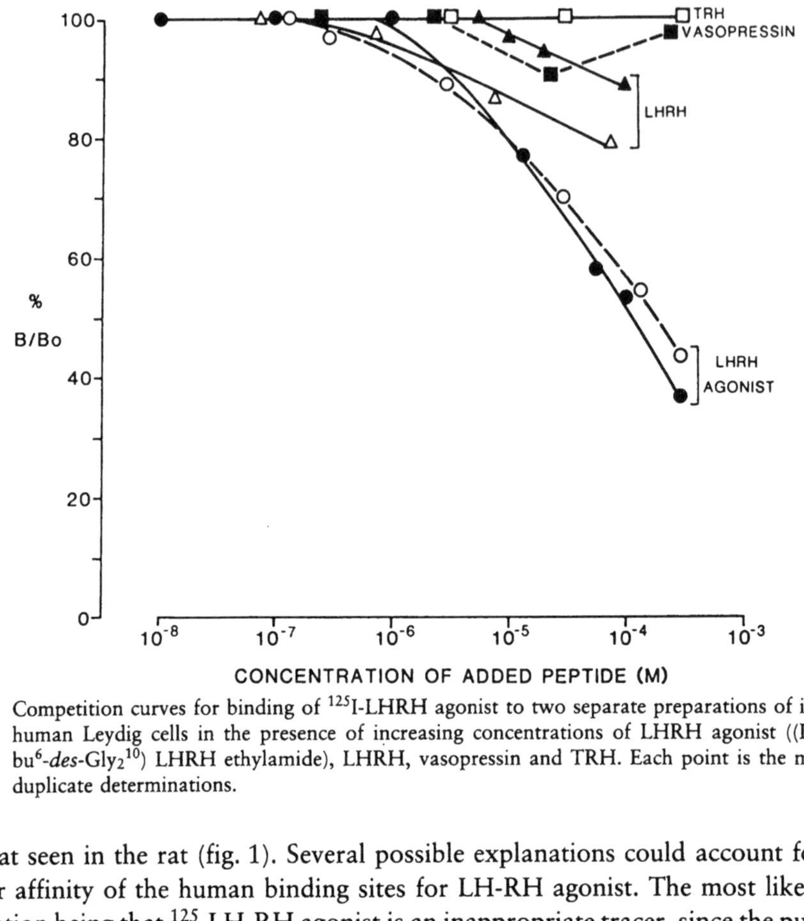

Fig. 5 Competition curves for binding of ^{125}I-LHRH agonist to two separate preparations of isolated human Leydig cells in the presence of increasing concentrations of LHRH agonist ((D-ser-t-bu^{6}-*des*-Gly2^{10}) LHRH ethylamide), LHRH, vasopressin and TRH. Each point is the mean of duplicate determinations.

to that seen in the rat (fig. 1). Several possible explanations could account for the lower affinity of the human binding sites for LH-RH agonist. The most likely explanation being that ^{125}-LH-RH agonist is an inappropriate tracer, since the putative endogenous ligand is likely to be non-identical to LH-RH agonist and may well have a greater affinity for the binding site. Alternatively, but unlikely, LH-RH agonist and LH-RH may be degraded at similar rates or the binding site may be the active site of an LH-RH-peptidase. Preliminary data would seem to rule out these alternatives, however (Bramley, in preparation).

The existence of specific binding sites for LH-RH in the human gonads and placenta raises the possibility that an endogenous molecule interacting with such binding sites is involved in paracrine regulation. LH-RH-like material has been reported in a variety of human sources from tumors [18] to milk [19]; however, evidence in favour of the existence of a gonadal LH-RH is slim in both rat [20] und human sources.

The evidence for placental LH-RH is, however, convincing as LH-RH-like acitivity has not only been detected in placental tissue [21], but more recently a peptide synthesized by placental tissue has been isolated, sequenced and found to be identical to hypothalamic LH-RH [22].

As regards the placenta, despite the presence of low affinity LH-RH binding sites a variety of evidence suggests a role for endogenous LH-RH in the control of placental function. *In vitro* studies on human placental cultures incubated with LH-RH have shown a stimulatory effect on hCG [23, 24] release and an inhibition of hCG release by an LH-RH antagonist [25]. However, other groups have failed to observe such a stimulation [26, 33]. It is also important to note that in *in vivo* studies in which LH-RH or its agonists have been administered to pregnant women, no alteration in plasma hCG levels has been demonstrated. We examined the effect of LH-RH and its agonist on hCG production by perfused placental tissue prepared from mixed chorionic villi or collaginase dispersed cells supported in Biogel columns. Inconsistent results were obtained, with stimulation of hCG release only occurring in response to some pulses of LH-RH and over 80% of pulses failed to significantly increase hCG release. Under the same conditions dispersed rat pituitary cells consistently and repeatedly released LH in response to LH-RH [33]. The physiological relevance of LH-RH in the control of placental function remains largely unsolved.

Evidence for direct gonadal actions of LH-RH in the human and primate remain slim. The reported absence of binding and direct effects using monkey corpus luteum tissue [27] contrasts with a recent report claiming LH-RH inhibition of progestrone production from granulosa cells isolated from FSH primed monkeys [28]. Similarly, in the human, LH-RH was reported to have no effect on steroidogenesis in isolated granulosa or luteal cells [29, 30]. However, one report suggested that LH-RH inhibited progesterone production from isolated human granulosa cells [31]. In addition for the male, indirect evidence from experiments with a Sertoli-Leydig cell tumor [32], suggests that LH-RH may be capable of influencing testosterone production.

The physiological significance of gonadal LH-RH in the human remains to be established, although the absence of binding to post-menopausal tissue and preliminary data suggesting changes in binding sites during the luteal phase are intriguing, and may suggest a role in the control of luteal function.

Finally, an important consideration regarding the clinical use of LH-RH and its analogs is whether exogenously administered hormone would be capable of interacting with these extrapituitary binding sites. Serum concentrations of LH-RH or LH-RH agonist would need to exceed 10^{-7} to achieve 50% occupancy of the extra pituitary binding sites. It is clearly unlikely therefore that the dose ranges of peptiedes used clinically would reach such circulating levels *in vivo*. Indeed, doses in excess of 1 mg intravenously would be needed to achieve such levels. It is therefore unlikely that extrapituitary actions of LH-RH could be invoked by exogenous administration of LH-RH for clinical purposes, unlesse exceedingly high doses were given. However, the presence of specific binding sites for LH-RH on gonadal tissue raises the possibility that LH-RH or an LH-RH-like peptide may be involved in the physiological paracrine regulation of gonadal function in the human.

References

[1] Clayton, R. N., J. P. Harwood, K. J. Catt: Nature (London) **282** (1979) 90–92.
[2] Jones P. B. C., P. M. Conn, J. Marian et al: Life Science **27** (1980) 2125–2132.
[3] Sharpe, R. M., H. M. Fraser: Biochem. Biophys. Res. Commun. **95** (1980) 256–262.
[4] Bourne, G. A., S. Regiani, A.–H. Payne et al: J. Clin. Endocrinol. Metab. **51** (1980) 407–409.
[5] Hsueh, A. J. W., P. B. C. Jones: Endocrine Reviews **2** (1981) 437–461.
[6] Sharpe, R. M.: J. Reprod. Fertil. **64** (1982) 517–527.
[7] Popkin, R., H. M. Fraser, J. Jonassen: Mol. Cell. Endocrinol. **29** (1983) 169–179.
[8] Sharpe, R. M., I. Cooper: Mol. Cell. Endocrinol. **26** (1982) 141–150.
[9] Fraser, H. M., R. M. Sharpe, R. M. Popkin: Volume 1 of Encyclopedia. In: Reproductive Health Care (Eds. B. H. Vickery, J. J. Nestor, Jr., E.S.E. Hafez). MTP Press, Boston (1983) in press.
[10] Naor, Z., M. Zilberstein, H. Zakur et al.: Mol. Cell. Endocrinol. **31** (1983) 261–270.
[11] Sharpe, R. M., H. M. Fraser: Mol. Cell. Endocrinol. (1983) in press.
[12] Ying, S. Y., R. Guillemin: Nature **280** (1979) 593–595.
[13] Fraser, H. M.: Br. Med. J. **285** (1982) 990–991.
[14] Yen, S. S. C.: Fertil. Steril. **39** (1983) 257–266.
[15] Massicotte, J., R. Velleux, M. Lavoie et al.: Biochem. Biophys. Res. Commun. **94** (1980) 1362–1366.
[16] Koos, R. D., K. E. B. Ahrén, P. O. Janson et al.: 64th Annual Meeting of Endocrine Society, Abstr. 395, 1982.
[17] Hunter, M. G., M. H. F. Sullivan, C. J. Dix et al.: Mol. Cell. Endocrinol. **27** (1982) 31–44.
[18] Seppälä, M., T. Wahlström: Int. J. Cancer **26** (1980) 267–268.
[19] Amarant, T., M. Fridkin, Y. Koch: Eur. J. Biochem. **127** (1982) 647–650.
[20] Esch, F., N. Ling, S. Y. Ying et al.: Role of peptides and protein in control of reproduction (Eds. S. M. McCann, D. S. Dhindsa), pp. 275–290. Elsevier Science Pub. Co. Inc., Amsterdam 1983.
[21] Khodr, G. S., T. M. Siler-Khodr: Fertil. Steril. **29** (1978) 523–526.
[22] Tan, L., P. Rousseau: Biochem. Biophys. Res. Commun. **109** (1983) 1061–1071.
[23] Khodr. G., T. M. Siler-Khodr: Fertil. Steril. **30** (1978) 301–304.
[24] Bützow, R.: Int. J. Cancer **29** (1982) 9–11.
[25] Siler-Khodr, T. M., G. S. Khodr, B. H. Vickery et al.: Life Sciences **32** (1983) 2741–2745.
[26] Hussa, R. O.: Endocrine Reviews **1** (1980) 268–294.
[27] Asch, R. H., M. V. Sickle, V. Rettori et al.: J. Clin. Endocrinol. Metab. **53** (1981) 215–217.
[28] Knecht, M., T. Ranta, Z. Naor et al.: Factors Regulating Ovarian Function (Eds. G. S. Greenwald, P. F. Terranova), pp. 225–243. Raven Press, New York 1983.
[29] Casper, R. F., G. F. Erickson, R. W. Rebar et al.: Fertil. Steril. **37**, 406–409.
[30] Tan, G. J. S., J. S. G. Biggs: J. Reprod. Fertil. **67** (1983) 411–413.
[31] Tureck, R. W., L. Jr. Mastroianni, L. Blasco et al.: J. Clin. Endocrinol. Metab. **54** (1982) 1078–1080.
[32] Lamberts, S. W. J., J. M. Timmers, R. Oosterom et al.: J. Clin. Endocrinol. Metab. **54** (1982) 450–453.
[33] Currie, A.: PhD Thesis. University of Edinburgh, 1983.
[34] Currie, A. J., H. M. Fraser, R. M. Sharpe: Biochem. Biophys. Res. Commun. **99** (1981) 332–338.
[35] Popkin, R., T. A. Bramley, A. Currie et al.: Biochem. Biophys. Res. Commun. **14** (1983) 750–756.

Influence of LH-RH and des-Gly^{10} [D-Ala^{6}]-LH-RH ethylamide on the biosynthesis of hCG in placental tissue culture

W. E. Merz, G. Hilf

Introduction

During evolution, the central nervous system, the immune and the endocrine system have developed up to a more complex degree than others. Especially, the reproduction of the species was a matter to be guaranteed with a high priority. For this purpose it was essential that the regulation of the reproductive organs by hormones became highly organized. The most complex peptide hormones known up today are included in this control system: the hypophyseal gonadotropins lutropin and follitropin as well as the placental hormone choriogonadotropin (hCG). Together with thyrotropin these hormones represent a superfamily of proteins which trace back to a common ancestor [1]. Like the other members of this hormone family, hCG is composed of two dissimilar, non covalently linked subunits, α und β, with molecular weights of 14 900 and 23 000, respectively.

Little is known about the biosynthesis of hCG and its regulation. In the present study the regulation of the biosynthesis of hCG in first trimester placental tissue is investigated.

Biosynthesis of human choriogonadotropin

Placental biosynthesis of hCG starts with the implantation of the fertilized ovum and reaches an optimum in the 8th–10th week of gestation. Thereafter, the rate of hCG biosynthesis is rapidly decreased to basal values, which persist up to the end of pregnancy. HCG, which is a biosynthetic product of the fetal part of the placenta, the syncytiotrophoblast, however, is also produced by a variety of tumors of trophoblastic and nontrophoblastic origin [2–4]. Biosynthesis of hCG is a process more complex than in case of most other hormones since it comprises not only the ribosomal synthesis of a preprotein and the processing of the polypeptide chain but also the glycosylation and the assembly of the subunits. The present conception is summarized in figure 1.

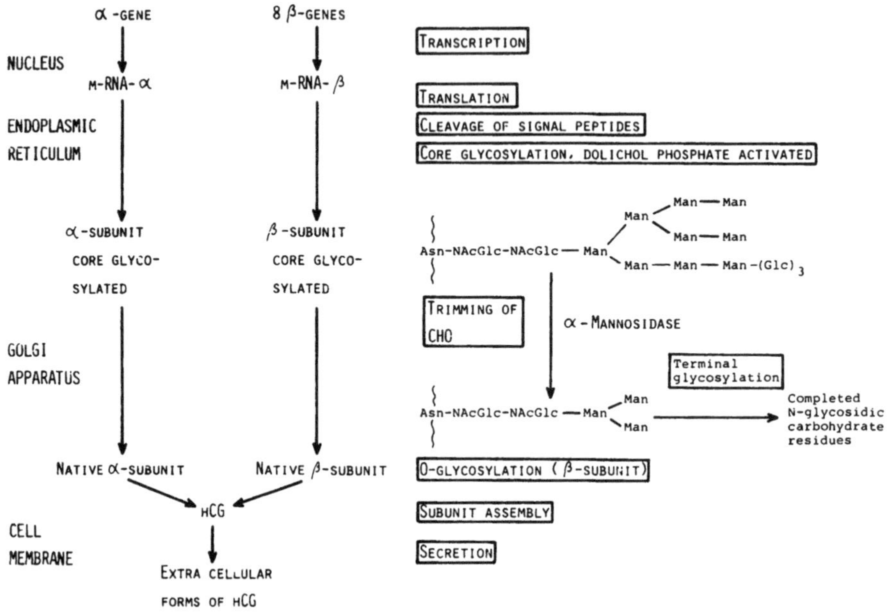

Fig. 1 Steps in the biosynthesis of hCG and their probable localization in different cellular compartments.

Recently Boorstein and coworkers [5] have shown that at least 8 genes exist which encode the β-subunit of hCG in comparison to one gene for the α-subunit. The subunits are translated as prepeptides which show NH_2-terminal elongations of 24 (α-subunit) and 20 (β-subunit) amino acid residues, respectively [6]. Like other signal peptides, these presequence regions contain a high content of hydrophobic amino acid residues. The preportions are cleaved at the sites of the NH_2-termini of the native subunits by signal peptidases during the translation process. In this early state of biosynthesis also N-glycosylation is started by the dolichol phosphate mediated attachment of high mannose oligosaccharide units to asparagine residues (52 and 78 in hCG-α and 13 and 30 in hCG-β). Thereafter, the subunits are transported to the golgi apparatus. There, the high mannose oligosaccharide units are trimmed by an α-mannosidase. Thise step has been suggested to be rate-limiting in the processing of the hCG-α-subunit when hCG biosynthesis was investigated in cultured choriocarcinoma (JAR) cells [7].

Our present knowledge of the following steps is rather small concerning their sequence as well as their intracellular localization. The reason for that may be the differences in the experimental models used. Three points should be kept in view:

1. The *vitro* experiments are certainly appropriate for some purposes, e.g. for obtaining the prepeptides, for others, however, like estimation of the rate of synthesis of α- and β-subunits other experimental models should be used. The ratio of the sub-

units obtained by biosynthesis *in vitro* seems to be influenced most sensitively by the experimental conditions: Using a magnesium concentration of 1.8 mM the α/β ratio was found to be 6:1, whereas at 1.5 mM the ratio was about 1:2 [8]. Therefore, only limited information is obtained from *in vitro* experiments about the complex biosynthesis of hCG.

2. Though closely related, the glycoprotein hormones show structural differences which may require variations in the biosynthetic pathways. At present it is not known e.g., whether the residues 115–145 which are present at the C-terminus of the hCG-β-subunit as an addition in comparison to the other members of the glycoprotein hormone family may influence the folding of the β-chain or the subunit assembly with respect to the sequence of the steps in biosynthesis. Furthermore, the influence of the carbohydrate moiety for correct processing, folding, and assembly of the subunits is not evaluated. The additional peptide region of the hCG-β-subunit mentioned above contains 4 serine residues (Ser 121, 127, 132, 138) which become glycosylated [9] during biosynthesis, whereas the other glycoprotein hormones show no O-linked oligosaccharide residues. The hypophyseal members of the hormone family seem to have oligosaccharide chains which may be sulfated [10, 11] whereas hCG carbohydrate moiety is not. In addition, species differences may exist.

3. The tissue which is used for investigation of hCG biosynthesis may be of great importance. In hCG *in vitro* translation experiments, qualitative as well as quantitative differences were observed between systems practiced with RNA which was derived from first trimester placenta and one obtained from term placenta [8]. Furthermore, in the biosynthetic process several differences between placental and tumor tissue seem to exist [7, 12]. In addition, even the structure of the hCG molecule may differ, in that tumor-derived hCG in some cases was observed to contain an unusual carbohydrate structure [13–15].

The precise sequence of events on hCG biosynthesis and their cellular localization following preparation of N-linked oligosaccharide chains for terminal glycosylation [16] is unknown at present. Some investigators claim that the assembly of the subunits occurs very early in biosynthesis prior to the processing of the asparagine-linked carbohydrate [17], whereas others have shown that the carbohydrate moiety does not increase the yield of correctly folded α-subunit but its ability do combine with the β-subunit [18, 19].

Action of LH-RH and des-Gly[10]-[D-Ala[6]]-LH-RH-ethylamide

In presence of LH-RH the amount of hCG secreted by cultured placental tissue is significantly increased ($p<0.01$) (fig. 2a). The optimum of hCG secretion is at day 3 of culture. It is not shifted in the presence of LH-RH. In contrast to the naturally occurring releasing hormone, the synthetic LH-RH agonist des-Gly[10]-[D-Ala[6]]-LH-

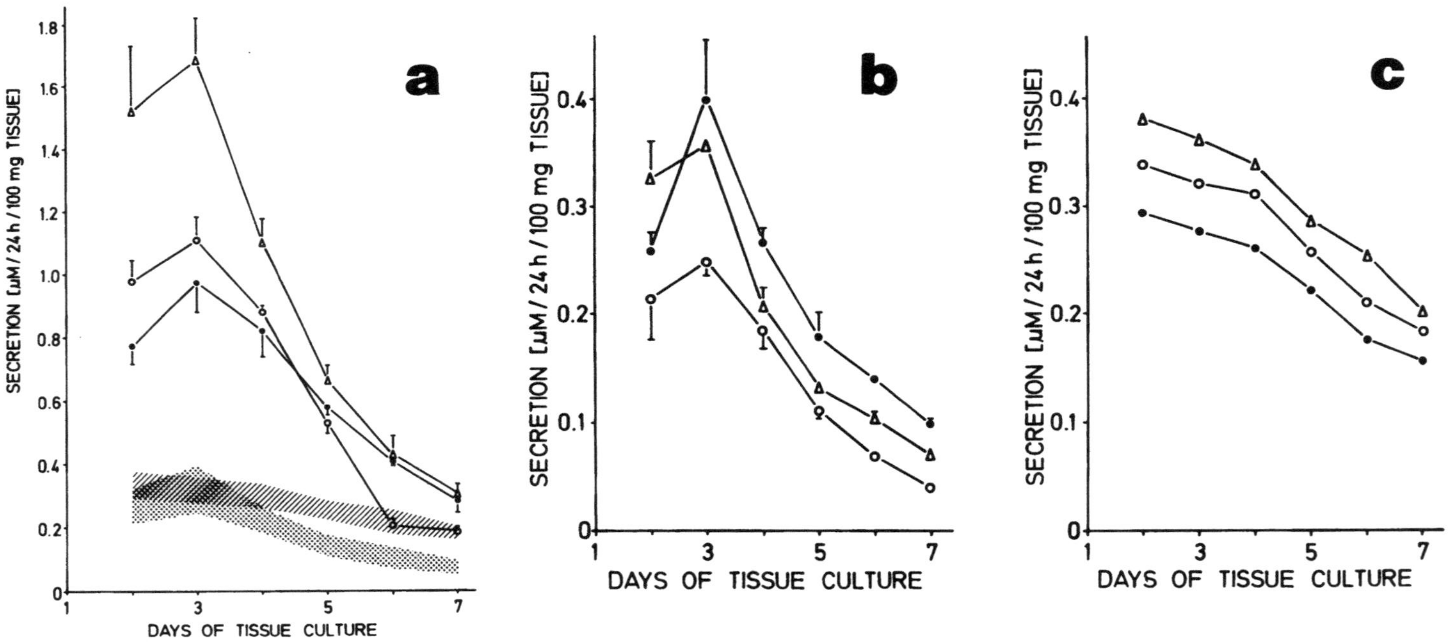

Fig. 2a) Influence of LHRH and the agonist des-Gly[10]-[D-Ala[6]]-LHRH ehtylamide on hCG secretion by placental tissue in culture.
HCG concentrations in the medium measured by radioimmunoassay in presence of 1 μM LHRH (△) or 1 μM des-Gly[10]-[D-Ala[6]]-LHRH ethylamide (○) and control cultures without addition of releasing hormones (●). Range of medium concentration levels of the isolated α-subunit (dotted area) an β-subunit (hatched area) in absence or presence of releasing hormones; for further details see b), c).
First trimester placental tissue (20–50 mg w.w.) was cultured in M199 containing per ml 1 μg insulin, 1 nmol dexamethasone, 120 μg penicillin, 200 μg streptomycin, 2.5 μg amphotericin B; 10% calf serum (newborn) was added. Tissue was cultured at 37 °C in 1.5 ml medium (Nunc multiwell plate) changed every 24 h and in an atmosphere of 5% CO_2 and 95% air.

RH ethylamide displays no effect on the amount of secreted hCG. This is noteworthy because in many other experimental systems the agonist shows higher potency than LH-RH [20, 21]. This is generally ascribed to the structural modifications introduced into the LH-RH molecule which prevents it from being rapidly degraded by exo- and endopeptidases. On the level of the isolated hCG subunits, however, LH-RH and the agonist seem to act in the same way: The amount of isolated β-subunit released into the culture medium is significantly increased ($p<0.01$) in presence of the releasing hormones (fig. 2b), whereas that of the α-subunit is decreased (except at day 2 in presence of LH-RH) (fig. 2c). The medium concentration of the isolated α-subunit shows an optimum which coincides with the optimum of hCG secretion irrespective of the culture conditions. The medium concentration of the isolated β-subunit is decreased with a constant rate during the observation time. These characteristic differences were also observed when hCG biosynthesis was stimulated by cAMP and cAMP derivatives [22, 23]. Considering the biosynthetic activity of the placental tissue at day 3 and e.g. day 7 of culture (figs. 2a–c), it is evident that the decrease in medium concentrations in that interval of hCG and of the α-subunit is more than twofold higher than that of the β-subunit (tab. 1). Therefore, it seems that a restriction of hCG biosynthesis is caused rather by the available amount of the α-subunit than of the β-subunit. This confirms the findings of Cole and coworkers [24] on hCG biosynthesis in tumor cell lines (DoT, CaSki) and our own investigations on the influence of cyclic nucleotides on placental hCG biosynthesis [22, 23, 25], whereas others have described a limitation of the hCG biosynthesis by the available amount of β-subunit [8].

At present it is not precisely known whether the medium concentrations of hCG and the isolated subunits also reflect the rate of biosynthesis. Preliminary studies have shown, however, that the stimulating activity of LH-RH is observed in experiments measuring the ^{3}H-proline incorporation into immunoreactive hCG (specific precipitation by anti-hCG), too. Furthermore, hCG does not seem to be stored in the cell prior to its secretion. The extracellular concentrations of the subunits, however, might result from biosynthesis of the peptide chains including the post- translational modifications and intracellular degradation of excessive subunits which have not assembled. A basis for such a subunit directed degradation might be the greater

Table 1 Ratios of medium concentrations of hCG and the isolated subunits at days 3 ÷ 7 of placental tissue culture

Conditions	Ratio of concentrations day 3 ÷ day 7		
	hCG	α	β
Control (no additions)	3.7	4.0	1.8
1 μM LH-RH	5.4	5.0	1.8
1 μM des-Gly[10]-[D-Ala[6]]-LH-RH ethylamide	5.8	5.0	1.8

resistance of hCG to proteases compared to the isolated subunits [22, 26–28]. In the case of biosynthesis of TSH, investigated by Chin et al. [29], the experimental findings suggest that the subunits initially are synthesized in equivalent amounts. Due to a faster intracellular degradation of the β-subunit, however, the medium concentration of the α-subunit was excessive.

Analysis of the medium concentration of the isolated subunits (fig. 3) demonstrates that the molar ratio β/α shows a higher increase in the presence of LH-RH and its agonist in comparison to the control. Considering this parameter, no differences exist between LH-RH and the agonist. In connection with the results presented in table 1 it is evident that the increase in the molar ratio β/α mainly is caused rather by a more rapid decrease of the amount of α-subunit released from the cell than of β-subunit. Furthermore, as shown in figures 2a and 2b, LH-RH induces a significantly higher yield of hCG and lower values for the isolated α-subunit in the medium.

Therefore, it is concluded from these experiments that LH-RH acts on hCG biosynthesis and secretion by a stimulation of the subunit assembly. At present it cannot be decided whether subunit assembly is promoted by the augentation of the available amount of finally processed subunits or perhaps by a direct regulation of the subunit assembly itself. It is completely unknown whether the assembly of subunits proceeds in a random, diffusion-controlled or in a regulated process. In comparison to LH-RH, the agonist seems to act stronger on the level of the α-subunit. However, no significant increase in hCG secretion is observed. Therefore, it cannot be excluded

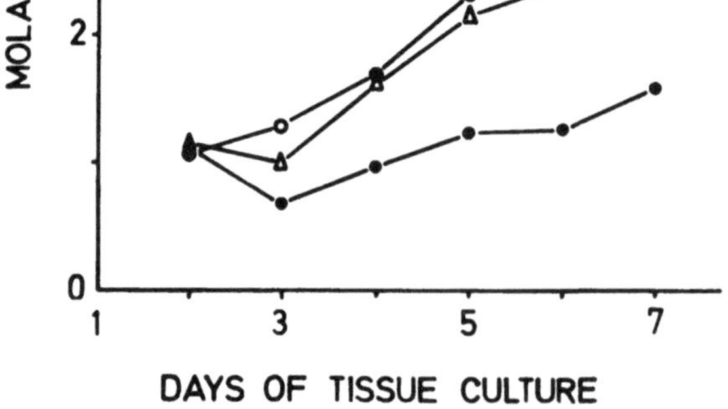

Fig. 3 Molar ratio of the hCG subunits β/α as determined by radioimmunoassay from the medium of placental tissue culture: Influence of LHRH (△) and des-Gly^{10}-[D-Ala^{6}]-LHRH ethylamide (○) in comparison to control (no releasing hormone added) (●).

that at least the agonist stimulates also the intracellular degradation of the α-subunit.

Concerning the possible physiological role of LH-RH in controlling placental functions, it should be added that LH-RH receptors as well as synthesis of an immunoreactive LH-RH-like peptide were recently demonstrated in placental tissue [30, 31].

Influence of inhibitors of prostaglandin biosynthesis

Neither the mode of action of LH-RH on the gonadotroph nor on the gonads is understood at present. The following preliminary results might give a hint on the mode of action of LH-RH on the biosynthesis of hCG in the placenta. Inhibition of prostaglandin biosynthesis on the level of cyclooxygenase reaction results in an increase in the amount of secreted hCG (Tab. 2). LH-RH might be able to counteract the inhibition of cyclooxygenase pathway by acetylsalicylate and indomethacin. The indomethacin concentration used in these experiments mainly blocks cyclooxygenase. At higher concentrations indomethacin inhibits also lipoxygenase [32]. An augmentation of LH-RH action by low doses of indomethacin as observed in the case of pituitary cells [33] does not seem to take place. LH-RH might act on placental hCG biosynthesis according to the principle of two reins, that is it may stimulate hCG biosynthesis but keeping the amount of synthesized hCG in a narrow range by stimulation of the biosynthesis of prostaglandins which may inhibit the placental output of the hormone. The significant influence of prostaglandins on placental hCG biosynthesis might also be of great clinical importance and needs further investigations as well as the possible interdependency with the action of LH-RH on the placenta. It is remarkable that LH-RH seems to be able to activate both the lipoxygenase and the cyclooxygenase pathway in different target organs like the pituitary and the ovary. In the pituitary, the LH-RH action seems to be mediated by products

Table 2 Effect of an inhibition of prostaglandin biosynthesis on the concentration of secreted hCG and on the action of LH-RH

Condition	HCG concentration in the medium nM/100 mg tissue/24 h ± S.D. Day 2 of culture	HCG concentration in the medium nM/100 mg tissue/24 h ± S.D. Day 3 of culture
Control (no additions)	136 ± 4	330 ± 8
10 µM Acetylsalicylate	225 ± 40	506 ± 50
27 µM Indomethacin	526 ± 126	914 ± 37
1 µM LH-RH	334 ± 31	412 ± 27
1 µM LH-RH ± 1 µM Acetylsalicylate	273 ± 27	443 ± 15
1 µM LH-RH ± 10 µM Acetylsalicylate	196 ± 49	427 ± 22
1 µM LH-RH ± 27 µM Indomethacin	707 ± 12	967 ± 28

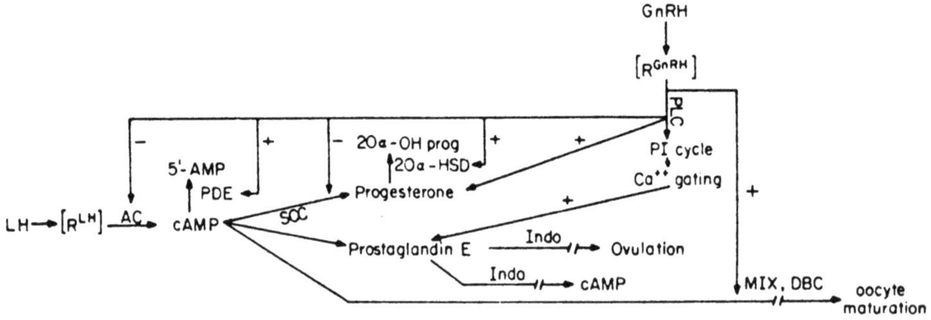

Fig. 4 Scheme of the mechanism of LH and LHRH action on the ovary prosed by Naor et al. [34]. R, receptor for LH and LHRH, respectively; PI, phosphatidyinositol; indo, indomethacin; MIX, 3-isobutyl-1-methylxanthine; DBC, dibutyryl-cAMP. (The figure was taken from [34] with permission by the Springer Verlag, Heidelberg.)

of the lipoxygenase pathway [33] and in the ovary, it stimulates probably prostaglandin E formation [34]. A very interesting model of the interaction of LH and LH-RH in the ovary was recently presented by Naor et al. [34] at a symposium in Heidelberg and is depicted in figure 4. Concerning the action of LH-RH the model comprises the stimulation of a phosphatidylinositol-specific phospholipase C by the LH-RH-receptor complex which results in the activation of the phosphatidylinositol cycle. By this, a calcium gating and the relase of arachidonic acid is effected and thus prostaglandin biosynthesis is stimulated. The results shown in table 2 do not yet provide strong evidence for LH-RH action on placental tissue as in the ovary; however, the weakening of the effect of inhibitors of cyclooxygenase by LH-RH might point into this direction. Furthermore, it fits into this model, that the concentration of cAMP in the medium of placental tissue cultures is decreased by a factor of 2.5 in the presence of LH-RH (1μM) at the optimum of hCG secretion (not shown).

Activity of α-Mannosidase

As pointed out above, there are some hints in literature that the available amount of α-subunit may be limiting for the biosynthesis of hCG. Ruddon et al. [7] have investigated the regulation of the hCG biosynthesis in cultured choriocarcinoma (JAR) cells. It turned out that the rate-limiting step in the biosynthesis of the α-subunit seems to be an α-mannosidase reaction. This enzyme performs the trimming of the high-mannose aparagine-linked oligosaccharide chains, which is a necessary prerequisite for the terminal glycosylation and therefore perhaps for the assembly of the subunits. For this reason, we investigated the α-mannosidase activity in placental tissue which was cultured under various conditions (tab. 3). It is evident from these data that the α-mannosidase activity is decreased in some cases, e.g. in presence of LH-RH and indomethacin or low doses of acetylsalicylate; however, that no corre-

Table 3 Activity of α-mannosidase in human placental tissue cultured in the presence of LH-RH and inhibitors of the prostaglandin biosynthesis

Condition	χ-Mannosidase activity at day 3 of culture pmol/min/mg protein ± S.D.	Control	HCG secreted at day 3 in relation to control
Control (no addition)	78.8 ± 6.3	1.00	1.00
10 μM Acetylsalicylate	58.3 ± 3.7	0.74	1.53
27 μM Indomethacin	61.6 ± 0.8	0.78	2.77
1 μM LH-RH	68.4 ± 3.2	0.87	1.25
1 μM LH-RH + 1 μM Acetylsalicylate	20.6 ± 2.1	0.26	1.34
1 μM LH-RH + 10 μM Acetylsalicylate	56.5 ± 2.7	0.72	1.29
1 μM LH-RH + 27 μM Indomethacin	27.9 ± 3.4	0.35	2.93

Activity of α-mannosidase in tissue homogenate at 30° C, pH 4.5 (0.5M sodium acetate) was determined fluorometrically from the amount of 4-methyl-umbelliferol formed by enzymatic cleavage of 4-methylumbelliferyl-α-D-mannopyranoside (Boehringer Mannheim, FRG) in presence of bovine serum albumin and $ZnSO_4$ according to Opheim and Touster [35] and Rosenthal and Saifer [36].

lation exists to the amount of secreted hCG. Especially, the augmentation of hCG biosynthesis and secretion seems not to be effected by a stimulation of the processing of the carbohydrate chains by α-mannosidase. In addition, it appears rather unlikely from these results that an α-mannosidase reaction is a rate-limiting step in biosynthesis of hCG by placental tissue.

Conclusions

LH-RH stimulates placental biosynthesis of hCG significantly. The agonist des Gly^{10}-[D-Ala^6]-LH-RH ethylamide does not increase the quantity of secreted hCG.

In the presence of LH-RH the extracellular concentrations of hCG and β-subunit are increased whereas that of α-subunit is decreased significantly. Therefore, one action of LH-RH may be the stimulation of hCG biosynthesis by promotion of subunit assembly.

Promotion of subunit assembly by LH-RH seems not to take place via processing of the carbohydrate moiety of the subunits by α-mannosidase.

The available amount of the α-subunit is a limiting factor for hCG biosynthesis.

LH-RH seems to countreract the inhibition of prostaglandin biosynthesis (inhibition of cyclooxygenase reaction). Therefore, part of the action of LH-RH on placental hCG biosynthesis may be the regulation of phospholipid metabolism as suggested for its action in the ovary by Naor [34].

Acknowledgements

These investigations were supported by the Deutsche Forschungsgemeinschaft, Bonn-Bad Godesberg.

References

[1] Hunt, L. T., M. O. Dayhoff: Atlas of Protein Sequences and Structure (Ed. M. O. Dayhoff), Vol. 5, Suppl. 2, pp. 113–145. Natl. Biomed. Res. Found., Washington, D.C., 1976.
[2] Braunstein, G. D., J. L. Vaitukaitis, P. P. Carbone et al.: Ann. Intern. Med. **78** (1973) 39–45.
[3] Vaitukaitis, J. L., G. T. Ross, G. D. Braunstein et al.: Rec. Progr. Horm. Res **32** (1976) 289–321.
[4] Baylin, S. B., G. Mendelson: Endocr. Rev. **1** (1980) 45–77.
[5] Boorstein, W. R., N. C. Vamvakopoulos, J. C. Fiddes: Nature **300** (1982) 419–422.
[6] Birken, S., J. Fetherstone, R. E. Canfield et al.: J. Biol. Chem. **256** (1981) 1816–1823.
[7] Ruddon, R. W., A. H. Bryan, C. A. Hanson et al.: J. Biol. Chem. **256** (1981) 5189–5196.
[8] Daniels – MC Queen, S., D. McWilliams, S. Birken: J. Biol. Chem. **253** (1978) 7109–7114.
[9] Kessler, M. J., T. Mise, R. D. Ghai et al.: J. Biol. Chem. **254** (1979) 7909–7914.
[10] Parson, T. F., J. G. Pierce: Proc. Natl. Acad. Sci. U.S.A. **77** (1980) 7089–7093.
[11] Hortin, G., M. Natowicz, J. G. Pierce et al.: Proc. Natl. Acad. Sci. U.S.A. **78** (1981) 7468–7472.
[12] Vaitukaitis, J. L., E. R. Ebersole: J. Clin. Endocrinol. Metab. **42** (1976) 1048–1055.
[13] Cox, S.: Cancer Res. **41** (1981) 3087–3094.
[14] Benveniste, R., M. C. Conway, D. Puett et al.: J. Clin. Endocrinol. Metab. **48** (1979) 85–91.
[15] Mann, K., J. J. Karl,: Cancer **52** (1983) 654–660.
[16] Kessler, M. J., M. S. Reddy, R. H. Shah et al.: J. Biol. Chem. **254** (1979) 7901–7908.
[17] Hoshina, H., I. Boime: Proc. Natl. Acad. Sci. U.S.A., **79** (1982) 7649–7653.
[18] Strickland, T. W., J. G. Pierce: J. Biol. Chem. **258** (1983) 5927–5932.
[19] Weintraub, B. D., B. S. Staunard, D. Linnekin et al.: J. Biol. Chem. **255** (1980) 5715–5723.
[20] Arimura, A., J. A. Vilchez-Martinez, D. H. Coy et al.: Endocrinology **95** (1974) 1174–1177.
[21] Coy, D. H., E. J. Coy, A. V. Schally et al.: Biochem. Biophys. Res. Comm. **57** (1974) 335–340.
[22] Merz, W. E.: In "Regulation of the Sekretion of Gonadotropins and their Action in Human: Physiology and Clinics" (Eds. B. Runnebaum, T. Rabe, L. Kiesel, W. E. Merz). Springer-Verlag, Berlin–Heidelberg, New York 1984, in preparation.
[23] Hilf, G., W. E. Merz: In "Peptide Hormones as Mediators in Immunology and Oncology" (Ed. R. D. Hesch). Acad. Press, New York 1984, in preparation.
[24] Cole, L. A., R. D. Hussa, C. V. Rao: Cancer Res. **41** (1981) 1615–1619.
[25] Hilf, G., W. E. Merz: Hoppe-Seyler's Z. Physiol. Chem. **364**, 1144–1145.
[26] Merz. W. E.: Eur. J. Biochem. **101** (1979) 541–553.
[27] Merz, W. E., M. Dörner: Hoppe-Seyler's Z. Physiol. Chem. **360** (1979) 1783–1797.
[28] Merz, W. E.: Hoppe-Seyler's Z. Physiol. Chem. **361** (1980) 302.
[29] Chin, W. W., F. Maloof, J. F. Habener: J. Biol. Chem. **256** (1981) 3059–3066.
[30] Hsueh, A. J. W., P. B. C. Jones: Ann. Rev. Physiol. **45** (1983) 83–94.
[31] Tan, L., P. Rousseau: Biochem. Biophys. Res. Comm. **109** (1982) 1061–1071.
[32] Siegl, M. I., R. T. McConnel, N. A. Porter et al.: Proc. Natl. Acad. Sci. U.S.A. **77** (1980) 308–312.
[33] Naor, Z., J. Y. Vanderhock, H. R. Lindner et al.: In "Advances in Prostaglandin, Thromboxane, and Leukotriene Research" (Eds. B. Samuelsson, R. Paoletti, P. Ramwell), **12**, pp. 259–263. Raven Press, New York 1983.

[34] Naor, Z., N. Dekel, J. Molcho et al.: In "Regulation of the Secretion of Gonadotropins and their Action in Human: Physiology and Clinics" (Eds. B. Runnebaum, T. Rabe, L. Kiesel, W. E. Merz). Springer-Verlag, Berlin–Heidelberg–New York 1984, in preparation.
[35] Opheim, D. J., O. Touster: In "Methods in Enzymology" (Ed. V. Ginsburg), 50, p. 495. Acad. Press, New York–San Francisco–London 1978.
[36] Rosenthal, A. L., A. Saifer: Analyt. Biochem. 55 (1973) 85–92.

The pharmacologic profile of [(ImBzl)-D-His[6],Pro[9]-NEt]-LH-RH (ORF 17070), an LH-RH agonist

D. W. Hahn, A. Phillips, J. L. McGuire

Introduction

Following the structural elucidation of LH-RH by the laboratories of Schally [18] and Guilleman [2] in 1971, LH-RH and hundreds of analogs of the decapeptide, both agonists as well as antagonists, have been synthesized and tested in biological assays. Agonistic analogs, many more potent and longer-acting than LH-RH itself, have been shown to stimulate as well as inhibit the reproductive endocrine system depending on the dosage and treatment regimen used.

This report describes the pharmacological characteristics of an LH-RH agonist, [(ImBzl)-D-His[6],Pro[9]-NEt]LH-RH (ORF 17070). This compound is a nonapeptide with an (Im-Bzl)-D-histidine residue in the 6-position (fig. 1) which has emerged as a potential therapeutic agent out of the research efforts of the laboratories of Rivier, Rivier and Vale at the Salk Institute [27, 33, 34] and our own laboratories [13, 14, 35]. ORF 17070 is being studied clinically [11] for a variety of disorders which respond to stimulation or inhibition of the reproductive endocrine system.

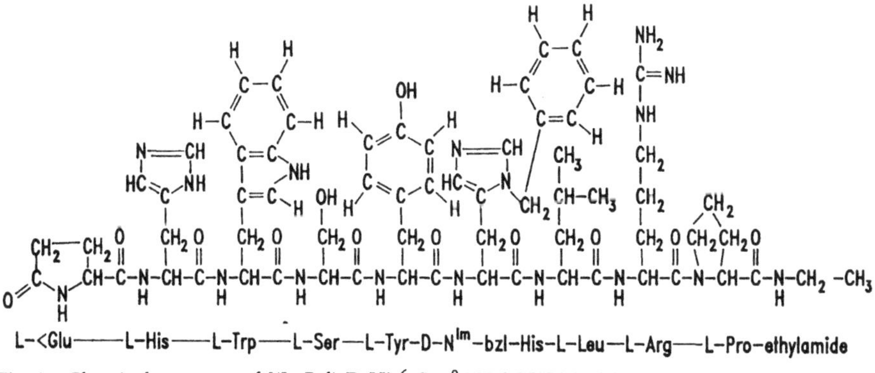

Fig. 1 Chemical structure of [(ImBzl)-D-His[6], Pro[9]-NEt] LHRH (ORF 17070).

Stimulation of the reproductive endocrine system

Agonists of LH-RH can either stimulate or inhibit the reproductive endocrine system depending on the dosage and frequency of administration. The studies below describe the ability of ORF 17070 to stimulate LH release *in vitro* and *in vivo* and to induce ovulation following acute administration in several animal models.

In vitro potency

When tested in standard *in vitro* assays, ORF 17070 is a potent LH-RH agonist (tab. 1). Vale *et al.* showed that it is 210 times more potent than LH-RH as a stimulator of LH release from enzyme dispersed rat pituitary cells in a monolayer culture [33, 34]. It is 55 times more potent than LH-RH when the binding affinity for pituitary LH-RH receptors is assessed by incubating the agonist with pituitary membranes [22, 23].

Table 1 Potency of [(ImBzl)-D-His^6,Pro^9-NEt]-LH-RH (ORF 17070) in two *in vitro* test systems

Peptide	Relative Potencies Secretion of LH *in vitro*	Radioligand Membrane Binding Assay
LH-RH	1	1
[(ImBzl)-D-His^6,Pro^9-NEt]LH-RH	210	55

In vivo stimulation of LH release

The ability of LH-RH agonists to stimulate the reproductive endocrine system is based on their ability to stimulate LH secretion from the pituitary gland. An intravenous injection of LH-RH or ORF 17070 (fig. 2) results in an elevation of serum LH levels in adult rats [35]. ORF 17070, at 5 μg/kg, caused a rise in serum LH levels which was evident at 30 minutes and which peaked at 3.0 hours after injection. Peak serum levels represented an 80-fold increase in serum LH over control level. A significant elevation of serum LH was still evident 8 hours after the injection whereas serum LH declined to baseline by 2.5 hours after an injection of the same amount of native LH-RH. Thus, in agreement with the *in vitro* data above, ORF 17070, when given *in vivo* is a more potent stimulator of LH secretion than is LH-RH, and it appears to be longer-acting than LH-RH.

Induction of ovulation

Acute administration of LH-RH or an agonist to females induces a release of pituitary LH followed by ovulation [6]. ORF 17070 and LH-RH were evaluated for their ability to induce ovulation in several animal models, including the rabbit, the nembutal-anesthetized proestrus rat, the androgen-sterilized rat [14], and the diestrus

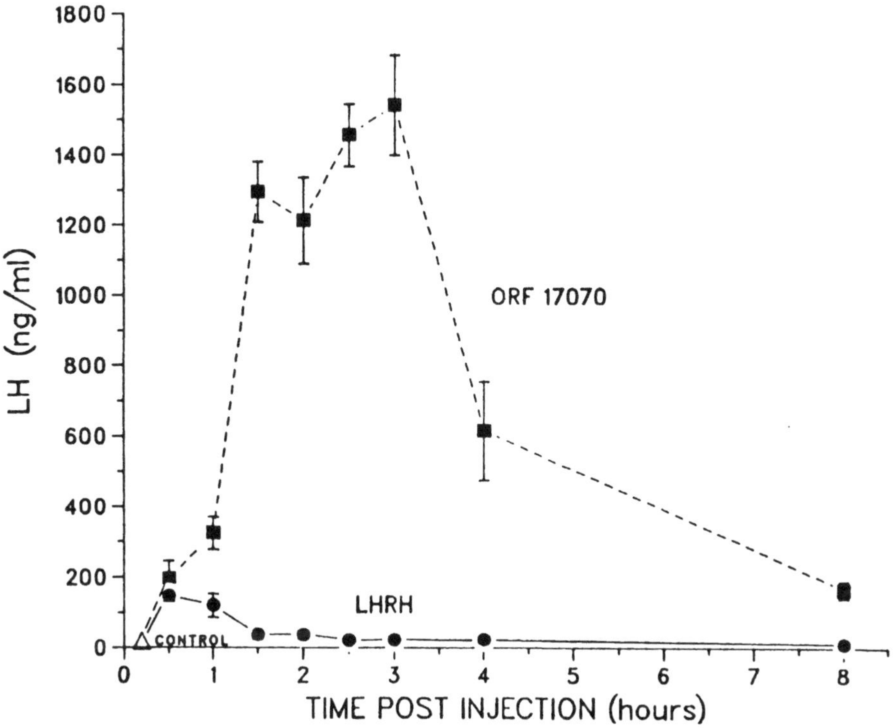

Fig. 2 ORF 17070 or LHRH was administered intravenously to conscious, restrained adult male rats at a dose of 5 μg/kg in 0.1 ml saline. Animals were decapitated at 0.5, 1, 1.5, 2, 2.5, 3, 4 or 8 hours post-injection and serum LH was measured by RIA. LH levels are expressed as ng NIAMDD rat LH-RP-1 ml serum. Each point represents the mean of six rats (± S. E. M.).

rat, mouse or hamster [13]. In all of these test systems, animals received a single subcutaneous or intravenous injection of LH-RH or ORF 17070 in saline. The following day the animals are sacrificed and the oviducts extracted and examined microscopically for the number of ova present. Figure 3 demonstrates the results obtained in one of these assays. In the androgen-sterilized rat model, ORF 17070 is 4.4 times more potent than LH-RH in inducing ovulation.

In other animal models measuring the induction of ovulation after acute administration, the potency estimate for ORF 17070 ranges from 1.8 to 9.2 times that of LH-RH (tab. 2). The varied values for the potency of ORF 17070 demonstrated in these different animal models and species are not unlike that which is found with other agonists of LH-RH and may be attributable to differences in drug absorption, drug metabolism, varied pituitary sensitivities or a combination of these effects.

Corbin and Bex [7] have shown that other agonists of LH-RH also exhibit different potencies when administered by different routes of administration. In studies eva-

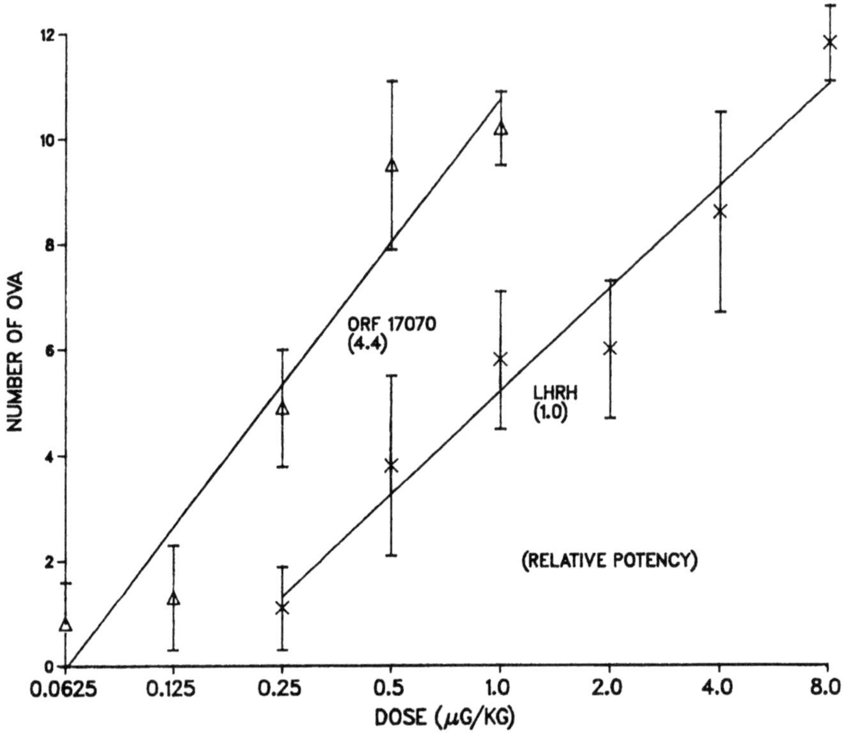

Fig. 3 Inducation of ovulation with ORF 17070 in androgensterilized rats. Animals received a single subcutaneous injection of LHRH of ORF 17070 in saline at 1400 to 1500 hr. The following day, they were sacrificed and their oviducts were examined microscopically for ova. Each point represents the mean of ten rats (± S. E. M.).

Table 2 Relative potency estimates of ORF 17070 in several animal models when administered in saline

Induction of ovulation	Relative Potency (95% CL) LH-RH = 1.0
Animal model	
Rabbit (s.c.)	1.8 (0.9– 6.0)
Rabbit (i.v.)	3.7 (2.0– 6.4)
Nembutal-Anesthetized Proestrus Rat (s.c.)	3.4 (2.4– 5.2)
Androgen-Sterilized Rat (s.c.)	4.4 (2.6– 6.9)
Diestrus Hamster (s.c.)	5.9 (3.7– 8.9)
Diestrus Mouse (s.c.)	7.7 (4.1–15.5)
Diestrus Rat (s.c.)	9.2 (6.1–14.7)

luating the ability of LH-RH and ORF 17070 to induce ovulation in rabbits by intravenous and subcutaneous routes of administration, we found that although LH-RH was equipotent by both routes of administration, ORF 17070 was 2.4 times more potent intravenously than when it was given subcutaneously (tab. 3). These differences may be related to different rates of absorption from the injection site or due to different degradation rates of these two peptides.

Table 3 A comparison of relative potencies of ORF 17070 and LH-RH when administered subcutaneously vs. intravenously in saline to rabbits for induction of ovulation. The relative potency of the agonist when given i.v. (2.4) is significantly different ($p < 0.05$) from when given s.c. (1.0)

Peptide	Relative Potency Estimates (95% CL) S.C.	I.V.
LH-RH	1.0	1.1 (0.5–2.9)
ORF 17070	1.0	2.4 (1.2–3.8)

Analogs of LH-RH, like many peptides, have been reported to be much less potent when given orally than when administered parenterally [21, 28]. The low oral potency of peptides is generally thought to be due to the rapid degradation of peptides in the gastrointestinal tract and serum [3, 16, 25]. When we compared the ability of ORF 17070 to induce ovulation in diestrus rats given either subcutaneously or orally (tab. 4), we found that the agonist was 945 times more potent by the subcutaneous than by the oral route of administration when given in a saline vehicle.

Table 4 Induction of ovulation in diestrus rats with ORF 17070 in saline using oral and subcutaneous routes of administration

Route	Dose	No. Rats Ovulating/Total	Number of Ova Mean ± SE	Relative Potency (95% CL)
Oral	0.10 mg/kg	1/10	1.6 ± 1.6	
Oral	0.15 mg/kg	2/10	1.8 ± 1.2	1.0
Oral	0.25 mg/kg	5/10	3.7 ± 1.6	
Oral	0.50 mg/kg	10/10	9.2 ± 0.9	
S.C.	0.12 µg/kg	1/10	0.5 ± 0.5	
S.C.	0.25 µg/kg	7/10	4.4 ± 1.5	945 (653–1402)
S.C.	0.50 µg/kg	10/10	9.4 ± 0.9	

In other studies, we tested ORF 17070 orally in a variety of different vehicles (tab. 5) and found we could enhance or reduce oral potency with different vehicles. These studies indicate that with a better understanding of the pharmacokinetics of these peptides and a development of alternate delivery systems, it may be possible to enhance the oral potencies of LH-RH analogs to a therapeutically useful level.

Table 5 Induction of ovulation in diestrus rats with orally administered ORF 17070 in different vehicles

Vehicle	Relative Potency (95% CL)
Saline	1.0 –
Sesame Oil	0.3 (0.1– 0.6)
40% Propylene glycol + Saline	1.8 (1.2– 2.6)
25% EtOH	5.2 (3.8– 7.4)
Propylene Glycol	7.2 (4.8–11.7)

Inhibition of the reproductive endocrine system

As shown above, acute administration of LH-RH or ORF 17070 stimulates LH release and induces ovulation. The studies below demonstrate the ability of chronically administered ORF 17070 to inhibit the reproductive endocrine system. Assays which measure this inhibition include the disruption of estrous cyclicity in rats, the inhibition of pregnancy in rats and the suppression of endometriosis in rabbits.

Disruption of estrous cyclicity

The first parameter used to assess the ability of ORF 17070 to inhibit the reproductive endocrine system was inhibition of estrous cyclicity in the female rat. In this standard assay system, mature, cycling female rats are injected once daily for 14 days beginning on the day of metestrus [13]. Daily monitoring of vaginal cytology shows that chronic treatment with ORF 17070 inhibits estrous cyclicity. Animals given saline cycled normally, exhibiting estrus vaginal cytology on day 4 of treatment, whereas animals given ORF 17070 exhibited a dose-related delay in the occurrence of estrus cytology (tab. 6).

Table 6 Effect of ORF 17070 administered in saline on estrous cyclicity in the rat. Animals (10 per group) were treated subcutaneously for 14 days beginning on the day of metestrus

Dose μg/kg/day	Day of Treatment First Estrus Occurred Mean ± SE
0	4.0 ± 0
0.156	4.5 ± 0.2
0.625	9.9 ± 1.4
1.25	14.0 ± 0

Inhibition of pregnancy

The second study used to assess the ability of ORF 17070 to inhibit the reproductive endocrine system was inhibition of pregnancy. In this assay system, rats are injected once daily on days 7 through 12 of pregnancy. A dose of 500 µg/kg of ORF 17070 given after implantation resulted in total inhibition of pregnancy (tab. 7). In studies not reported, a dose of 1000 µg/kg of ORF 17070 given before implantation was needed for total inhibition of pregnancy.

Table 7 Effect of ORF 17070 on pregnancy in rats when given after implantation. Animals were injected subcutaneously daily with ORF 17070 in saline on days 7 through 12 of pregnancy

Dose µg/kg	% Non-Viable Implants Mean ± S.E.
0 (vehicle control)	1.2 ± 1.2
5	4.4 ± 2.8
25	60.0 ± 24.4
50	55.8 ± 26.0
100	73.8 ± 16.2
500	100.0

Animal models predictive of clinical utility

LH-RH agonists are currently being studied clinically for regulation of fertility and treatment of various endocrine-related disorders including endometriosis, precocious puberty, polycystic ovarian disease, benign prostatic hypertrophy, hormone-dependent tumors and hypogonadism. ORF 17070 is active in animal models of several of these disorders.

One striking demonstration of the effect of ORF 17070 in animal models believed predictive of clinical utility is its effect in a new animal model for endometriosis. Endometriosis, which is often associated with pelvic pain and infertility, is characterized by the aberrant occurrence of endometrial tissue in various locations of the pelvic cavity. This condition can be surgically-induced in rabbits using a technique developed by Schenken and Asch [29]. In this model, a section of one uterine horn is surgically removed and cut into pieces. The pieces are then sutured into various sites on the contralateral side of the reproductive tract and allowed to grow for a period of 7 weeks. In the study described here, the endometriotic implants grew from a mean weight of 10.7 mg to 89.0 mg (tab. 8). In the next 4 weeks, these rabbits received a daily subcutaneous injection of either ORF 17070 or vehicle. By the end of this treatment period, the implants in the control group had grown to a mean of 135.1 mg. Four weeks of treatment with ORF 17070 resulted in a visually evident (fig. 4) reduction in mean endometriotic implant weight to 21.7 mg (tab. 8).

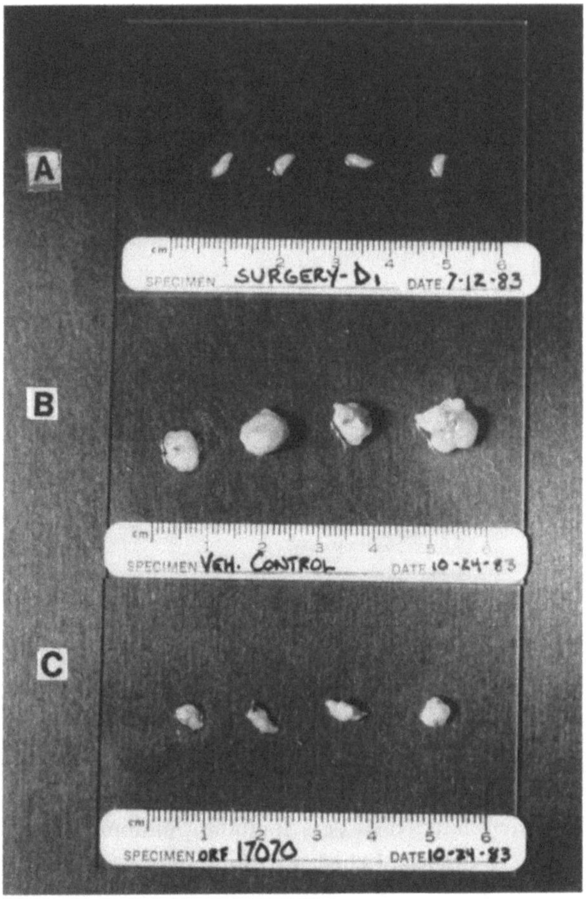

Fig. 4 Endometrial implants (A) at the time of surgical implantation, (B) after 11 weeks of growth with 4 weeks of vehicle administration or (C) with 4 weeks of chronic treatment with ORF 17070 at 0.1 mg/kg/day.

Table 8 The weight of endometrial implants in rabbits at the time of implantation, following 7 weeks of growth, and after 4 weeks of treatment with ORF 17070. The implant weight of 21.7 mg is significantly different from 135.1 mg ($p < 0.01$)

Treatment	Weeks after Surgery	No. Animals	Mean (± SE) Implant Wt. (mg)
None	0	17	10.7 ± 0.4
None	7	5	89.0 ± 11.6
Sesame Oil	11	6	135.1 ± 20.5
ORF 17070	11	6	21.7 ± 2.3

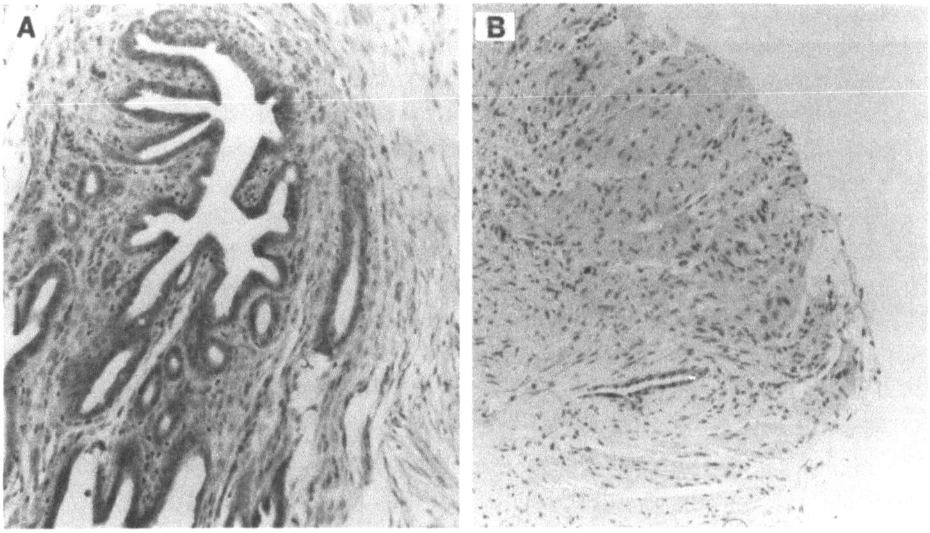

Fig. 5 Photomicrographs of endometrial implants after (A) 4 weeks of vehicle administration or (B) 4 weeks of treatment with ORF 17070 at 0.1 mg/kg/day. Note the reduction in gland size and thinning of stroma following ORF 17070 treatment (H & E×100).

Histological evaluation of endometriotic implants from vehicle control rabbits revealed an endometrial proliferation with well-developed glandular epithelial and dense stroma (fig. 5A). Treatment with ORF 17070 caused a regression of the endometrial glands and a thinning of the stroma (fig. 5B).

Discussion

Preclinical studies presented here demonstrate that ORF 17070 is a potent LH-RH agonist which, like other agonists, can stimulate as well as inhibit the reproductive endocrine system depending on the dosage and treatment regimen used. ORF 17070 binds to LH-RH receptors of the pituitary. It stimulates the release of LH from pituitary cells *in vitro* and elevates serum LH when given acutely *in vivo*. ORF 17070 induces ovulation in several animal models with an average *in vivo* potency of about 5 times greater than that of native LH-RH when given acutely. Chronic administration of ORF 17070, as measured indirectly by its effects on estrous cyclicity and pregnancy in rats, inhibits the reproductive endocrine system.

It is important to note that biopharmaceutic factors, such as the choice of vehicle, can influence potency estimates of LH-RH analogs. For example, in a previous report, we showed that another LH-RH agonist stimulated uterine growth in immature mice when given in sesame oil but not when administered in saline [12], indicating that these vehicles may provide different release rates. This agonist did stimulate uterine growth when given in saline in divided injections daily. Similar results were obtained by Rivier et al. [26] when [D-Trp^6-NEt]-LH-RH was evaluated in saline and sesame oil for its ability to inhibit pregnancy in the rat. In studies not reported here we found certain similar effects with ORF 17070. For example, it was a more potent inhibitor of pregnancy in rats when given in sesame oil than when administered in saline. However, no potency differences were seen with these vehicles when ORF 17070 was tested as an inhibitor of estrous cyclicity in rats. These studies with ORF 17070 and those reported previously with other LH-RH agonists [12, 26] indicate that a prolonged elevation of serum LH-RH agonist levels, as may be provided with a vehicle such as sesame oil, is an important factor in the activity of LH-RH agonists in some test systems. These biopharmaceutic factors, which may play an important role in clinical medicine, suggest that certain drug delivery systems for LH-RH agonists may not only provide a more acceptable mode of administration for the patient, but also more effective therapy for clinical disorders.

The mechanism by which LH-RH agonists inhibit the reproductive endocrine system when given chronically is still the subject of ongoing investigations in many laboratories. In clinical studies, suppression of endometriosis or prostatic carcinoma with LH-RH agonists was accompanied by a decrease in serum estrogen or testosterone levels [20, 32]. Because of this, it has been stated that chronic administration of LH-RH agonists results in a clinical effect similar to "medical castration". However, it is not known at which level of the hypothalamic-pituitary-gonadal axis chronically administered LH-RH agonists exert their action leading to an inhibition of the reproductive endocrine system. Several theories have been hypothesized. First, it has been proposed that inhibition of the reproductive endocrine system may be the result of "down-regulation" of LH-RH receptors in the pituitary caused by over-stimulation by the agonists [11, 17]. Second, down-regulation of gonadal LH receptors may occur in response to elevated LH blood levels [5, 24]. Third, agonists may act directly on gonadal cells [15]. It should be noted that other studies suggest that LH-RH analogs may directly interfere with steroid action on target tissues such as uterus or prostate [31].

In clinical studies, pulsatile administration of LH-RH has been shown to induce ovulation in women with an LH-RH deficiency [8, 30] and stimulate reproductive functioning in hypogonadal males [9]. Chronic administration of LH-RH agonists has been reported to provide effective therapy for endometriosis [19, 20], prostatic carcinoma [1, 32] and precocious puberty [4]. Preclinical studies presented here demonstrate that ORF 17070 is a potent LH-RH agonist with potential as a therapeutic agent 1. for long-term suppression of gonadal function due to chronic therapy as treatment of a variety of disease states dependent on ovarian or testicular function and 2. if administered as pulsatile doses, for stimulation of ovarian function in certain types of infertility.

Acknowledgements

We wish to thank W. Vale and J. Rivier of the Salk Institute, H. L. Judd and D. R. Meldrum of the Department of Obstetrics and Gynecology at UCLA, W. Crowley of Massachusetts General Hospital, and M. E. Rosenthale, R. M. Cohn and R. Murphy of our laboratories for their helpful discussions and suggestions; R. Foldesy and R. Homm for providing us with data from their studies; R. Carraher, E. Ericson, S. Klimek, M. T. Lai and M. Vanderhoof for their technical assistance; and M. Westlake and K. Daniels for the preparation of this manuscript.

References

[1] Ahmed, S. R., S. M. Shaley, P. J. C. Brooman et al.: The Lancet. **8347** (1983) 415–419.
[2] Amoss, M., R. Burgus, R. Blackwell: Biochem. Biophys. Res. Commun. **44** (1971) 205.
[3] Chang, W. C., A. J. Rao, C. H. Li: Int. J. Peptide Protein Res. **11** (1978) 93–94.
[4] Comite, F., G. B. Cutler Jr., J. Rivier et al.: N. Engl. J. Med. **305** (1981) 1546–1550.
[5] Conti, M., J. P. Harwood, A. J. W. Hsueh et al.: J. Biol. Chem. **251** (1976) 7729–7731.
[6] Corbin, A., C. W. Beattie, J. Tracy et al.: Int. J. Fert. **23** (1978) 81–92.
[7] Corbin, A., F. J. Bex: In "Peptides as Female and Male Contraceptives" (Eds. G. I. Zatuchni, J. D. Shelton, J. J. Sciarra), p. 68. Harper and Row, Philadelphia 1981.
[8] Crowley, Jr., W. F., J. W. McArthur, J. Donnelly et al.: In "The Gonadotropins: Basic Science and Clinical Aspects in Females" (edited by C. Flamigni and J. R. Givens), pp. 457–469. Academic Press, New York 1982.
[9] Crowley, Jr., W. F., W. W. Vale, J. Rivier et al.: In LH-RH Peptides as Female and Male Contraceptives" (edited by G. I. Zatuchni, J. D. Shelton and J. J. Sciarra), pp. 321–333. Harper and Row, Philadelphia 1981.
[10] DeFazio, G., J. K. H. Lu, W. Vale et al.: Endoc. Res. Commun. (in press).
[11] Fraser, H. M., N. C. Laird, D. M. Blakely: Endocrinology **106** (2) (1980) 452–457.
[12] Hahn, D. W., A. Phillips, J. L. McGuire: Endocr. Res. Commun. **8** (1981) 273–283.
[13] Hahn, D. W., A. Phillips, M. T. Lai et al.: Endocr. Res. Commun. (1984). In Press.
[14] Hahn, D. W., J. L. McGuire: Endocrinology **102** (6) (1978) 1741–1747.
[15] Hsueh, A. J. W., C. Wang, G. F. Erickson: Endocrinology **106** (6) (1980) 1697–1705.
[16] Kastin, A. J., C. Nissen, A. V. Schally et al.: Brain Res. Bull. **1** (1976) 583–589.
[17] deKoning, J., J. A. M. J. van Dieten, G. P. van Rees: J. Endoc. **79** (1978) 311–318.
[18] Matsuo, H., Y. Baba, R. M. G. Nair: Biochem. Biophys. Res. Commun. **43** (1971) 1334.
[19] Meldrum, D. R., R. J. Chang, J. Lu et al.: J. Clin. Endocr. Metab. **54** (1982) 1081–1083.
[20] Meldrum, D. R., W. M. Pardridge, W. G. Karow et al.: Ob. Gynecol. **62** (4) (1983) 480–485.
[21] Nekola, M. V., A. Horvath, D. H. Coy et al.: Science **218** (1982) 160–161.
[22] Perrin, M., J. Rivier, W. Vale: Endocrinology **106** (1980) 1289–1296.
[23] Perrin, M. H., J. M. Vaughn, J. E. Rivier et al.: Life Sci. **26** (1980) 2251–2255.
[24] Rao, M. C., J. S. Richards, A. R. Midgley et al.: Endocrinology **101** (1977) 512–523.
[25] Redding, T. W., A. J. Kastin, R. M. G. Nair et al.: Biochem. Pharmacol. **22** (1973) 1915–1919.
[26] Rivier, C., J. Rivier, W. Vale: Endocrinology **103** (1978) 2299–2305.
[27] Rivier, J., W. W. Vale: Patent No. 4244946 Issue date: Jan. 13, 1981.
[28] Rivier, C., J. Rivier, M. Perrin et al.: Biol. Reprod. **29** (1983) 374–378.

[29] Schenken, R. S., R. H. Asch: Fert. Steril. **34** (6) (1980) 581–587.
[30] Seibel, M. M., M. Kamrava, C. McArdle et al.: Ob. Gyn. **61** (1983) 292–298.
[31] Sundaram, K., Y-Q. Cao, N-G. Wang et al.: Life Sci. **28** (1981) 83–88.
[32] Tolis, G., D. Ackman, A. Stellos et al.: Proc. Natl. Acad. Sci. **79** (1982) 1658–1662.
[33] Vale, W., G. Grant, M. Amoss et al.: Endocrinology **91** (1972) 562–572.
[34] Vale, W., C. Rivier, M. Brown et al.: In "Hypothalamus and Endocrine Functions" (edited by F. Labrie, J. Meites and G. Pelletier), pp. 397–429. Plenum Press, New York 1976.
[35] Vanderhoof, M. M., R. G. Foldesy, D. W. Hahn: Federation Proceedings (Submitted).

Reversible pharmacologic castration of the female: implications for endometriosis, contraception and ovulation induction

G. D. Hodgen, L. B. Werlin, D. Kenigsberg, B. A. Littman, M. P. Platia, R. S. Schenken

Introduction

The agonists or antagonists of GnRH (LH-RH) allow reversible pharmacologic castration by transient functional obliteration of the hypothalamic-pituitary-ovarian axis. These conditions may be desired for a number of medical objectives. Among them are: 1. contraception through the prevention of ovulation or implantation; 2. hypoestrogenism for the involution of ectopic endometrium (endometriosis); and 3. management of individual response to exogenous gonadotropin therapy for *in vitro* fertilization or ovulation induction. Each of these will be considered in turn.

Endometriosis or contraception

Numerous studies have indicated the effectiveness of daily GnRH agonist administration on the suppression of ovulation. These reports have stimulated interest in GnRH analogs as possible agents for medical treatment of endometriosis or as a means of contraception [1].

Frequently, endometriosis is a disease of ovulating women. Thus, medical therapy has been directed toward preventing follicular maturation in order to avoid a steroidal milieu that stimulates ectopic endometrial tissue. Previously, this condition has been accomplished through the administration of various preparations containing progestins, as well as danazol [2–4]. Despite wide utility, these medications have not been uniformly satisfactory. Recently, it has been suggested that GnRH agonists may be useful in treating endometriosis by achieving a transient state of medical ovariectomy [5].

One study was designed to test the efficacy of a long-acting GnRH agonist for inhibition of ovulation and menses in monkeys as well as suppression of mild to moderate endometriosis through an individualized, intermittent regimen [1]. Our principal objectives were to evaluate a brief course of individualized, intermittent treatment that may minimize potential side effects and allow prompt resumption of fertile menstrual cycles. The dose and/or frequency of administration of the GnRH analog were increased in accordance with persistence or cessation of the ovarian/menstrual cycle.

Surgical induction of endometriosis

Although endometriosis occurs spontaneously in monkeys [6], our studies required that the disease be induced for practical reasons. On day 24 of the normal menstrual cycle, endometrial tissue was obtained by a transfundal incision; the tissue was minced in a few drops of saline using a scalpel. The minced tissue was seeded over the peritoneal surfaces, including the uterine incision [6]. After resting the monkeys for one intervening menstrual cycle, all underwent laparotomy to verify the presence of viable ectopic endometrial tissue. These assessments were both visual and histological (biopsy). The severity of endometriosis was assessed according to recognized clinical criteria [7]. Once persistent endometriosis was documented, monkeys were assigned randomly to either the treatment ($n = 15$) or control ($n = 6$) protocol.

Intermittent GnRH agonist therapy

Initially, all 15 monkeys received the GnRH agonist (leuprolide, D-Leu^6-Pro^9-Net-LH-RH, Abbott Laboratories, North Chicago, IL; 10 μg/kg, sc) once every 7 days. If menstrual flow was detected during administration of the GnRH analog, laparotomy was performed to assess ovarian status. When ovulation had occurred, the dose of GnRH agonist was increased by 50% (15 μg/kg, once every 7 days). Finally, if evidence of cyclic ovarian function persisted (menses and/or a corpus luteum) despite the higher dose of GnRH agonist, the interval between doses was changed to once every 4 days. In all, the treatments spanned 84 days, approximating 3 idealized menstrual cycles. At the cessation of GnRH agonist injections, all monkeys (treated and control) underwent inspection at laparotomy.

Hormonal measurements in circulation

Blood (3.5 ml) was drawn from the femoral vein daily (at ~ 0600 h) from days 1–28 of the treatment regimen. The monkeys were not bled from days 29–56; thereafter, blood was collected daily until day 84, concurrent with cessation of GnRH agonist therapy. Sera were frozen until RIA for FSH, LH, 17β-estradiol, and progesterone, as described previously [6, 8].

Resumption of the ovarian/menstrual cycle and fertility tests

Beginning with the first menstrual flow after ending GnRH agonist treatments (or after 90 days in controls), daily rapid serum estradiol determinations were used to predict the next ovulation (estradiol, > 200 pg/ml for 2 days). On this basis, all monkeys were mated to males of established fertility, except when signs (menses and the preovulatory estrogen surge) of cyclic ovarian function were absent. CG tests for pregnancy [8] were performed during the third week after each mating, and the results were confirmed by manual palpation. This study was limited to the initial 90 days after termination of GnRH agonist therapy. Statistical comparisons were made by a two-way analysis of variance at the 5% and 1% levels of confidence.

Hormonal responses

Intermittent administration of the GnRH agonist led to highly individualized responses. For example, figure 1 illustrates the relative sensitivity of a representative monkey to only 10 μg/kg GnRH analog weekly. Note the near concurrence of estradiol and LH elevations in circulation during the first month of treatment. That ovulation was blocked is indicated from consistent low serum progesterone values, as well as the onset of amenorrhea.

In contrast, one monkey manifested profound resistance to suppression of the ovarian cycle, even when the GnRH agonist regimen was increased to 15 μg/kg every fourth day. Her serum hormonal patterns suggested persistent follicular maturation and corpus luteum function, consistent with our observations at laparotomy.

Most striking throughout was the instability of serum estradiol levels. It is apparent that the ovarian cycles of some individuals were not fully suppressed in the first month by a regimen of 10 μg/kg, once every 7 days; indeed, the lower serum estradiol and progesterone values ($P < 0.05$) in the third month of treatment, as well as the absence of a dominant follicle or corpus luteum and menses, indicated that the hypothalamic-pituitary-ovarian axis gradually was coming under the inhibitory influence of weekly injections of the long-acting GnRH agonist.

Posttreatment assessments of endometriosis and resumption of fertility

Table 1 summarizes: 1. menstrual and ovarian responses during and after GnRH agonist administration; 2. the status (before and after) of ectopic endometrial tissue; and 3. the time course of resumption of fertile menstrual cycles. For 9 of the 15 monkeys, GnRH agonist therapy was increased in dose and/or frequency because ovarian function was not inhibited fully in the first or second months of treatment. After 84 days of treatment, marked improvement in the extent of endometriosis was noted in 12 of the 15 monkeys undergoing serial laparotomy. Favorable outcomes were characterized by complete resolution of ectopic endometrium; even among unresolved cases, ectopic tissue involuted.

The intervals from the cessation of GnRH agonist therapy until the first menstrual flow and ovulation were brief in 14 of 15 cases (21.6 ± 3.2 and 33.2 ± 3.6 days, respectively; tab. 1). More importantly, 6 of the 15 monkeys became pregnant within 90 days after termination of GnRH agonist injections (an interval sufficient

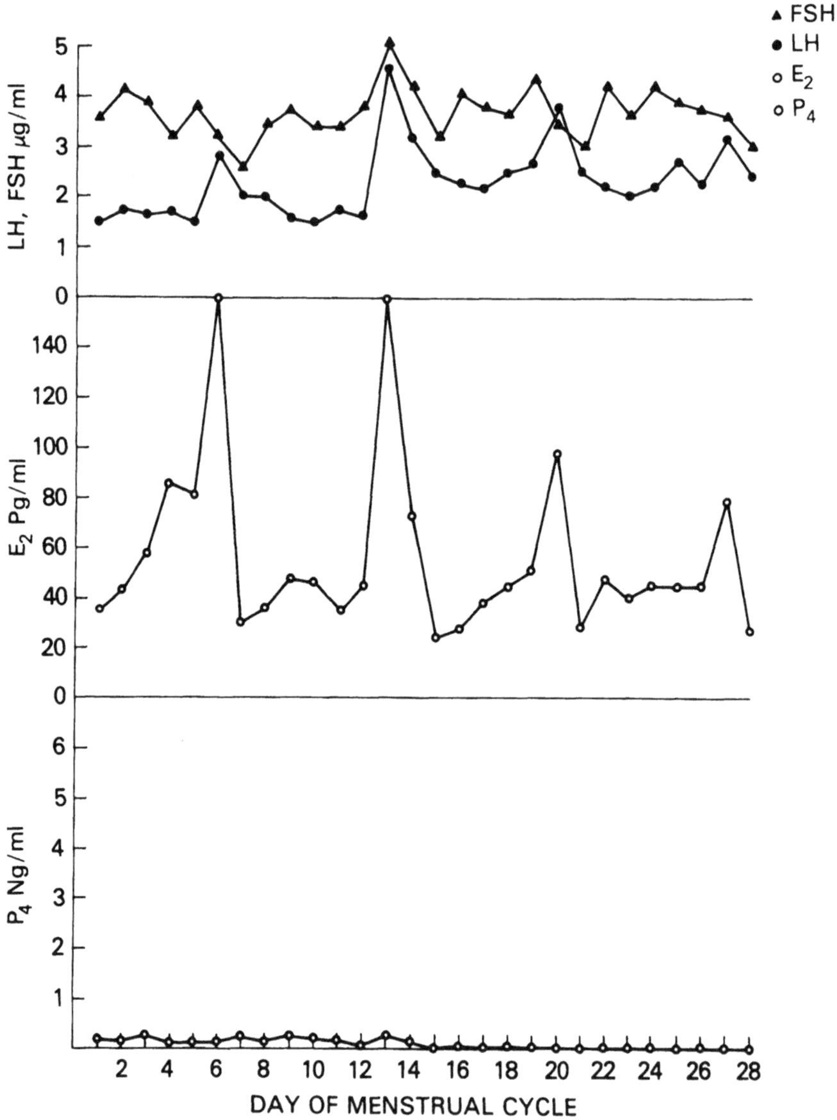

Fig. 1 Representative serum concentrations of LH, FSH, estradiol (E_2) and progesterone (P_4) in a highly responsive monkey receiving (↓) the long-acting GnRH agonist (Leuprolide; 10 µg/kg weekly, sc) for treatment of endometriosis in the first cycle (month). (With permission from [1].)

for approximately 2 ovulatory cycles), although 2 early abortions followed. This is not an unusual rate of pregnancy loss in our primate colony; we do not suggest any effect of the GnRHα in these abortions.

In contrast, timely menses and apparent ovulations continued in the six control monkeys (untreated endometriosis). They, too, were mated during the 90 days after

Table 1 Resumption of the ovarian/menstrual cycle and fertility after intermittent GnRH agonist therapy (leuprolide, D-Leu[6]-Pro[9]-Net-LHRH, Abbott Laboratories) in monkeys with induced endometriosis

GnRH agonist therapy[a]			Assessments at serial laparotomy				Posttreatment		
Monkey No.	Dose (μg/kg,sc)	Frequency (days)	Before[b]			After	Resumption of menses (days)	Resumption of ovulation (days)	Fertile menstrual cycles within 90 days
1	10	7	Stage I	(mild)	3 pts	Resolved	11	24	Pregnant, aborted
2	10	7	Stage II	(mod)	6 pts	Resolved	18	32	Pregnant
3	10	7	Stage I	(mild)	3 pts	Resolved	41	53	Pregnant
4	10	7	Stage I	(mild)	3 pts	Resolved	34	50	Pregnant
5	10	7	Stage I	(mild)	3 pts	Mild (2 pts)	24	34	Not pregnant
6	10	7	Stage I	(mild)	3 pts	Mild (1 pt)	36	Anovulation	Not mated
7	15	7	Stage I	(mild)	2 pts	Resolved	30	40	Pregnant, aborted
8	15	7	Stage II	(mod)	12 pts	Resolved	29	39	Not pregnant
9	15	7	Stage I	(mild)	3 pts	Resolved	5	20	Not pregnant
10	15	7	Stage I	(mild)	4 pts	Resolved	23	39	Pregnant
11	15	7	Stage I	(mild)	3 pts	Mild (1 pt)	17	26	Not pregnant
12	15	4	Stage I	(mild)	3 pts	Resolved	1	13	Not pregnant
13	15	4	Stage I	(mild)	3 pts	Resolved	9	22	Not pregnant
14	15	4	Stage II	(mod)	7 pts	Resolved	35	48	Not pregnant
15	15	4	Stage I	(mild)	3 pts	Resolved	13	25	Not pregnant
16[c]	0	0	Stage II	(mod)	6 pts	Mod (7 pts)	3	18	Not pregnant
17	0	0	Stage I	(mild)	3 pts	Mild (3 pts)	17	31	Not pregnant
18	0	0	Stage II	(mod)	11 pts	Mod (10 pts)	11	24	Not pregnant
19	0	0	Stage I	(mild)	4 pts	Mild (4 pts)	21	37	Not pregnant
20	0	0	Stage II	(mod)	6 pts	Mod (6 pts)	5	17	Pregnant
21	0	0	Stage II	(mod)	9 pts	Mod (8 pts)	12	27	Not pregnant

[a]) Treatment regimen, followed by cessation of ovulation and menses.
[b]) Classification of endometriosis: mild, 1–5 points; moderate (mod), 6–15 points (6).
[c]) Monkeys 16–21 are untreated controls.
(With permission from [1].)

the GnRH agonist was withdrawn from the treatment group (an interval sufficient for approximately 3 ovulations each). One control monkey with moderate endometriosis became pregnant; the remaining 5 maintained mild-moderate endometriosis and failed to conceive. The small sample size (15 treated and 6 control) precludes an adequate statistical comparison of pregnancy rates at this time.

Whether these treatment effects resulted from loss of pituitary sensitivity to endogenous GnRH, insensitivity of the ovaries to pituitary gonadotropins, or some direct inhibition of ovarian function by the GnRH agonist is not known with certainty. However, our preliminary data [1] may suggest ovarian desensitization, rather than pituitary refractoriness, after intermittent GnRHα treatments. We have previously reported that an untimely hCG injection during the monkey follicular phase can interrupt the ovarian cycle [9]; here, perhaps, the intermittent GnRHα-induced LH elevations cause a similar hiatus of follicular maturation. Also, a direct action of the GnRH analog on the ovaries and/or ectopic endometrium is possible. It is clear that intermittent GnRH treatments can accomplish "medical ablation" of the dominant follicle in successive follicular phases, thereby blocking ovulation.

That consistent improvement in the extent of endometriosis was observed here without achieving maximal suppression of serum estradiol, such as after castration (< 15 pg/ml), may be of interest. Indeed, amenorrhea frequently persists in the intact state so long as the tonic serum estradiol level remains below 30–40 pg/ml [10]. Our data indicate that a sufficient hypoestrogenic state was reached to negate proliferation of endometrial tissue; this may explain the observed atrophy of ectopic implants.

Others have achieved a state of medical ovariectomy in women by daily administration of a GnRH agonist [5]. Although full suppression of ovarian estrogen secretion may be required to effectively treat endometriosis, both approaches (individualized, intermittent administration vs. a daily regimen) deserve consideration. These find-

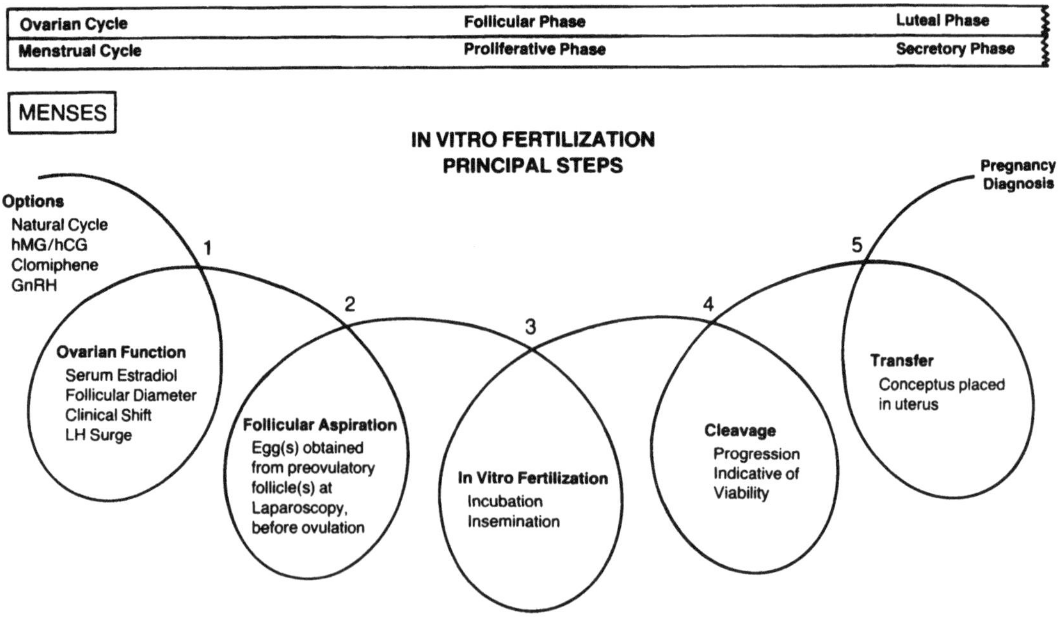

Fig. 2 Principal steps in an in vitro fertilization/embryo transfer protocol. Among the options for ovarian stimulation, exogenous gonadotropins may be employed to increase the number of oocytes collected.

ings may encourage clinical investigations employing GnRH agonists for medical treatment of endometriosis or for fertility control.

Stimulation of the ovarian cycle

Ovarian stimulation via exogenous gonadotropins for *in vitro* fertilization therapy (fig. 2) is notoriously difficult to manage, in part because of the marked individual variability in response to injected agents (fig. 3). Endogenous hypothalamic-pituitary functions may be principal sources of this variation. In an effort to explore the etiology of this individualism and to control or reduce variable response patterns, we

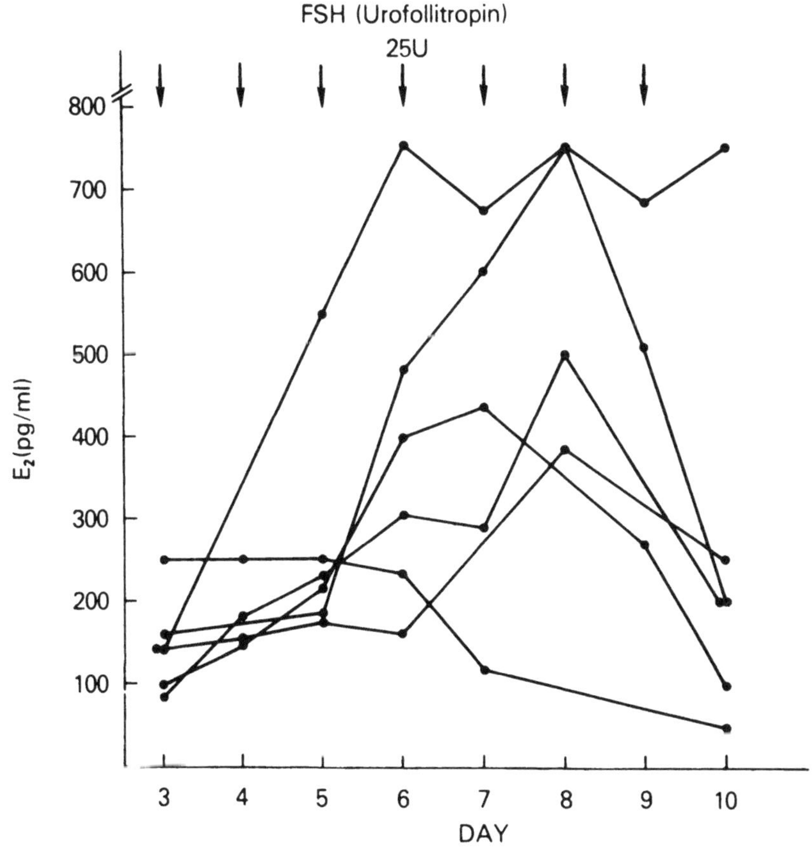

Fig. 3 Administration of "pure" FSH to normal cycling monkeys on days 3 to 9 after the onset of menses. Note the great individuality of estrogen secretory pattern even when the FSH dose was constant at 25 IU (im) daily [Serono, Urofollitropin].

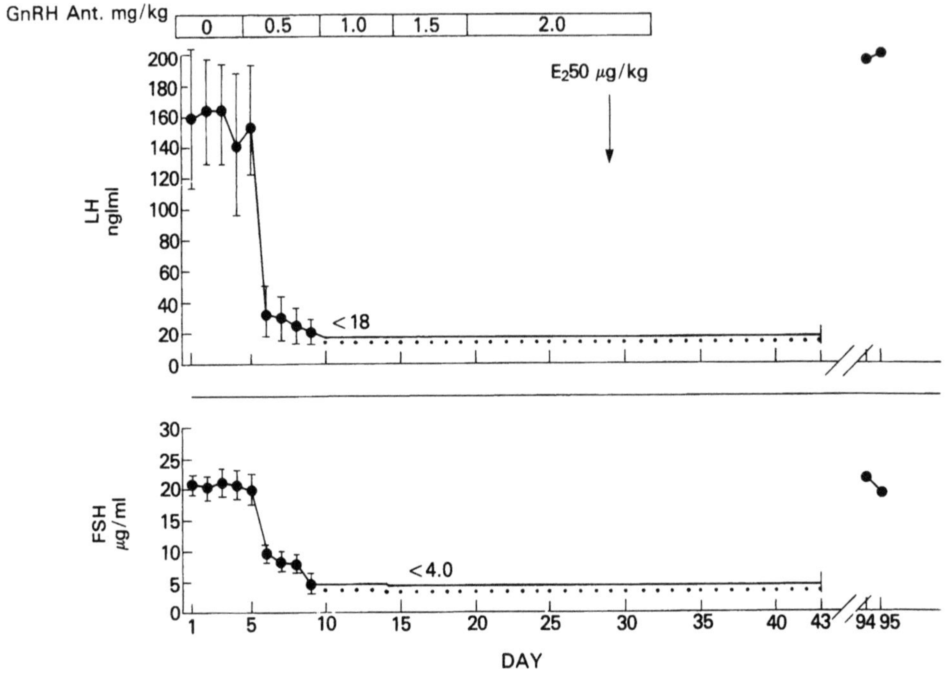

Fig. 4 GnRH antagonist [(Ac-pClPhe^{1},pClDPhe^{2},DTryp^{3},DArg^{6}, DAla^{10})-GnRH HCl] suppresses FSH and LH levels in serum to below limits of assay detection. Long-term ovariectomized monkeys did not respond to an estrogen challenge test. Note full recovery of gonadotropin secretion by 2 months after cessation of treatment.

performed a "medical hypophysectomy" (with regard to gonadotropin secretion) by use of a potent GnRH antagonist [(Ac-pClPhe^{1},pClDPhe^{2},DTrp^{3},DArg^{6},DAla^{10})-GnRH HCl] (a generous gift from the Contraceptive Development Branch, CPR, NICHD) in order to eliminate endogenous pituitary FSH and LH secretion (fig. 4). Superimposed on this treatment, we administered hMG (n=15, Pergonal, Serono) or "pure" FSH (n=5, Urofollitropin, Serono) to stimulate ovarian follicular maturation in otherwise normal cynomolgus monkeys [11]. Control groups received either hMG (n=15) or "pure" FSH (n=15) alone. All groups received a fixed regimen of gonadotropin treatment for 7 consecutive days (25 IU/day/im, cycle days 3–9) followed by hCG (1000 IU/im) on cycle day 10.

Our preliminary observations [11] suggest that the variability in response to hMG treatment was less in the group treated with GnRH antagonist (fig. 5). The patterns of estradiol rise in serum and the appearance of the ovaries at laparotomy were more uniform when endogenous gonadotropin secretion was suppressed. Surprisingly, the regimen employing "medical hypophysectomy" plus "pure" FSH promoted maturation of multiple ovarian follicles (fig. 6); further, these follicles were ovulated by hCG

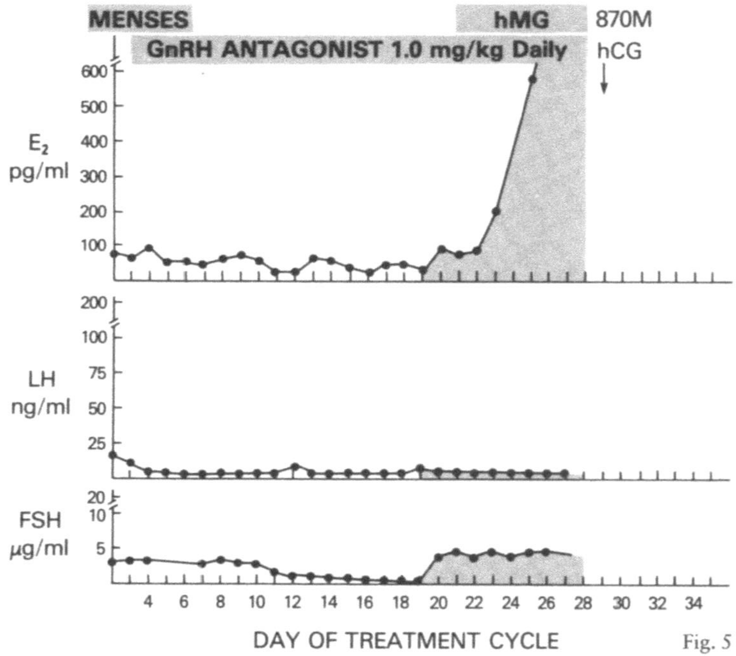

Fig. 5

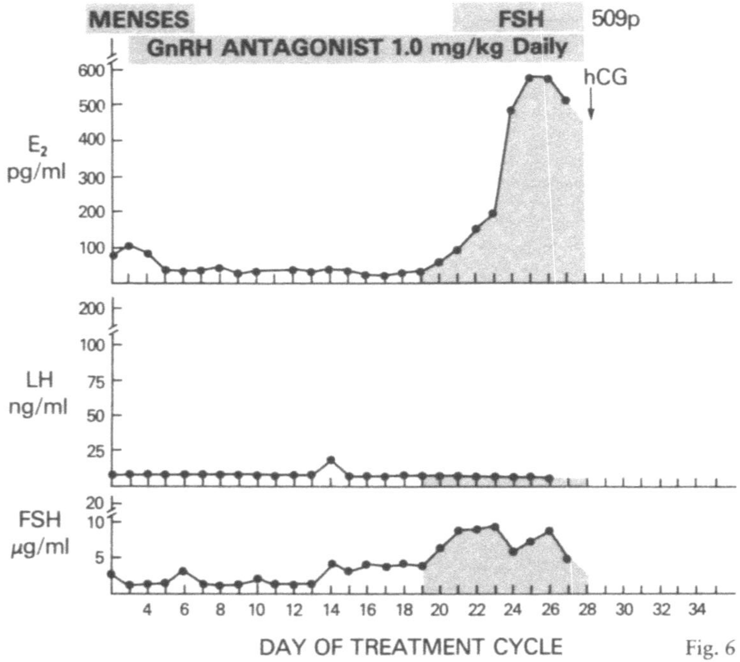

Fig. 6

Fig. 5 GnRH antagonist [AC-pClPhe[1],pClDPhe[2],DTryp[3],DArg[6],DAla[10])-GnRH HCl] followed by hMG therapy in intact cycling monkeys. Note suppression of endogenous gonadotropin secretion and ovarian responsiveness to hMG treatments, as indicated by elevation of estradiol (E_2) in serum.

Fig. 6 GnRH antagonist [(Ac-pClPhe[1],pClDPhe[2],DTryp[3],DArg[6],DAla[10])-GnRH HCl] followed by FSH therapy is intact cycling monkeys. Note suppression of endogenous gonadotropin secretion and ovarian responsiveness to FSH treatments, as indicated by elevations of estradiol (E_2) in serum.

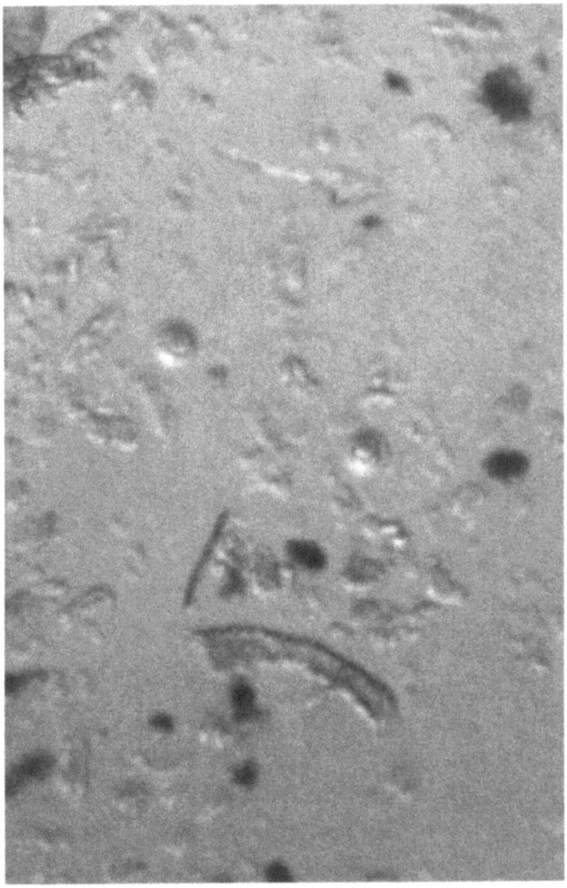

Fig. 7 Two-cell embryos collected from the fallopian tubes of a monkey given GnRH antagonist with "pure" FSH, mated and undergoing lavage 72 hours after hCG injection. The treatment regimen was that illustrated in figure 6.

with subsequent recovery of 2–cell embryos (fig. 7). To our knowledge this is the first demonstration that ovarian follicular maturation can be promoted by FSH in the absence of detectable levels of LH in serum. Ovulation was also achieved in 9 of 15 control monkeys treated with "pure" FSH.

Clearly, FSH is the principal stimulus for follicle growth in the primate ovarian/menstrual cycle; conversely, LH may be much less important than previously regarded in the follicular phase (fig. 8), until the midcycle LH surge for ovulation [11, 12].

We suggest that a condition of "medical hypophysectomy", achieved by administration of a GnRH antagonist, may be a useful adjunct for improving patient management during gonadotropin therapy by reducing individual variability of ovarian response [13, 14].

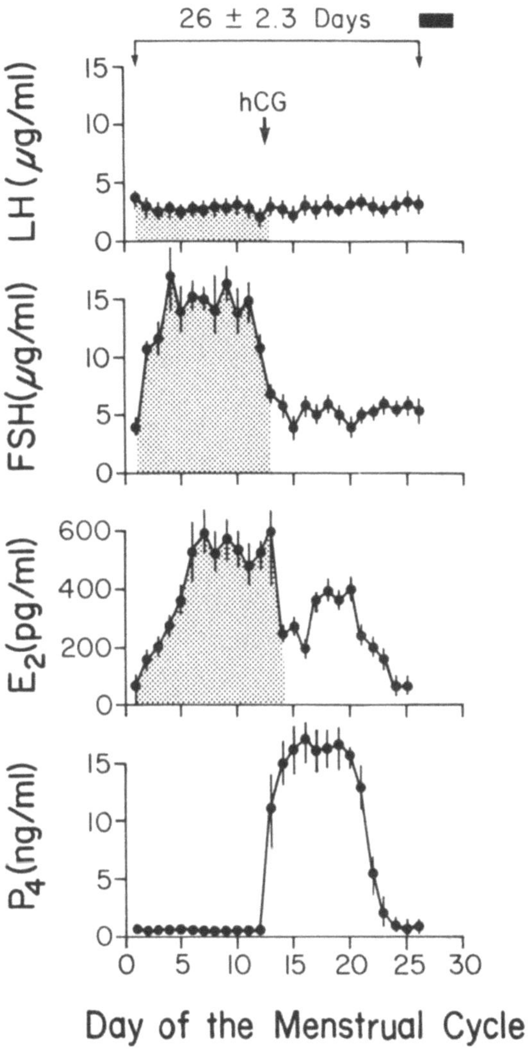

Fig. 8 Mean pattern of circulating pituitary gonadotropins and ovarian steroids before and after "pure" FSH administration (shaded zone) to 3 monkeys on days 1–11 of the menstrual cycle (50 IU/day, im). Human chorionic gonadotropin (hCG) was administered (1000 IU im) on day 12. Cycle length was ~ 26 days. Vertical bars indicate ± SE. (With permission from [12].)

References

[1] Werlin, L. B., G. D. Hodgen: J. Clin. Endocrinol. Metab. **56** (1983) 844–848.
[2] Hammond, C. B., A. F. Haney: Fertil. Steril. **30** (1978) 497.
[3] Andrews, W. C., D. Larson: Am. J. Obstet. Gynecol. **118** (1974) 643.
[4] Greenblatt, R. B., W. P. Dmowski, V. B. Mahesh et al.: Fertil. Steril. **22** (1971) 102.

[5] Meldrum, D., J. Chang, J. Lu et al.: J. Clin. Endocrinol. Metab. **54** (1982) 1081.
[6] diZerega, G. S., D. L. Barber, G. D. Hodgen: Fertil. Steril. **33** (1980) 649.
[7] American Fertility Society: Fertil. Steril. **32** (1979) 649.
[8] Hodgen, G. D., W. W. Tullner, J. L. Vaitukaitis et al.: J. Clin. Endocrinol. Metab. **39** (1974) 417.
[9] Williams, R. F., G. D. Hodgen: Fertil. Steril. **33** (1980) 64.
[10] Hodgen, G. D.: Fertil. Steril. **38** (1982) 281.
[11] Kenigsberg, D., B. Littman, G. D. Hodgen: Annual Meeting of the American Fertility Society, New Orleans, Louisiana, Abstract (1984).
[12] Schenken, R. S., R. F. Williams, G. D. Hodgen: Fertil. Steril. (submitted), (1984).
[13] Garcia, J. E., G. S. Jones, A. A. Acosta et al.: Fertil. Steril. 39 (1983) 174.
[14] Fleming, R., A. H. Adam, D. H. Barlow et al.: Brit. J. Obstet. Gynecol. **89** (1982) 80.

Metabolism and pharmacokinetics of LH-RH agonists

J. Sandow, G. Jerabek-Sandow, M. Schmidt-Gollwitzer †

Introduction

The structural analysis and synthesis of LH-RH [27, 45] provided the incentive to investigate physiology and pharmacology of this hypothalamic peptide, and initiated numerous studies on its localization, metabolism and enzyme inactivation (see reviews [11, 25]). The organ distribution in laboratory animals and the plasma elimination in animals and in man were studied [9, 34, 35, 40], using biological assays for LH-RH activity in plasma as the end point, and by monitoring the radiolabelled compound (^{3}H-LH-RH, ^{125}I-LH-RH). When incubated with plasma *in vitro*, a gradual loss of LH-RH bioactivity was found, whereas radioimmunoassay indicated different rates of plasma inactivation depending on the specificity of the LH-RH antiserum employed in measurement [17]. This was traced to the limited specificity of many LH-RH antisera, which recognize the intact LH-RH decapeptide, together with inactive C-terminal metabolites like the (3–10)octapeptide, a typical degradation product in plasma. The enzyme mechanisms involved in LH-RH degradation were elucidated [1, 12, 20, 22] with tissue homogenates, and studies of LH-RH agonist analogues [21, 26] disclosed significant differences in degradation pattern and rate of degradation depending on the chemical substitution, in particular in amino acids 6 (glycine) and 10 (glycine-amide). The increased biological activity was attributed to enzyme resistance. In view of binding and degradation studies in isolated pituitary cells [24], it is still disputed whether receptor affinity is the key factor for increased biological activity, or whether enzyme stability explains enhanced agonist activity.

The pharmacokinetics of LH-RH are difficult to evaluate even with highly sensitive radioimmunoassays, due to the limited specificity of the available antisera, to the high rate of metabolic inactivation, and to rapid plasma elimination. It is clearly possible to detect secretory episodes of LH-RH by measurement in portal plasma samples of rats, sheep and monkeys [6]. Minute concentrations are found in plasma after therapeutic doses. The pulses of LH-RH in plasma after bolus injections of 5–10, ug can be measured, but monitoring the biological effect (LH release) is more practical for control of pulsatile LH-RH therapy. Immunoreactive LH-RH metabolites are excreted in the urine [3, 18], and ^{3}H-LH-RH metabolites were found in the urine of animals and man [34, 35]. A correlation of the urinary excretion of LH-RH metabolites with the functional state of the hypothalamic-pituitary system was established in the human [4, 5].

With the investigation of LH-RH agonists in numerous clinical conditions requiring reversible pituitary-gonadal suppression, and with their extensive application in contraception, it became necessary to investigate the pharmacokinetics of these hormone analogues, and to study the mechanisms involved in drug disposition and metabolism. In our own studies [39, 43], we have investigated LH-RH(1–9)nonapeptide-ethylamide agonists, in particular /D-Ser$(Bu^t)^6$/LH-RH(1–9)nonapeptide-ethylamide (buserelin, Hoe 766). The experimental studies in animals were performed with biologically active/^{125}I-Tyr^5/ labelled peptides, with identification of metabolites by thin layer chromatography (TLC), high performance liquid chromatography (HPLC), and specific radioimmunoassays. The biological activity of metabolites found in plasma and urine samples after peptide administration was monitored by bioassay in rats (LH release).

Pharmacokinetics in animals

After intravenous injection, LH-RH agonists are rapidly cleared from plasma (initial half-life about 5 min). There is a progressively decreasing rate of elimination (terminal half-life about 60–90 min), when buserelin is measured by RIA in serum of ovariectomized rats (fig. 1). Significant differences are found between estimates of plasma elimination by bioassay, by thin layer chromatography in plasma extracts [43], and by radioimmunoassay [47] both for LH-RH and for buserelin. After intravenous injection of LH-RH in rats and dogs, the LH-releasing activity monitored by bioassay in serum or plasma decreases rapidly, with a half life of 4–5 min [40]. A rapid decline in biological activity to nondetectable levels is also observed within 15–30 min after i.v. injection of LH-RH agonists, depending on the dose injected. In the dog, bioactive buserelin in plasma decreases to levels below 10 ng/ml about 60 min after an i.v. dose of 5 mg. Bioassay of LH-RH activity in serum or plasma is performed in male rats by LH release after a two hours infusion of each serum sample. This method requires a dose of 1–2 ng buserelin, or 20–40 ng LH-RH per sample to detect LH-RH activity. For pharmacokinetic monitoring by bioassay, it is necessary to inject a high test-dose of unlabelled agonist, and to concentrate the LH-releasing activity in serum or plasma by adsorption on silicates (octadecasilyl, SEP PAK C18 cartridges, Waters), elution with appropriate organic solvents, and reconstitution after evaporation in physiological saline.

The immunoreactive peptide in serum or plasma measured by RIA decreases much more slowly. A highly specific RIA method has been reported for one agonist [50]. In our own experience, all buserelin antisera exhibit some crossreactivity with metabolites, and HPLC purification of plasma samples is mandatory for an estimate of intact agonist in rats, and in humans.

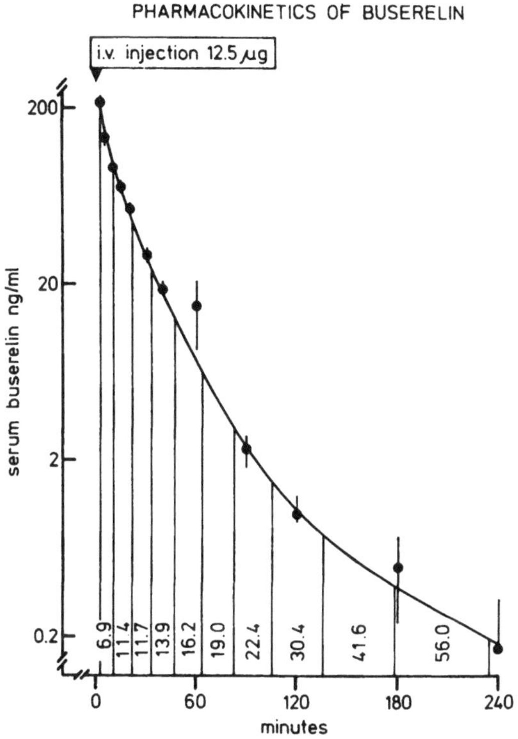

Fig. 1 Plasma elimination of buserelin in adult ovariectomized rats: buserelin 12.5/µg was injected i.v., and the serum level was determined by RIA (antiserum AS-639). Means and standard error of 10 rats/group. The calculated half-life for successive phases of plasma elimination is indicated from 0–240 min after injection.

In contrast to rapid elimination after intravenous injection, plasma elimination is considerably prolonged when a steady state is obtained by infusion, and the half-life is estimated after termination of the infusion. Prolonged plasma elimination was found in rats at the end of an infusion of buserelin at a rate of 60/µg/day, and after termination of an infusion of /D-Trp^6/LH-RH in men, where the half-life estimate was 17.3 min [2].

The rate of plasma elimination after intravenous injection of buserelin is unaffected by an increase of the peptide dose over a wide dose range [39]. In a study with a tracer dose of 50 ng ^{125}I-buserelin (2/µCi), the simultaneous injection of an excess dose of 50/µg unlabelled peptide did not change the rate of tracer elimination from plasma. Similar findings have been obtained with other LH-RH agonists. The experimental conditions can significantly affect the half-life estimate. In urethane-anaesthetized rats, plasma elimination is decreased by interference of urethane with renal clearance of LH-RH agonists. In patients with renal or hepatic failure, the response to an LH-RH test injection is augmented due to reduced degradation, and the plasma half-life is prolonged [33].

There is some controversy about agonist binding to plasma proteins. LH-RH and D-Leu^6-ethylamide are not bound to more than 19% of proteins [49]. Our own results (equilibrium dialysis) indicate a plasma protein binding of the same order for buserelin.

Identification of the peptide fragments circulating in serum after i.v. or s.c. injection of LH-RH agonists requires separation of metabolites and intact peptide. The ratio of metabolites over intact peptide increases with time. In one of our studies in rats, 125-I-buserelin was injected i.v., and radiolabelled metabolites were concentrated by ethanol extraction of serum samples. Intact buserelin was identified by thin layer chromatography, and by antiserum binding. The ethanol extract of serum taken 5 min after injection of 125-I-buserelin contained intact buserelin, whereas serum taken 60 min later was devoid of any radiolabelled peptide material, despite an elevated concentration of 125-I in serum. This nonpeptide material was identified by

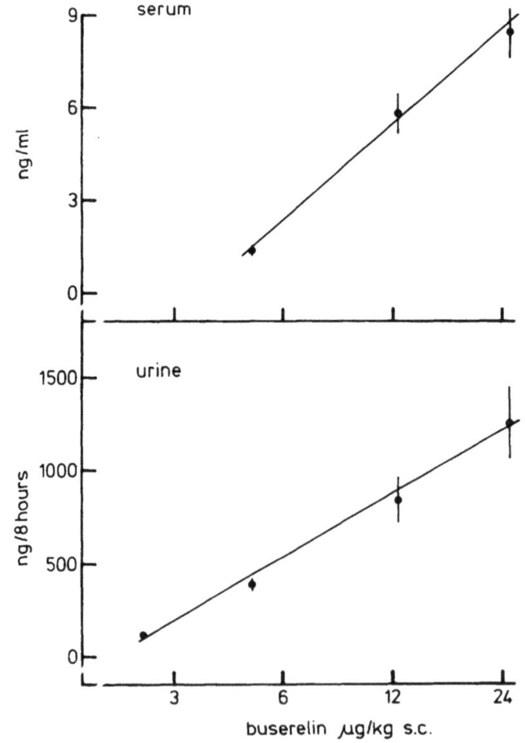

Fig. 2 Dose-dependent increase in immunoreactive buserelin in serum and urine of rats during long-term treatment with doses of 2.5–25 µg/kg s.c. once daily. Means and standard error of 10 rats/group. Serum level is non-detectable at the lowest dose, but urinary excretion can be measured.

its adsorption characteristics on aluminium oxide, and by absence of binding to buserelin antisera. It consists of 125-I resulting from metabolic inactivation and de-iodination of the buserelin tracer preparation.

Buserelin metabolites are detected by RIA in plasma for 2–6 hours after i.v. injection in dogs or in cows, depending on the initial dose. The half-life estimate for the terminal half-life is low if a specific antiserum recognizing intact buserelin is used, and high with antisera crossreacting with C-terminal metabolites. We tested the specificity of antisera by infusion of synthetic buserelin metabolites in rats, and found, that with one antiserum (AS-639) the (3–9)heptapeptide and (4–9)hexapeptide induced a marked increase in the plasma level, whereas a more specific antiserum (AS-14) did not measure these metabolites. The method of choice for analysis of metabolites in plasma samples is extraction on octadecasilyl cartridges (Waters), separation by HPLC and detection of the individual metabolites by RIA. Extraction of plasma samples of 4 ml results in recoveries of 90–95% buserelin.

In the rat and small experimental animals, measurement of the plasma level of LH-RH or LH-RH agonists is of limited value, when low stimulatory doses are investigated. The problems of obtaining sufficiently high sample volumes cannot be overcome. At higher suppressive doses, the plasma level is useful for monitoring of drug absorption, and for dosage control in pharmacological and toxicological studies. In rats, both the plasma concentration of buserelin, and the urinary excretion are time- and dose-dependent [44], and provide a valuable control of drug absorption under experimental conditions, when secretion of gonadotrophins and gonadal steroids is increasingly suppressed (fig. 2).

Organ distribution studies

Numerous studies have been performed with ^{3}H-LH-RH, ^{125}I-LH-RH and ^{125}-I-labelled agonists [9, 28, 34, 36, 38, 41], indicating a similar pattern of distribution, but with significant quantitative differences. Labelled peptide accumulate in liver and kidneys (main inactivating organs), and a small quantity is found in the anterior pituitary (specific LH-RH receptors, biological target organ). The thyroid gland concentrates ^{125}I resulting from metabolic breakdown of LH-RH or agonists, accumulation can be prevented by pretreatment with unlabelled iodine. The tissue/plasma ratio of radiolabelled peptide found in anterior pituitary tissue increases with chemical stability of LH-RH agonists. Enhanced biological activity is correlated with prolonged time of pituitary accumulation [36, 43], and with enzyme resistance [16, 42]. In studies of organ distribution and metabolic inactivation in male rats, 60 min after i.v. injection of ^{125}I-LH-RH (10/μCi/50 ng peptide), the liver contained 1.61% of the dose injected, the kidneys 1.33%, and anterior pituitary accumulation was no longer detectable (maximum at 15 min after injection). The thyroid gland contained 0.27% of the ^{125}I dose. After i.v. injection of a similar dose of ^{125}I-buserelin, the liver contained 21% of the dose, the kidneys 5.3%, and the anterior pituitary 0.025%. In the thyroid gland, 0.24% of the radiolabel were recovered. Increased pituitary accumulation of potent LH-RH agonists is correlated with enhanced receptor binding affinity [7, 8]. In contrast, LH-RH is only transiently accumulated in the pituitary gland, and biologically inactive agonist metabolites do not reach significant tissue/plasma ratios indicative of pituitary accumulation [38].

In liver and kidneys, the organ distribution of 125-I-buserelin is not modified by a high dose of unlabelled peptide. However, there is significant competitive inhibition of tracer accumulation in the anterior pituitary gland, indicating pituitary binding of the high affinity, low capacity type. Both LH-RH and agonists are metabolized and excreted by the kidneys [3, 18, 39, 46]. In organ distribution studies, a significant amount of radiolabelled peptide is found in the urine. Identification by TLC, HPLC and RIA indicates excretion of C-terminal metabolites. In studies with buserelin, the biological activity of the peptide material excreted in rat urine is low, about 1/400 in

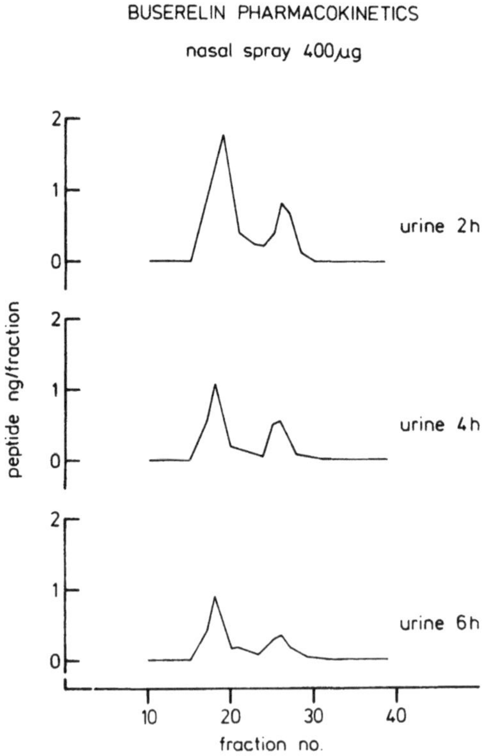

Fig. 3 Excretion of immunoreactive buserelin metabolites in urine of male test persons after a nasal spray dose of 400 µg buserelin. Urine was collected in fractions of 2 hours, and metabolites were separated by HPLC and identified by RIA (antiserum AS-639). There are two distinct metabolites, different from intact buserelin.

comparison with intact buserelin. By HPLC, the immunoreactive peptide material excreted in urine consists of two or more different metabolites (fig. 3), with an increasingly complex pattern after high suppressive doses.

Identification of metabolites *in vivo*

When male rats are treated with a near-physiological dose of buserelin (10/uCi/50 ng ^{125}I-buserelin) by i.v. injection, a sufficient amount of radiolabelled metabolites can be extracted from the inactivating tissues (liver, kidney, anterior pituitary) for identification by TLC, HPLC, enzyme digestion with specific enzymes (pyroglutamyl-aminopeptidase, chymotrypsin), and binding to buserelin antisera. Metabolism of LH-RH *in vivo* is much more rapid than that of buserelin. After i.v. injection of rats with ^{125}I-LH-RH (10/uCi/50 ng), no intact peptide material can be recovered from either liver or kidney, at autopsy 60 min after treatment. After ^{125}I-buserelin injection, extracts of liver and kidneys obtained 60 min after treatment contain several metabolites which can be identified on TLC after enzyme digestion with pyroglutamyl-peptidase and chymotrypsin [43]. In the anterior pituitary, a characteristic metabolite MI is found, which is not present in liver, kidney or thyroid gland. This metabolite, the buserelin (2–9)octapeptide, is also observed *in vitro* after incubation of ^{125}I-buserelin with a rat anterior pituitary enzyme preparation. Liver and kidney extracts do not contain metabolite MI, whereas a different group of metabolites is identified, which are not susceptible to enzyme degradation with pyroglutamyl-peptidase. These metabolites are C-terminal fragments, like the (3–9)heptapeptide, and (4–9)hexapeptide. They retain their affinity for buserelin antisera, and are susceptible to chamotrypsin degradation.

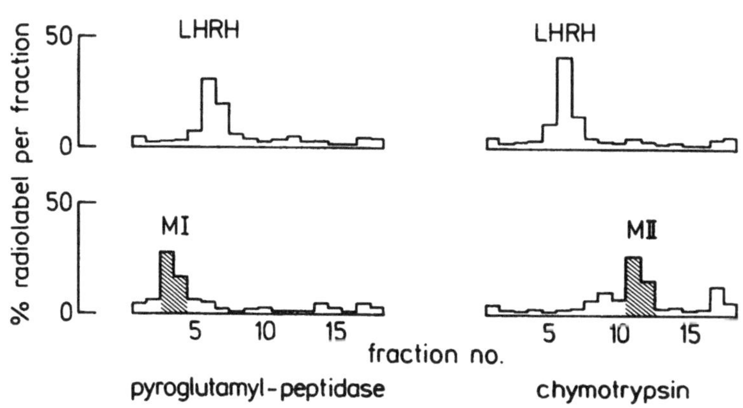

Fig. 4 Identification of LHRH metabolites after enzyme digestion with pyroglutamyl-peptidase or chymotrypsin by thin layer chromatography (silica plates in butanon: pyridin: water: acetic acid, 70:15:15:2, by vol.). The metabolites MI and MII are characteristic degradation products.

An advantage of LH-RH nonapeptide-ethylamide agonists for metabolic studies is their characteristic behavior on thin layer chromatography and HPLC upon incubation with pyroglutamyl-peptidase, which provides unequivocal identification of intact nonapeptide. This is also the case for LH-RH. As an example, the incubation products of 125-I-LH-RH with either pyroglutamyl-paptidase or chymotrypsin are clearly detected by TLC on silica plates (fig. 4). Pyroglutamyl-peptidase (EC 3.4.11.8) is an enzyme found in mammalian pituitary and liver [32, 48].

Metabolism of LH-RH agonists *in vitro*

In vitro degradation studies with homogenates of various organ tissues are helpful in determining the potential LH-RH-inactivating organs. Peptidases present in homogenates of hypothalamus, anterior and posterior pituitary and cerebral cortical tissue rapidly abolish the biological activity of LH-RH [1, 12, 22, 23]. When the LH-RH concentration in incubation media is measured by bioassay (LH release in ovariectomized, oestrogen-progesterone blocked rats), it can be shown that LH-RH is also rapidly inactivated by enzymes contained in the 10,000 x g supernatant fraction of liver and kidney homogenates, as well as by homogenates of ovarian and testicular tissue [37].

There is a good correlation between biological activity and enzyme stability. The weakly active /Arg^4/LH-RH is rapidly inactivated by homogenates of liver, kidney, hypothalamus, anterior pituitary and muscle tissue (40,000 x g supernatant fraction). LH-RH is more resistant to degradation by these enzyme preparations, and the potent agonist, /D-Glu^6/LH-RH is mainly degraded by liver homogenate, whereas degradation by the other tissues is negligible (fig. 5).

In studies on degradation of buserelin, two enzymes are of particular relevance. After incubation of 125-I-userelin with purified pyroglutamyl-peptidase, the buserelin(2–9)octapeptide (primary metabolite of buserelin) is separated from the intact nonapeptide by thin layer chromatography on silica plates in a system of butanone:pyridine:water:acetic acid (70:15:15:2, by vol.). Subsequent treatment with chymotrypsin abolishes this metabolite, by cleavage of the His-Ser, and to a lesser extent of the Trp-D-Ser(Bu^t) bonds [43]. The presence of intact buserelin in tissue extracts is assessed by sequential treatment with pyroglutamyl-peptidase, generating the (2–9)octapeptide (MI), followed by incubation with chymotrypsin, which abolishes the characteristic peak of the (2–9)octapeptide (fig. 6). An identical degradation pattern is found upon incubation of buserelin with pituitary homogenates, pituitary plasma membranes, pyroglutamyl-peptidase, or in pituitary tissue extracts from rats treated with 125-I-buserelin. In the anterior pituitary, cleavage by pyroglutamyl-peptidase is the predominant mechanism of inactivation. A neutral endopeptidase different from chamotrypsin has been isolated [15]. LH-RH is also inactivated by the post-prolin cleaving enzyme [19], present in pituitary and other tissues. This inacti-

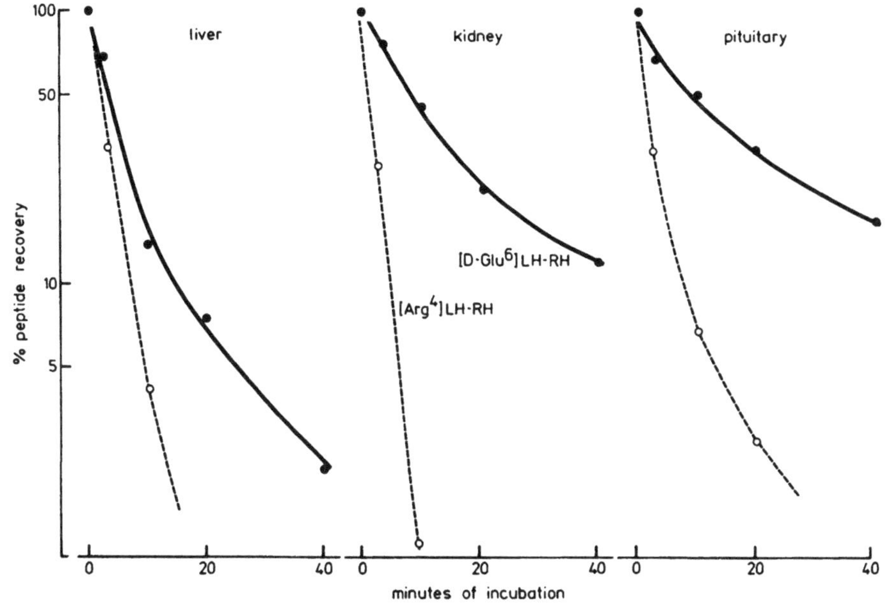

Fig. 5 Degradation of two LHRH agonists *in vitro* by homogenate of liver, kidney or anterior pituitary gland. The weakly active /Arg^4/LHRH is degraded rapidly. /D-Glu^6/LHRH, a potent agonist, is degraded slowly, mainly by liver homogenate. Incubation at + 37 °C for 40 min, % peptide recovery measured by specific LHRH-RIA, four determinations per point.

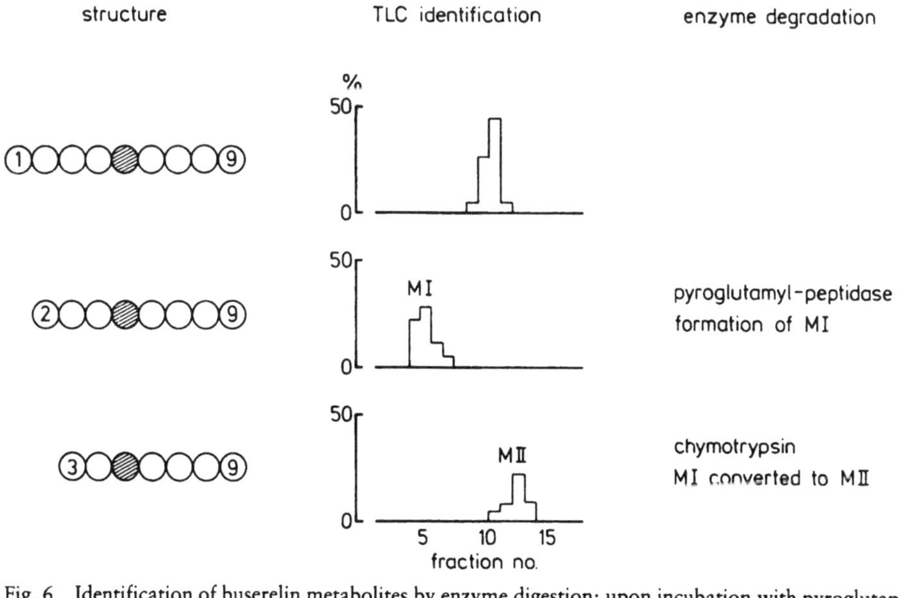

Fig. 6 Identification of buserelin metabolites by enzyme digestion: upon incubation with pyroglutamyl-peptidase, a characteristic metabolite MI is observed by thin layer chromatography (compare Figure 3). The (2–9)octapeptide (MI) is converted to the (3–9)heptapeptide MII by subsequent incubation with chymotrypsin.

vation site is protected in LH-RH-ethylamide agonists. Additional cleavage sites (Gly^6-Leu^7 bond) have been identified [13, 14]. Analysis of LH-RH degradation *in vitro* by serum, plasma or subcellular fractions using an HPLC method has been highly effective [29, 30, 31]. Synaptosomal enzymes in hypothalamus and cortex cleave LH-RH in the Trp^5-Gly^6 and Pro^9-Gly^{10} positions.

Pharmacokinetic monitoring by radioimmunoassay

Highly specific antisera recognizing LH-RH nonapeptide-ethylamide agonists but not LH-RH can be raised due to the chemical difference in C-terminal structure. We developed a radioimmunoassay for the measurement of buserelin in biological fluids and tissue extracts [41]. Rabbits were immunized by intradermal injection of buserelin conjugated to different carrier proteins [10]. The antigenic determinant of the antisera was evaluated by displacement curves of synthetic fragments of buserelin containing the C-terminal sequence Leu-Arg-Pro-ethylamide, structurally related nonapeptides substituted with different amino acids instead of D-Ser(Bu^t)^6, nonapeptides substituted with different C-terminal residues instead of Pro-ethylamide, and synthetic fragments of LH-RH. Buserelin was iodinated by the chloramine-T method, and the /mono-^{125}I-Tyr^5/buserelin fraction was used at a specific activity of about 1,000/uCi//ug. Antisera of high titre with selective specificity for buserelin, or C-terminal buserelin metabolites, were obtained. Endogenous LH-RH secretion was evaluated separately by suitable antisera. The RIA was applied to buserelin determination in serum, plasma and urine samples of clinical studies.

The estimates of immunoreactive (IR) buserelin as determined by the RIA, were controlled by bioassay for buserelin, if sufficiently high concentrations were present. In general, it was necessary to separate metabolites from intact buserelin by HPLC, to obtain an estimate for the ratio of bioactive buserelin, and inactive metabolites. Buserelin can be measured both in unextracted plasma or urine, and in extracts. For analysis of tissue extracts, the contaminating peptidase activity has to be eliminated by boiling, to avoid tracer and sample degradation during the assay. Since buserelin is inactivated rapidly *in vivo* by the liver and kidneys, the biologically active fraction in serum declines exponentially. For concentration of buserelin in samples, solvent extraction is unsatisfactory due to protein co-precipitation, whereas adsorption on silicates (e.g. silicic acid, glass powder, or octadecasilyl cartridges) provides reproducible dose-dependent recovery.

The application of the buserelin RIA to pharmacokinetic monitoring was validated by long-term infusion in rats (14 days), and longterm injection in rats (from 2 weeks to 12 months). Infusions were administered from osmotic minipumps implanted into the subcutaneous tissue, and injections were given daily s.c. in isotonic saline containing 0.1% gelatine. Unrestrained male rats were placed in metabolism cages, on steel grids, to collect the urine in fractions of 8 to 24 hours. Plasma was taken by retroorbital punction or from the jugular vein under light ether anaesthesia. In anaesthetized adult male rats, silastic catheters were implanted into the jugular vein, and heparinized blood was withdrawn continuously by a peristaltic pump.

During daily injections, there was a reproducible dose-dependent increase of the serum level of IR-buserelin, and of buserelin metabolites excreted into the urine. A serum level of 0.97 ± 0.06 ng/ml was measured 1 hour after a dose of 2.5 μg/kg s.c., whereas the urinary excretion after this dose was 123 ± 9.8 ng within 8 hours after treatment. After i.v. or s.c. injection, there was an early peak increment followed by a time-dependent decrease in urinary excretion of buserelin, with a return to nonde-

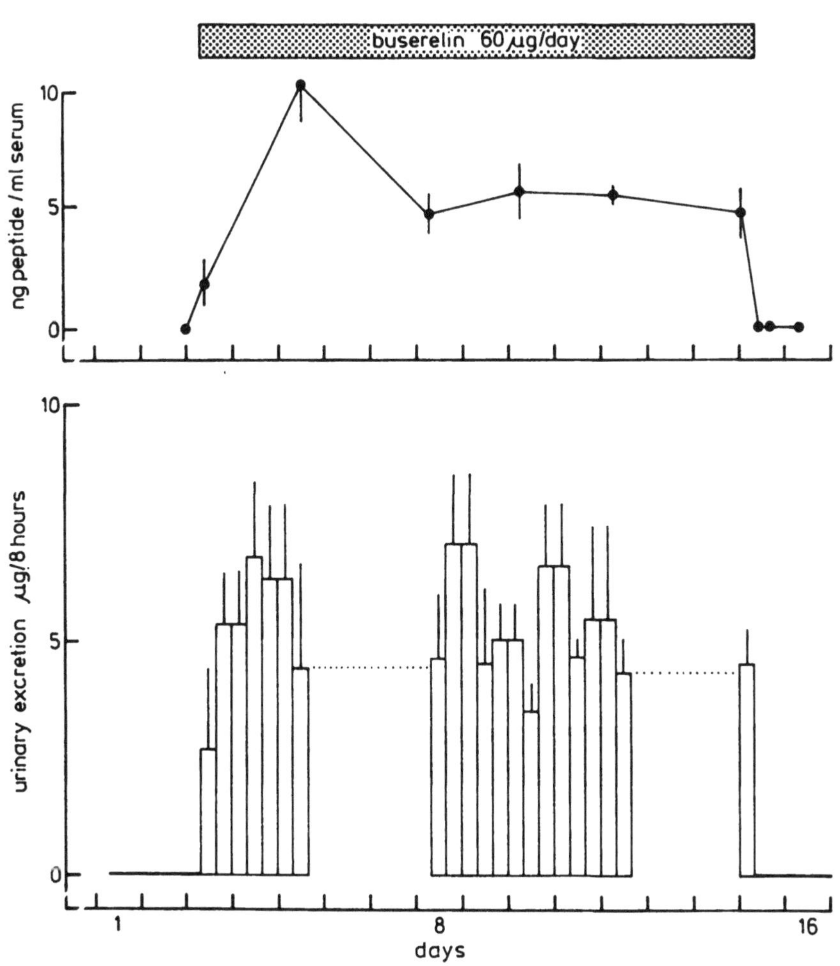

Fig. 7 Pharmacokinetic monitoring of buserelin in serum and urine: continuous infusion of buserelin 60 μg/day for 14 days in conscious unrestrained rats. Determination of buserelin by RIA (urine collected in three fractions of 8 hours/day, means and standard error of 4 rats).

tectable levels after 6–10 hours depending on the dose administered. In rats receiving a 14 days s.c. infusion from minipumps, buserelin in serum reached a stable level of 6.23 ± 1.03 ng/ml between 4 and 14 days of infusion. The urine was collected in three fractions of 8 hours per day, the average urinary excretion was 5.94 ± 0.24 µg/8 hours (fig. 7). During daily s.c. injections, the highest urinary level was found in the first 8 hours after treatment, with a subsequent decline during the second and third 8 hours' sampling period. When the total excretion of LH-RH and buserelin were compared, a striking difference was found between the total excretion of immunoreactive buserelin in urine, which averaged 30% of the daily dose of 60 µg, and the excretion of urinary LH-RH, which averaged only 0.23% at the same dose. This difference reflects the relative stability of buserelin metabolites circulating in plasma, whereas LH-RH is rapidly metabolized to peptide fragments not detected by the conventional LH-RH antisera directed against the C-terminal LH-RH sequence.

Human pharmacokinetic studies

LH-RH agonists stimulate pituitary function at low doses, but gradually lead to a loss of pituitary sensitivity (desensitization). At higher doses, the initial stimulation phase is followed by progressive inhibition of gonadotrophin secretion and gonadal steroid production. The onset and extent of the individual response to suppression may be variable. In dose-finding studies, monitoring of peptide levels in plasma and urine provides valuable information about drug absorption, and helps to define the doses required to maintain suppression under continuous release of agonist by infusion or sustained-delivery devices. In clinical trials, determination of agonist excretion is useful for the control of therapy and patient compliance.

Pharmacokinetic studies in phase I clinical trials with low doses of buserelin indicate that the urinary excretion of buserelin metabolites is a more sensitive parameter than the serum level. After an intravenous dose of 15 µg in normal test persons, the maximal urinary excretion of buserelin is measured during the first hour (total excretion 2 µg/hour), with an exponential decrease over the next 8 hours. In serum, there is only a brief increase of buserelin with a peak at 5 min., lasting for 15–20 min after intravenous injection. A similar pattern of urinary excretion is found after an intranasal dose of 400 µg (equivalent to an injection of 10 µg s.c.). There is a rapid increase of FSH and LH, sustained over more than 6 hours, while the level of buserelin in unextracted plasma remains low, barely reaching the limit of detection of 30 pg/ml serum. In contrast, the urinary excretion is significant and time-dependent. During the first sampling period (0–2 hours), total excretion is 448 ± 42 ng buserelin, followed by a progressive decrease (263 ± 21 ng during the second sampling period from 2–4 hours, and 160 ± 12 ng during the 3rd sampling period from 4–6 hours). At low doses of 10–15 µg i.v. or s.c., the pattern of metabolites in urine

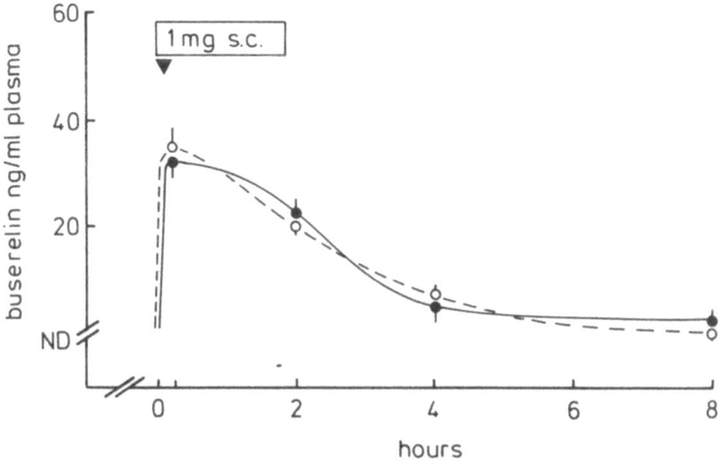

Fig. 8 Buserelin serum level in treatment of endometriosis: after s.c. injection of 1 mg, the maximum concentration is found 15 min after treatment, with a decrease to low levels after 4 hours.

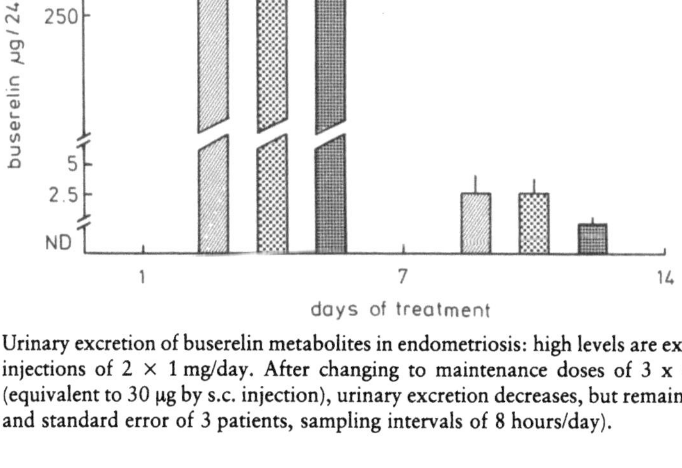

Fig. 9 Urinary excretion of buserelin metabolites in endometriosis: high levels are excreted during initial injections of 2 × 1 mg/day. After changing to maintenance doses of 3 x 400 µg nasal spray (equivalent to 30 µg by s.c. injection), urinary excretion decreases, but remains detectable (means and standard error of 3 patients, sampling intervals of 8 hours/day).

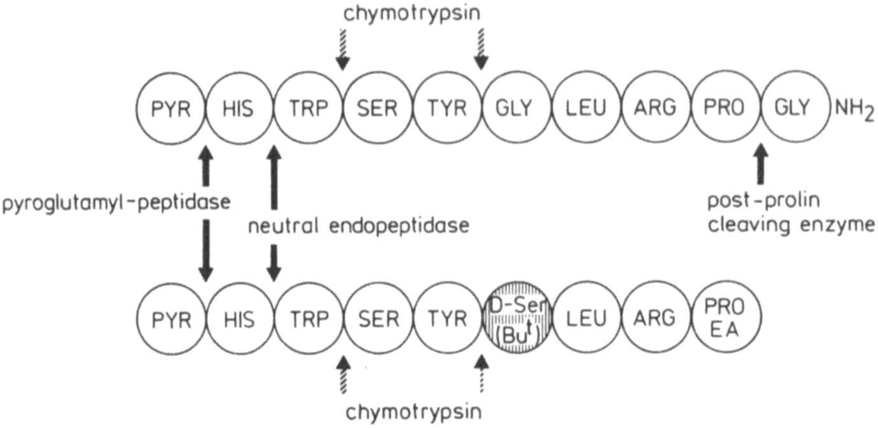

Fig. 10 Enzymes involved in degradation of LHRH and agonists: cleavage sites by pyroglutamyl-aminopeptidase, pituitary neutral endopeptidase and chymotrypsin indicated by arrows. LHRH is also inactivated by the post-prolin cleaving enzyme.

extracts analysed by HPLC and RIA is consistent with two major metabolites, which decrease time-dependently. The pattern of metabolites found in four test persons was identical.

In therapeutic studies, buserelin levels in serum and urine were monitored in patients with endometriosis and with prostate carcinoma. Treatment in endometriosis was initiated with injections of 2 x 1000 µg s.c. every 12 hours, to achieve rapid suppression of oestradiol secretion. Serum levels increased to about 35 ng/ml after 15 min and progressively declined over the next 4 hours; detectable levels persisted until 8 hours (fig. 8). In 3 patients, the pattern of urinary excretion of buserelin was highly reproducible, with a total excretion of 300–400 µg IR-buserelin within 24 hours. When these patients changed to a maintenance regimen of 3 x 400 µg nasal spray (equivalent to s.c. injections of 3 x 10 µg), urinary excretion fell to 2–2.5 µg buserelin/24 hours (fig. 9).

Summary

The biological inactivation of LH-RH and of LH-RH agonists is rapid and leads to biologically inactive metabolites. The main inactivating organs are the liver and kidney; they determine the amount of intact peptide persisting in the circulation and available to the pituitary LH-RH receptors. The anterior pituitary gland metabolises LH-RH agonists by receptor-associated enzymes, regulating duration of hormone action. The quantitative contribution of pituitary enzymes to inactivation is negligible. *In vitro*, organ homogenates of liver, kidney, hypothalamus, anterior and posterior pituitary, brain, testes and ovaries inactivate LH-RH agonists, depending on their relative enzyme stability. In rats *in vivo* 60 min after i.v. injection of 125-I-buserelin, the highest fraction of labelled metabolites is found in liver and kidney. These peptides are identified by thin layer chromatography, high performance liquid chromatography, sequential enzyme digestion with pyroglutamyl-peptidase/chymotry.psin, and binding to specific buserelin antisera. The peptides extracted from liver and kidney are C-terminal buserelin metabolites of negligible biological activity. In the anterior pituitary, a specific metabolite, MI, is identified as the buserelin (2–9) octapeptide. This metabolite is also found after *in vitro* degradation of buserelin with pituitary homogenate, anterior pituitary plasma membranes, or pyroglutamyl-aminopeptidase.

Pharmacokinetic studies with LH-RH agonists at low doses are difficult due to the analytical problems imposed by minute plasma concentrations. Classical pharmacokinetics using radioimmunoassays are not applicable, because at low doses the plasma level of buserelin does not reflect hormone action, the binding and prolonged accumulation by anterior pituitary receptors. In order to establish methods for clinical monitoring of buserelin absorption and excretion, a specific RIA was developed for buserelin in serum or plasma and urine. At low stimulatory doses, the serum level decreases rapidly, and the urinary excretion is the more practical parameter for monitoring therapy. At high suppressive doses, both the sustained serum level and the urinary excretion are suitable for dosage control, and calculation of absorption rates. Immunoreactive (IR) buserelin is dose-dependently elevated in serum and urine samples of patients treated with buserelin injections or nasal spray for endometriosis, or prostate carcinoma. The pattern of metabolites in urine in phase I dose-finding studies and during therapy was analysed by HPLC and RIA. In endometriosis, after s.c. injection of 1000 μg s.c., highest serum levels are reached after 15 min, declining exponentially. The highest urine concentration is found during the first two hours after treatment. When patients are transferred to a maintenance regimen with lower doses of nasal spray, urinary excretion remains detectable. In prostate cancer, similar dose-related findings of urinary buserelin excretion are obtained under infusion, injection or maintenance with buserelin nasal spray. It is concluded that pharmacokinetic monitoring of LH-RH agonists in serum, and in urine, is a valuable parameter for control of absorption rates and compliance in clinical studies.

References

[1] Bauer, K., B. Horsthemke, H. Knisatschek et al.: Hoppe-Seyler's Z. Physiol. Chem. **360** (1979) 229.

[2] Barron, J., R. P. Millar, I. Wegener: In "Neuropeptides: Biochemical and Physiological Studies" (Ed. R. P. Millar), pp. 207–213. Churchill Livingstone, Edinburgh 1981.

[3] Bolton, A. E.: J. Endocrinol. **63** (1974) 255–256.

[4] Bourguignon, J. P., P. Franchimont: Acta Endcrinol. **86** (1977) 15–24.
[5] Bourguignon, J. P., C. Hoyoux, A. Reuter et al.: J. Clin. Endocr. Metab. **48** (1979) 78.
[6] Carmel, P. W., S. Araki, M. Ferin: Endocrinology **99** (1976) 243.
[7] Clayton, R. N., K. J. Catt: Endocr. Reviews 2 (1981) 186–209.
[8] Clayton, R. N., R. A. Shakespear, J. A. Duncan et al.: Endocrinology **105** (1979) 1369–1376.
[9] Dupont, A., F. Labrie, G. Pelletier et al.: Neuroendocrinology **16** (1974) 65–73.
[10] Fraser, H. M., J. Sandow, B. Krauss: Acta Endocrinol. **103** (1983) 151–157.
[11] Griffiths, E. C.: Hormone Res. 7 (1976) 179–191.
[12] Griffiths, E. C., K. C. Hooper, C. R. N. Hopkinson: Acta Endocr. **74** (1973) 49–55.
[13] Hazum, E., M. Friedkin, T. Baram et al.: FEBS Lett. **123** (1981) 300.
[14] Hazum, E., M. Friedkin, T. Baram et al.: FEBS Lett. **127** (1981) 273.
[15] Horsthemke, B., K. Bauer: Biochemistry **19** (1980) 2867.
[16] Horsthemke, B., H. Knisatschek, J. Rivier et al.: Biochem. Biophys. Res. Commun. **100** (1981) 753–759.
[17] Jeffcoate, S. L., D. T. Holland: J. Endocrinol. **62** (1974) 333.
[18] Jeffcoate, S. J., D. T. Holland: Acta Endocrinol. **78** (1975) 232–238.
[19] Knisatschek, H., K. Bauer: J. Biol. Chem. **254** (1979) 10936–10943.
[20] Koch, Y., T. Baram, P. Chobsieng et al.: Biochem. Biophys. Res. Commun. **61** (1974) 95–102.
[21] Koch, Y., T. Baram, E. Hazum et al.: Biochem. Biophys. Res. Commun. **74** (1977) 488–491.
[22] Kochmann, K., B. Kerdelhue, U. Zor et al.: FEBS Lett. **50** (1975) 190–194.
[23] Leblanc, P., E. Pattou, A. L'Heritier et al.: Biochem. Biophys. Res. Commun. **96** (1980) 1457–1465.
[24] Loumaye, E., Z. Naor, K. J. Catt: Endocrinology **111** (1982) 730–736.
[25] Marks, N.: In "Peptides in Neurobiology" (Ed. H. Gainer) pp. 221–238. Plenum Press, New York 1977.
[26] Marks, N., F. Stern: Biochem. Biophys. Res. Commun. **61** (1974) 1458–1463.
[27] Matsuo, H., Y. Baba, R. C. M. Nair et al.: Biochem. Biophys. Res. Commun. **43** (1971) 1334–1339.
[28] Mayar, M. Q., G. K. Tarnavsky, J. J. Reeves: Proc. Soc. Exp. Biol. Med. **161** (1979) 216–219.
[29] McDermott, J. R., A. I. Smith, J. A. Biggins et al.: Regulatory Peptides **2** (1981) 69.
[30] McDermott, J. R., A. I. Smith, J. A. Biggins et al.: Regulatory peptides **3** (1982) 257–269.
[31] McDermott, J. R., A. I. Smith, P. R. Dodd et al.: Peptides **4** (1983) 25–30.
[32] Mudge, A. W., R. E. Fellows: Endocrinology **93** (1973) 1428–1434.
[33] Pimstone, B., S. Epstein, S. M. Hamilton et al.: J. Clin. Endocr. Metab. **44** (1977) 356–360.
[34] Redding, T. W., A. V. Schally: Life Sci. **12** (1973) 23–32.
[35] Redding, T. W., A. J. Kastin, D. Gonzales-Barcena et al.: J. Clin. Endocr. Metab. **37** (1973) 626–631.
[36] Reeves, J. J., G. K. Tarnavsky, S. R. Becker et al.: Endocrinology **101** (1977) 540.
[37] Sandow, J.: In "Basic Applications and Clinical Uses of Hypothalamic Hormones", pp. 113–123. Excerpta Medica, Amsterdam 1975.
[38] Sandow, J., W. König: J. Endocrinol. **81** (1979) 175–182.
[39] Sandow, J., R. N. Clayton: In "Hormone Biochemistry and Pharmacology", Vol. 2 (Eds. M. Briggs, A. Corbin), pp. 63–106. Eden Press, Montreal 1983.
[40] Sandow, J., W. Heptner, H. G. Vogel: In "Hypothalamic Hypophysiotropic Hormones: Physiological and Clinical Studies" (Eds. C. Gual, E. M. Rosenberg), pp. 64–67. Excerpta Medica, Amsterdam 1973.
[41] Sandow, J., W. von Rechenberg, W. König et al.: In "Hypothalamic Hormones: Chemistry, Physiology and Clinical Applications" (Eds. D. Gupta, W. Voelter) pp. 307–325. Verlag Chemie, Weinheim 1978.
[42] Sandow, J., H. Kuhl, B. Krauss: J. Endocrinol. **81** (1979) 157P–158P.

[43] Sandow, J., G. Jerabek-Sandow, B. Krauss et al.: In "LH-RH Peptides as Female and Male Contraceptives, PARFR Series on Fertility Regulation" (Eds. G. I. Zatuchni, J. D. Shelton, J. J. Sciarra), pp. 338–354. Harper & Row, Philadelphia 1981.
[44] Sandow, J., W. v. Rechenberg, G. Jerabek-Sandow et al.: Arch Pharmacol. Suppl. 319 R-54, Abstract No. 14 (1982).
[45] Schally, A. V., A. J. Kastin, A. Arimura: Vitamins and hormones **30** (1972) 83–164.
[46] Stetler-Stevenson, M. A., D. C. Yang, A. Lipkowski et al.: J. Med. Chem. **24** (1981) 688.
[47] Swift, A. D., D. B. Crighton: J. Endocrinol. **80** (1979) 141–152.
[48] Szewczuk, A., J. Kwiatkowska: Eur. J. Biochem. **15** (1970) 92–96.
[49] Tharandt, L., H. Schulte, G. Benger et al.: Horm. Metab. Res. **11** (1979) 391.
[50] Yamazaki, I., H. Okada: Endocr. Jap. **27** (1980) 593.

Studies on controlled release systems for LH-RH analogues

B. H. Vickery, L. M. Sanders

Introduction

More than a decade ago, knowledge of the key role that luteinizing hormone releasing hormone (LH-RH) plays in the reproductive cascade was used to forecast that it would become the treatment of choice for primary infertility and that competitive antagonists would be synthesized that would become a new generation of contraceptives useful in both men and women [1]. In the intervening time it has become apparent that potent LH-RH agonists, by virtue of receptor down-regulation and thus deprivation of the gonads from their source of gonadotropins, can interrupt both gametogenesis and steroidogenesis. LH-RH analogues, whether agonistic or antagonistic, are therefore now expected to have a wide variety of applications. They are under evaluation for utilities as diverse as male and female contraception; therapy for endometriosis, metastatic mammary and prostatic carcinoma; regression of precocious puberty and adjunctive treatment in growth hormone replacement; and protection of the gonads from the cytotoxicity due to cancer chemotherapeutic agents.

LH-RH analogues have very little oral activity, requiring 400–10 000 x the dose by this route as by injection [2, 3]. However, while for acute diagnostic or challenge purposes an injection is acceptable, daily chronic treatment by this route would be poorly tolerated and result in low compliance in other than life threatening situations. Non-invasive parenteral routes of administration such as nasal insufflation and vaginal tablets have been explored but presently again require daily or more frequent placement and, at up to only 5% relative bioavailability, require considerably greater amounts of compound than does the injectable route.

An attractive alternative would be the development of biocompatible, controlled release formulations which could be injectable, implantable or even with proper design and structural integrity, be placed intravaginally. There exists substantial literature on the preparation and utility of such formulations with lipophilic drugs, particularly steroids [4]. However, in the main, water-soluble materials such as peptides are insufficiently soluble in or permeable through the traditional silicone elastomer or other similar carrier polymers to allow formulation of simple diffusion-controlled or membrane-limited devices. There is, however, an emerging literature on other approaches to controlled release of water-soluble materials of higher molecular weight. This includes the use of hydrogels which are permeable to hydrophilic compounds such as narcotic antagonists [5], and polymeric matrices with peptides or proteins, for example insulin incorporated in an ethylene-vinyl acetate matrix [6].

With this background, then, we began to explore controlled release formulations of LH-RH analogues. Early studies evaluated the possibility of using sparingly soluble salts and complexes emulsified into stabilized thixotropic gels [7]. Although durations of release of [D-Trp^6, Pro^9-NHEt]LH-RH, evaluated by bioassay, could be extended to means of 124 days following single injection of such formulations, the range from animal to animal was unacceptably great. The more classical implant systems of fixed geometry such as compacted cholesterol pellets with incorporated LH-RH analogues gave more acceptable delivery efficiencies and more tolerable range of duration of biological efficacy. Although the impracticability of reproducible mass fabrication of such devices, together with non-linear release kinetics, proved insurmountable problems, such devices were an extremely useful experimental tool [8–15]. The results of such studies, together with those using sustained administration from implantable osmotic pumps (Alzet® minipumps), have suggested that qualitatively different effects may accrue from continuous administration versus intermittent or pulsatile administration of LH-RH agonist analogues [16–18].

Our more recent work has concentrated on the development of shorter term 30–90 day bioerodable systems and on longer term systems with life expectancies of 1 year or more, both designed to deliver nafarelin acetate ([D-Nal(2)^6]LH-RH; RS-94991).

There are a number of prerequisites for preparation of a controlled release implantable or injectable system. Firstly, the compound should be sufficiently potent that when the quantity necessary for efficacy over the required duration is incorporated into the dosage form, the total mass is of acceptable size. Secondly, the compound should be stable both under the conditions of device fabrication and in the *in vivo* environment in which it will dwell for an extended length of time. The loading level, the solubility and the diffusivity of the compound in the chosen carrier material must be compatible with the required release mechanism and kinetics. Finally, it is a clear advantage if the compound has a high therapeutic ratio, since this will not only preclude any concern for the potential for 'dose dumping' on administration of the material, but makes the requirement for linear or 'zero order' compound release less critical.

Bioerodable injectable systems

Naferelin acetate is an agonist analogue of LH-RH whose potency is 200 x the native hormone in rats [19] and possibly greater in other species, including man. Therapeutic doses for daily administration are in the microgram range so that it becomes feasible to incorporate the compound into bioerodable systems at relatively low loading levels with release rate then governed by the erosion rate of the polymer.

Manufacture

Accordingly, nafarelin acetate has been microencapsulated at a level of 1% into microspheres of poly (d, 1 lactide-co-glycolide). PLGA, by a phase separation or coacervation process [20], as shown in figure 1. An aqueous solution of nafarelin acetate is co-emulsified by high-speed stirring with an organic solution of PLGA, to form a water-in-oil emulsion. A non-solvent for the polymer is then added, causing the PLGA to precipitate out around the aqueous droplets. The resulting suspension of semi-formed microspheres is then run into a larger volume of non-solvent to harden and complete their formation. They are then washed, screened and dried.

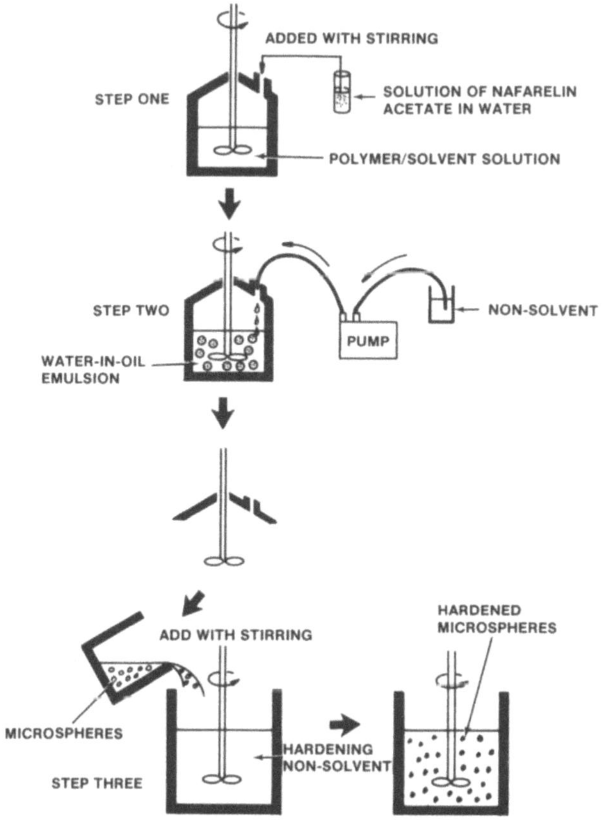

Fig. 1 Flow diagram of phase-separation microencapsulation process for nafarelin acetate in PLGA (from [20] with permission).

The resulting microspheres are homogeneous, range in size from 20 to 50 μ in diameter (fig. 2) and after suspension in an appropriate vehicle may be injected via an 18 gauge needle. The vehicle commonly used is aqueous and contains 0.1% surfactant (Tween 80), 0.5% of a viscosity enhancer (carboxymethylcellulose) and sodium chloride as isotonicifier.

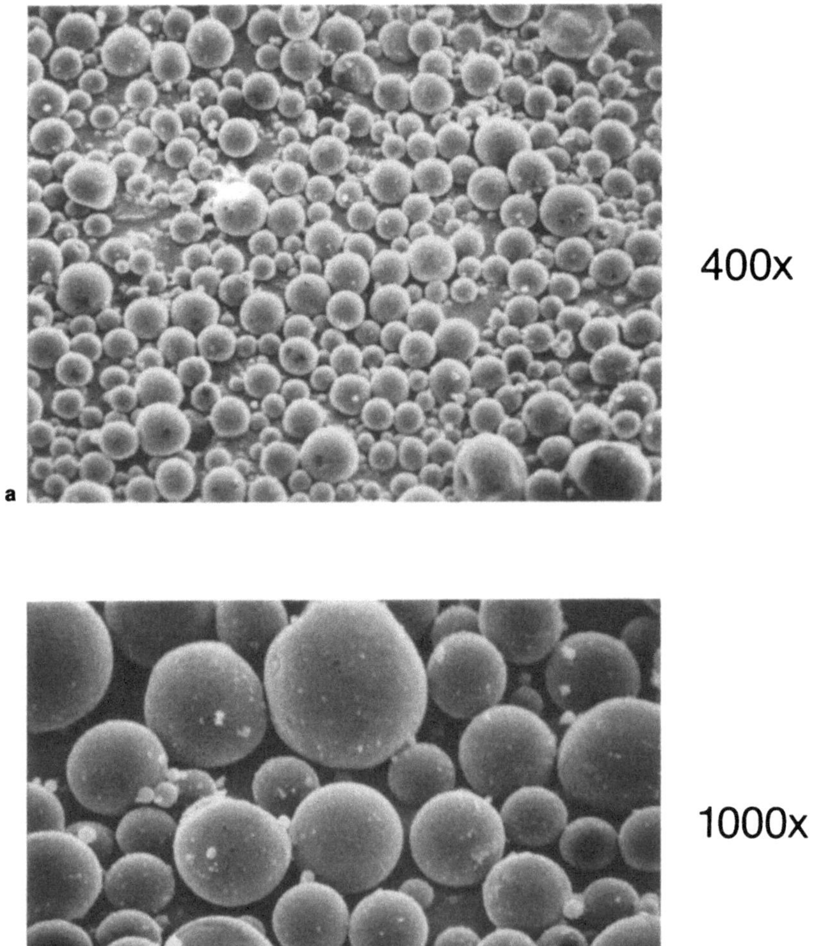

Fig. 2 Scanning electron micrographs of microspheres of 50:50 PLGA containing 1% nafarelin acetate a) x 400; b) x 1000.

Bioassay

A convenient bioassay with which to assess the performance of such loaded microspheres is the effect on vaginal cytology in cycling female rats. Suppression of the pituitary-gonadal axis is indicated by the occurrence of persistent vaginal diestrus. Unfortunately nafarelin acetate is not sufficiently stable in the blood of rats to allow quantitation of blood levels of compound. However, it has been determined that continuous estrus suppression will result from a daily dose of 0.4 μg or more of nafarelin acetate delivered on a continuous basis from a subcutaneously implanted minipump. Thus, persistent diestrus resulting from administration of microspheres indicates delivery of at least 0.4 μg per day of nafarelin acetate. It has also been demonstrated that after removal of an adequately dispensing minipump, the rats will return to synchronized estrus 4–5 days later, a timing consistent with little carryover effect of dosing and with the 4–5 day length of the rat estrous cycle. Doses lower than 0.4 μg per day interfere with the regularity of cycling. Thus the interval to the return of regular estrous cycles, less 4–5 days, gives an indication of the duration of release of nafarelin acetate from a given formulation.

This estrus suppression assay has been used to evaluate the impact of varying the monomer ratio (lactic:glycolic monomer units) in the polymer and also of molecular weight (measured as inherent viscosity) of polymer on the release of nafarelin acetate. It was found that the duration of release was markedly affected by changes in monomer ratio (fig. 3) but less affected by inherent polymer viscosity or dose within the ranges of these parameters studied [20].

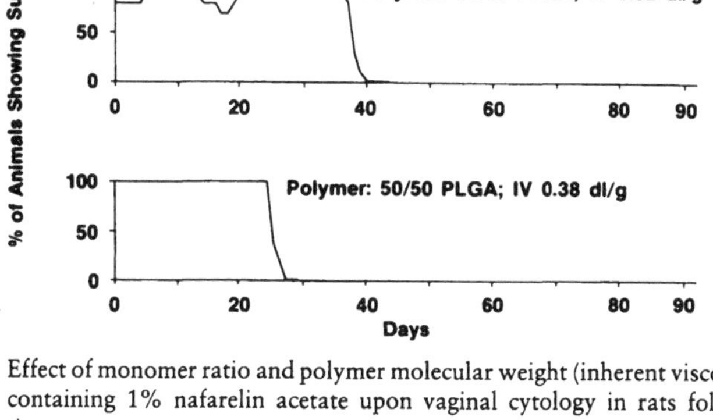

Fig. 3 Effect of monomer ratio and polymer molecular weight (inherent viscosity) of PLGA microspheres containing 1% nafarelin acetate upon vaginal cytology in rats following subcutaneous injection.

The changes in monomer ratio affect not only duration of release but also the release profile. The profile can be monitored by assay of compound remaining at the site of injection [21] and if great enough, by biological effect (fig. 3). The data so far are compatible with a triphasic release profile. An early high release rate is probably due to relatively rapid leaching of compound from the surface of the microspheres. The second phase is of low release rate and occurs while the polymer is hydrating and decreasing in molecular weight but still remaining insoluble in biological fluids. When the molecular weight decreases sufficiently, fragments of the polymer become water soluble and the contained compound is then released at a higher rate as the polymer dissolves. The kinetics of degradation are controlled by factors such as the monomer unit ratio and the degree of crystallinity of the polymer. The molecular weight of the polymer determines the extent of hydrolysis necessary to render a significant fraction of the polymer water soluble. The duration of the second phase is affected by these factors and may be undetectably short, as is the case for a 55:45 PLGA ratio. The fact that the release of compound is subservient to polymer erosion as opposed to simple diffusion is well illustrated by the narrow range of distribution routinely observed in the time of return to normal estrous cyclicity in individual rats.

For ultimate use the microspheres have to be sterile. The sterilization method of choice is γ irradiation in the final container. The disadvantage to this technique is that exposure to sterilizing doses of γ irradiation brings about a decrease in molecular weight by random chain scission [22] as evidenced by a decrease in intrinsic viscosity of the polymer. This affects the duration of efficacy in a manner predictable by the described release mechanism (fig. 4).

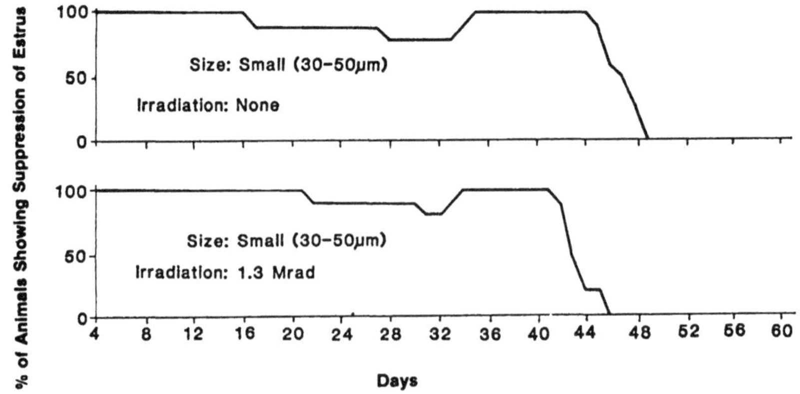

Fig. 4 Effect of 1.25 Mrad of γ irradiation of 50:50 PLGA microspheres containing 1% nafarelin acetate on vaginal cytology in rats following subcutaneous injection.

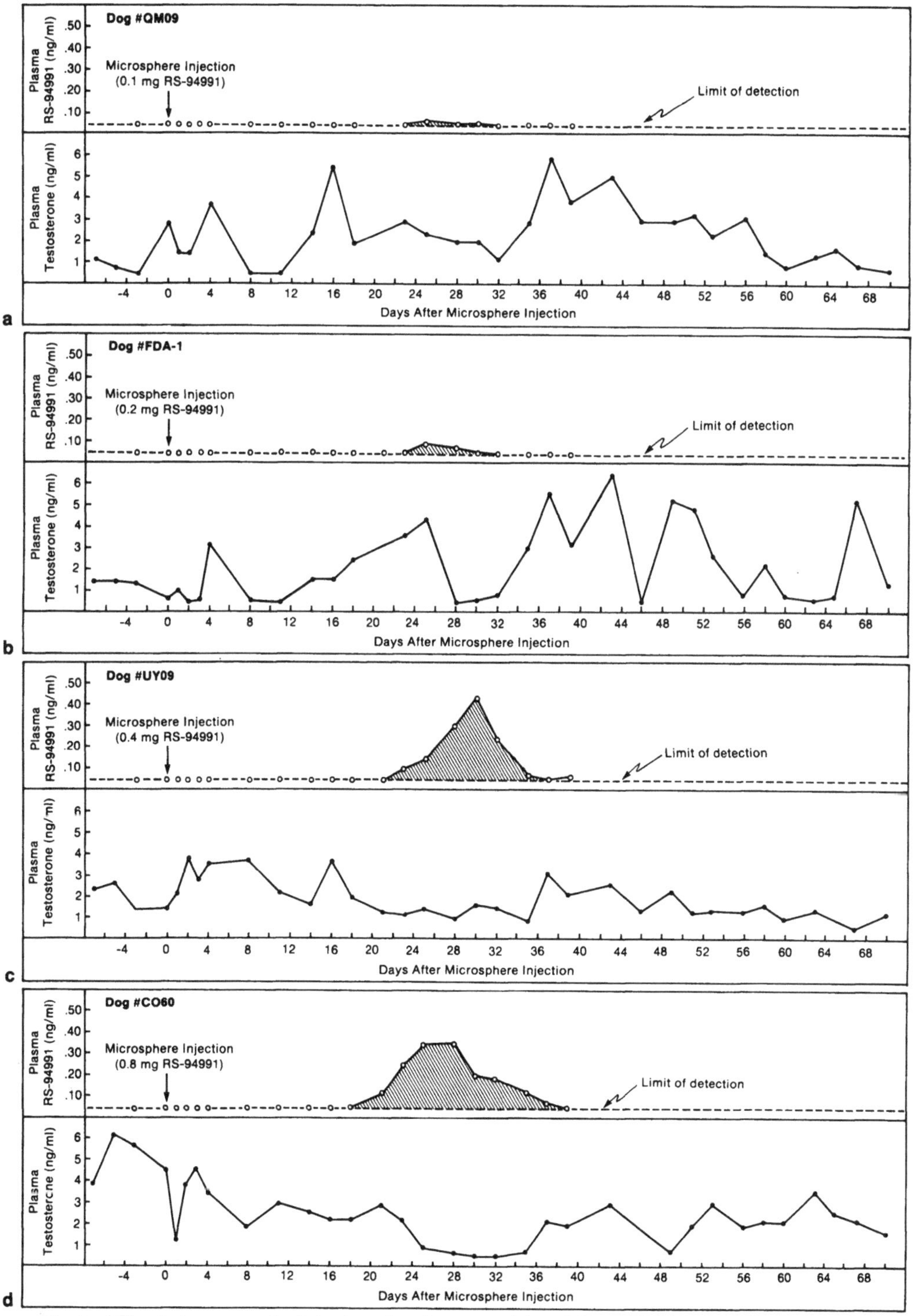

Fig. 5 Effect in intramuscular injection of various quantities of 50:50 PLGA microspheres containing 1% nafarelin acetate (RS-94991) upon circulating levels of nafarelin acetate and testosterone in male beagle dogs. Panels depict injection of a) 10; b) 20; c) 40; d) 80 mg of polymer.

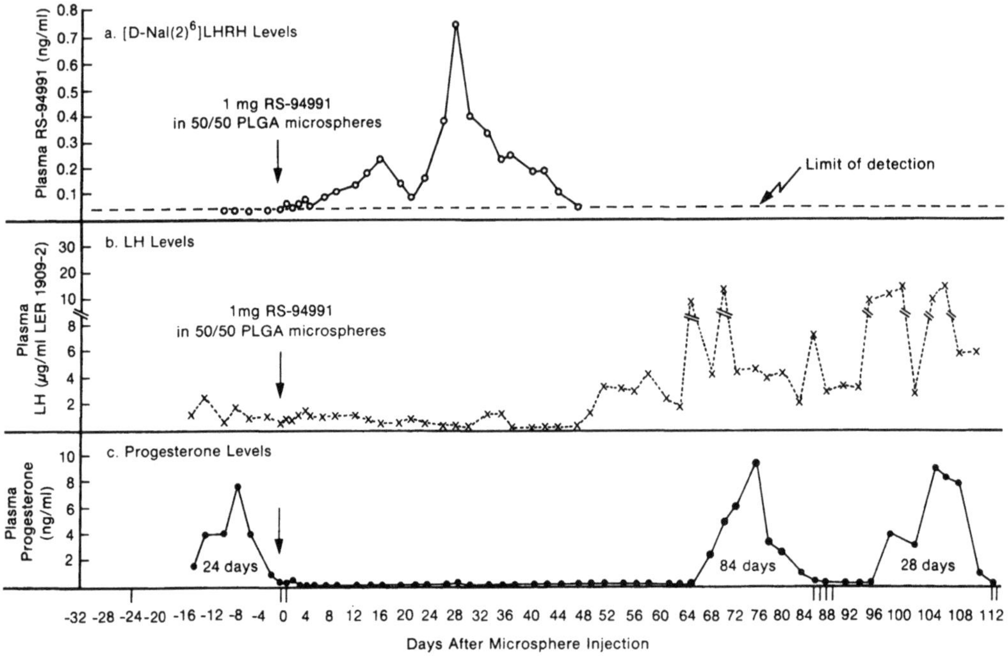

Fig. 6 Effect of intramuscular injection of 1 mg of nafarelin acetate ([D-Nal (2) [6]LHRH; RS-94991) incorporated in microspheres of 50:50 PLGA (100 mg) upon circulating levels of a) nafarelin acetate; b) luteinizing hormone (LH); c) progesterone, in a female rhesus monkey.

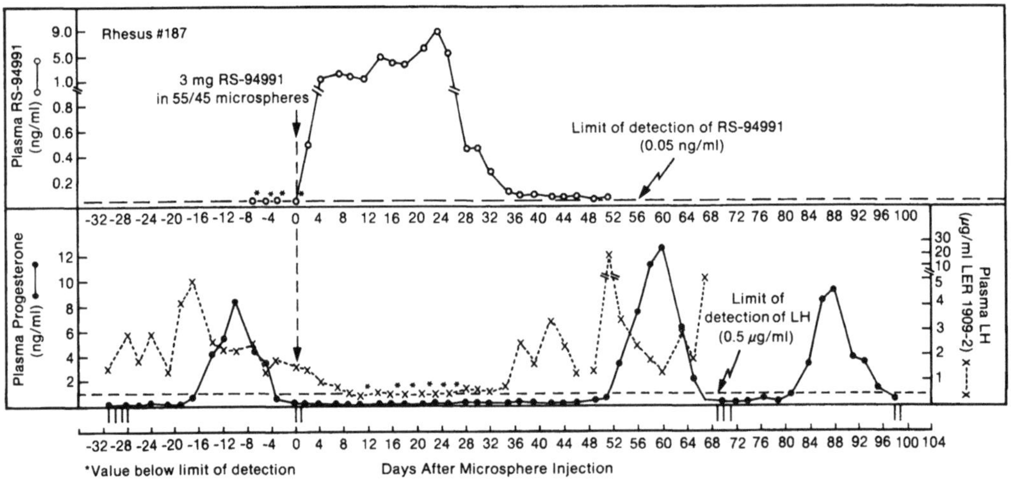

Fig. 7 Effect of intramuscular injection of 3 mg of nafarelin acetate (RS-94991) incorporated in microspheres of 55:45 PLGA (300 mg) upon circulating levels of nafarelin acetate (upper panel) and luteinizing hormone (LH) and progesterone (lower panel) in a female rhesus monkey.

Release rate studies and effects in larger animals

As mentioned earlier, nafarelin acetate is unstable in the plasma of rats and therefore it is not possible to correlate plasma levels of compound with biological effect. For these correlations it has been necessary to extend the studies to other species, such as the dog and monkey, in the plasma of which the compound is stable.

Dose response studies have been conducted in male dogs with a 50:50 PLGA ratio polymer. In these studies the primary phase of nafarelin release was not detected, either by circulating levels of nafarelin or by effect on circulating levels of testosterone using sensitive and specific radioimmunoassays. However, in the tertiary phase, there was good correlation between detectable levels of nafarelin and a decline in testosterone values (fig. 5).

Similar studies have been conducted in female rhesus macaques. Injection of 1 mg or more of nafarelin acetate in a 50:50 PLGA microsphere formulation extended the intermenstrual interval by a predictable 50 days due to inhibition of ovulation. Assay of circulating levels of nafarelin acetate showed two peaks of compound, again compatible with a triphasic release profile (fig. 6). There was a remarkably good correlation between detectable amounts of circulating nafarelin acetate and lowered levels of circulating LH. LH levels returned into the normal range following disappearance of nafarelin from the blood and the normal events of the menstrual cycle were rapidly entrained.

Injection of 3 mg nafarelin acetate incorporated into 55:45 PLGA microspheres gave a different release profile (fig. 7). Circulating nafarelin levels rapidly rose to ten-fold higher values than for 50:50 microspheres and were maintained high for the duration of release. The tendency for a correlated decline in plasma levels of LH noted for the 50:50 formulation was dramatic for the 55:45 formulation, with LH levels being at or below limits of detection of the assay for 24 days. The continued presence of high circulating levels of nafarelin acetate thus causes qualitative differences in effect from that achievable with daily, high dose injection which merely abolishes the LH surge [17]. The greater suppressive effect of controlled release of LH-RH analogues may have profound implications for the treatment of gonadal hormone sensitive syndromes.

Bioerodable implantable systems

In certain situations, it might be advantageous to be able to terminate administration of compound from such a controlled release formulation. This of course would not be possible following injection of microspheres. However, retrieval of a solid implant, even of bioerodable materials, would be possible for at least part of the life of the formulation. For this reason we have evaluated the use of monolithic implantable preparations of PLGA containing nafarelin acetate.

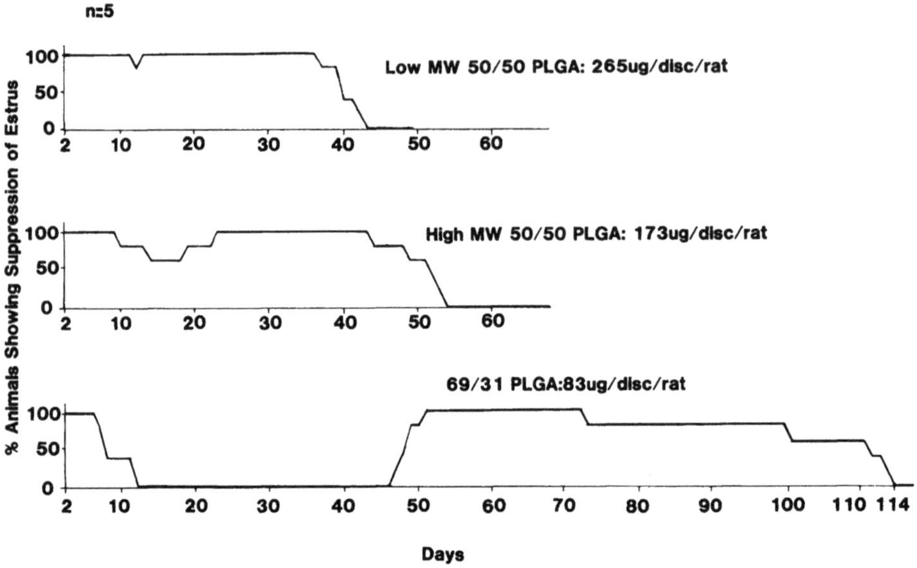

Fig. 8 Effect of subcutaneous implantation of discs of varying molecular weight and monomer ratio PLGA containing nafarelin acetate upon vaginal cytology in female rats. All discs were of equal size (0.3×6.3 mm). Upper panel shows the effect of 50:50 low molecular weight (inherent viscosity = 0.38 dl/g) acetate. Middle panel shows the effect of high molecular weight (inherent viscosity = 1.52 dl/g) 50:50 PLGA discs containing 173 μg of nafarelin acetate. Lower panel shows the effect of 69:31 PLGA discs (inherent viscosity = 0.97 dl/g) containing 83 μg of nafarelin acetate.

Manufacture

In initial studies 1% compound was melt blended with 50:50 PLGA. The formulation was then melt compressed to a flat sheet from which discs, measuring 0.6 x 6.3 mm, were punched out. When assayed for effects on estrous cyclicity following subcutaneous implantation into female rats it was noted that the duration of action was extended, although release profiles were qualitatively similar when compared to microspheres of the same polymer composition (fig. 8). Following this demonstration of feasiblity, a more practical method of manufacture was developed. The method of choice at present is melt extrusion or mold injection of the PLGA-nafarelin blend in the shape of a rod.

Bioassay

The rat estrus suppression assay has been used to evaluate the effects of manipulation of a) the ratios of lactide:glycolide, b) the molecular weight of the polymer and c) the loading level of the drug. The implants appear to have a similar triphasic release profile as do the microspheres. However, by appropriate adjustment of the critical parameters of the polymer, the secondary phase can be minimized to a point undetectable *in vivo* (fig. 9) and the duration of the tertiary phase can be extended to many months.

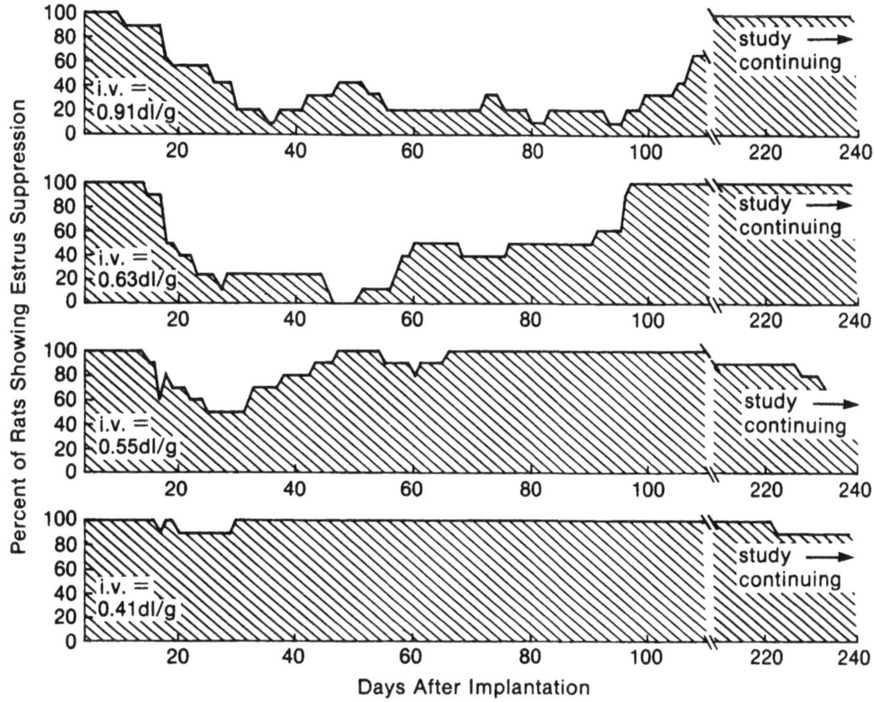

Fig. 9 Effect of subcutaneous implantation of rods of 90:10 PLGA of varying molecular weight (inherent viscosity) containing 3 mg of nafarelin acetate upon vaginal cytology in rats. Each rat received on rod measuring 3.2×6.4 mm.

Concluding remarks

The high potency and therapeutic ratio of LH-RH analogues, together with their chemical and physical properties, well suit them for incorporation into these erosion-controlled systems. The capacity for adjustment of duration and kinetics of compound release by adjustment of the nature of the polymer makes these systems very versatile, and of broad potential applicability. Indeed, the development of systems such as those described may be a critical factor in the overall development of LH-RH analoques for therapeutic and other indications.

Acknowledgements

Our thanks to Karen Vitale and Brian Kell for preparation of the controlled release formulations, to Georgia McRae, Anne Worden, Bryan Roberts and David Donahue for the biological studies, to Agnes Bajka, William Briones and Dorothy Tallentire for radioimmunoassay of steroids and gonadotropins and to Clinton Nerenberg and JoAnn Foreman for radioimmunoassay of nafarelin acetate.

References

[1] Schally, A. V., A. J. Kastin: Drug Ther. **1** (1971) 29–32.
[2] Saito, M., T. Kumasaki, Y. Yaoi et al.: Fertil. Steril. **28** (1977) 240–245.
[3] Nekola, M. V., A. Horvath, L-J. Ge et al.: Science **218** (1982) 160–162.
[4] Roseman, T. J.: In "Controlled Release of Biologically Active Agents" (Eds. A. C. Tanquary, R. E. Lacey), pp. 99–115. Plenum Press, New York 1974.
[5] Abrahams, R. A., S. H. Ronel: J. Biomed. Mater. Res. **9** (1975) 355–366.
[6] Creque, H. M., R. Langer, J. Folkman: Diabetes **29** (1980) 37–40.
[7] Vickery, B. H., G. I. McRae, L. M. Sanders et al.: In "Long Acting Contraceptive Delivery Systems" (Eds. G. I. Zatuchni, J. D. Shelton, J. J. Sciarra). Harper & Row, Philadelphia 1984 (in press).
[8] Vickery, B. H., G. I. McRae: J. Reprod. Fert. **60** (1980) 399–402.
[9] Herschler, R. C., B. H. Vickery: Am. J. Vet. Res. **42** (1981) 1405–1408.
[10] Vickery, B. H., G. I. McRae: Int. J. Fertil. **25** (1980) 171–178.
[11] Vickery, B. H., G. I. McRae: Int. J. Fertil **25** (1980) 179–184.
[12] Vickery, B. H., G. I. McRae: Life Sci. **27** (1980) 1409–1415.
[13] Vickery, B., G. I. McRae, J. Rowland: 6th Int. Congr. Endocrinol, Melbourne, Australia, February 1980.
[14] Vickery, B. H., G. I. McRae, H. Bonasch: The Prostate **3** (1983) 123–130.
[15] Vickery, B. H., G. I. McRae, V. C. Stevens: Fertil. Steril. **36** (1981) 664–668.
[16] Vickery, B. H.: In "LH-RH Peptides as Female and Male Contraceptives" (Eds. G. I. Zatuchni, J. D. Shelton, J. J. Sciarra), pp. 109–125. Harper & Row, Philadelphia 1981.
[17] Vickery, B. H., G. I. McRae, D. Tallentire: Fertil. Steril. **39** (1983) 417.
[18] Bint Akhtar, F., G. R. Marshall, E. J. Wickings et al.: J. Clin. Endocrinol. Metab. **56** (1983) 534–540.
[19] Nestor, J. J. Jr., T. L. Ho, R. A. Simpson et al.: J. Med. Chem. **25** (1982) 795–801.
[20] Kent, J. S., L. M. Sanders, T. R. Tice et al.: In "Long Acting Contraceptive Delivery Systems" (Eds. G. I. Zatuchni, J. D. Shelton, J. J. Sciarra). Harper & Row, Philadelphia 1984 (in press).
[21] Sanders, L. M., J. S. Kent, G. I. McRae et al.: Contr. Del. Systems. **3** (1982) 60.
[22] Sanders, L. M., J. S. Kent, G. I. McRae et al.: J. Pharm. Sci. (1984) in press.

Comparative reproductive pharmacology of LH-RH agonist and antagonist: contraceptive, therapeutic and safety aspects

A. Corbin, F. J. Bex, R. C. Jones

Introduction

The significant advances regarding the reproductive development of the LH-RH peptides have yielded a novel pharmacologic approach to the control of fertility and the therapy of steroid-dependent disorders of the reproductive tract.

The synthesis and preliminary biologic evaluation of over 1600 LH-RH analogues have resulted in the availability of numerous selected agonists and antagonists that are undergoing extensive pre-clinical, safety and clinical evaluation [26, 34, 38, 39].

The early availability of highly potent LH-RH agonists ("super" agonists) resulting from a few but critical modifications of the LH-RH molecule has produced a burgeoning literature on the reproductive properties and mechanisms of action of this chemical subclass, in both sexes, of several animal species, including man.

In contrast, the LH-RH antagonists paced behind the agonists, since major structural modifications of the LH-RH molecule were required to yield congeners that possessed sufficient potency to enable their detailed and extensive biologic characterization [3].

The primary profertility (conceptive) and paradoxical antifertility (contraceptive) properties of LH-RH and agonists have been welldocumented [3, 5, 26, 34, 38, 50]. It suffices to state that the agonists produce their initial antireproductive effects in both females and males via inappropriate, acute hyperactivation of pituitary gonadotropin/gonadal steroid secretion. Continuous or repeated administration in a non-pulsatile fashion and at non-"physiologic" doses ultimately leads to inhibition of the pituitary-gonadal-target organ axis. The spectrum of events results in gonadal gonadotropin receptor down-regulation, pituitary LH-RH receptor down-regulation, desensitization of pituitarygonadal function, reduced gonadotropin secretion, impeded steroidogenesis and gametogenesis, and consequent retardation of target organ function. Such effects are fully reversible with rapid return to normal fertility patterns upon cessation of treatment. Additionally, the agonists may act directly on extrapituitary reproductive end organs (e.g. gonad, uterus, ventral prostate) thereby contributing to the syndrome of reproductive abeyance; this event occurs most notably in the rat, whereas in other species (e.g. monkey, man), the existence of this phenomenon is questionable [21, 22].

On the other hand, the LH-RH antagonists appear to inhibit, at the onset, reproductive function simply by competitively blocking pituitary LH-RH receptors, thereby eliminating access of endogenous LH-RH or exogenously administered agonists to their requisite recognition sites. Consequently, pituitary LH and FSH secretion is inhibited with subsequent ovulatory and spermatogenic blockade and reduced steroid output. While, at least in the rat, LH-RH antagonists do bind to gonadal LH-RH receptors, they produce no biologic event at this level per se; however, they can once again interfere with the direct gonadal, extrapituitary effects of LH-RH agonists in a competitive manner [2, 3, 37].

Thus, from the array of antifertility (contraceptive) effects visualized in both males and in cycling and pregnant female laboratory species, it was realized that such effects could be translated into the therapeutic management of gonadal steroid-dependent disorders of the reproductive tract (e.g. endometriosis, breast and prostatic cancer). However, it was thought that, because the LH-RH agonists produce an initial gonadal (steroidal) stimulatory effect (thereby bearing the potential for an acute exacerbation of the disease state) prior to the desired therapeutic effects, the antagonists might be the agents of choice; this would be based on the antagonist's ability immediately to produce a unidirectional antireproductive effect with no attendant initial stimulatory phase. This premise is based on the supposition that the antagonist possesses an activity and potency equivalent to those documented for the agonists.

This report will relate our laboratory experiences with a highly potent LH-RH agonist and antagonist in terms of their comparative contraceptive and therapeutic utility, and safety.

The major compounds employed in the comparative studies carried out in female and male rats are:

Agonist: Wy-40,972 (Lutrelin) D-Trp^{6}-N$^{\alpha}$MeLeu^{7}-DesGly^{10}-Pro^{9}-NHEt-LH-RH.

Antagonist: Wy-45,760 (obtained from the Salk Institute) [Ac-βDNAL(2)^{1},4FD-Phe^{2},D-Trp^{3},D-Arg^{6}]-LH-RH (NAL-ARG Antagonist) [32a].

Contraceptive evaluation

Ovulation induction/ovulation inhibition in rat

Earlier studies [6–8, 12] established the fact that the LH-releasing and ovulation-inducing activity and potency of the LH-RH agonists were predictive of their pregnancy-terminating and estrouscycle-disrupting properties. Thus, this primary profertility screen served as an activity and dose marker for the paradoxical antifertility effects that eventually were to be observed in both female and male animal models. In the primary screen for agonist activity the spontaneous ovulatory LH surge is prevented with nembutal on the afternoon of proestrus; the test material is then administered by a variety of routes; blood samples are withdrawn at appropriate times and oviductal ova are sought the following morning (estrus).

The primary screen for an antagonist is the inhibition of ovulation in the unanesthetized cyclic proestrous rat. Once effective ovulatory and antiovulatory doses are determined for each analog class, respectively, more detailed evaluation can proceed. Table 1 lists the doses of Wy-40,972 and Wy-45,760 that are 100% active in their respective primary screens. While both compounds are equipotent administered subcutaneously (SC), the agonist is considerably more potent than the antagonist [32a] when delivered either intranasally (IN) or orally (PO) (figs. 1 and 2). In crossover studies, in which each representative compound is tested in the opposite screen, no activity could be detected at doses in considerable excess of those active in the relevant homologous test (tab. 1).

Studies were carried out in cyclic rats to determine the duration of activity of either analog administered subcutaneously. Since the agonist is capable of causing LH release on each day of the cycle and of inducing ovulation in 100% of recipients on each day of the cycle at the same dose (except estrus) (fig. 3), serum LH levels were employed to monitor the chronology of the event during the period of time encompassing the natural LH surge (i.e. afternoon of proestrus). The data in figure 4 demonstrate the very large LH surge induced by Wy-40,972 during proestrus, in considerable excess of that produced by exogenous LH-RH or during the spontaneous event. Additionally, the peak LH rise produced by Wy-40,972 was advanced by 3 hours compared to the control surge values. Serum LH levels still were significantly elevated even at approximately 9 hours post-Wy-40,972 administration.

With regard to Wy-45,760, SC administration of the antagonist can prevent ovulation on individual days of the estrous cycle, except estrus (fig. 5). The greatest potency (i.e. lowest dose required for 100% ovulatory blockade) was detected on proestrus (0.50 µg/rat); in contrast, diestrus 1 and 2 required 50 and 10 µg/rat, respectively, whereas 100 µg/rat on estrus had no effect. Thus, the antagonist can prevent ovulation when given approximately 50 hours in advance of the ovulatory LH surge but higher doses are required, perhaps reflecting time-related binding

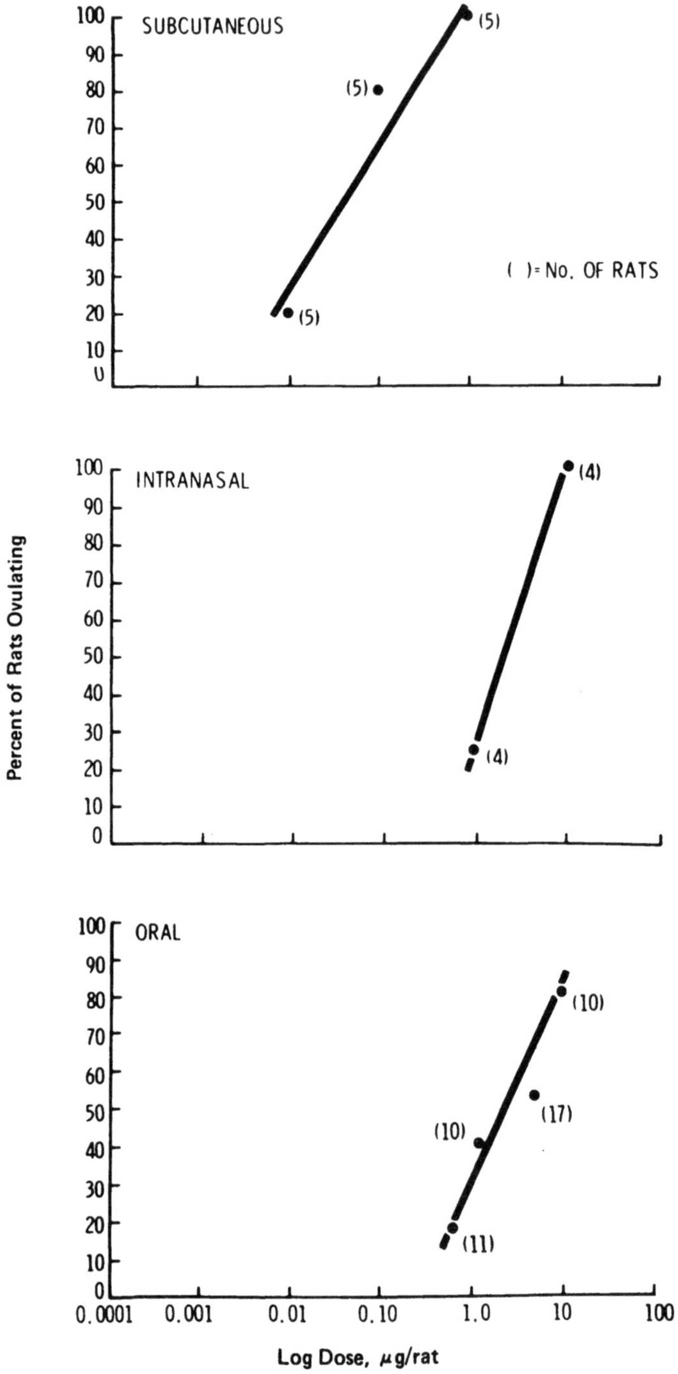

Fig. 1 Wy-40,972: Ovulation induction in nembutalized proestrous rats via various routes of administration.

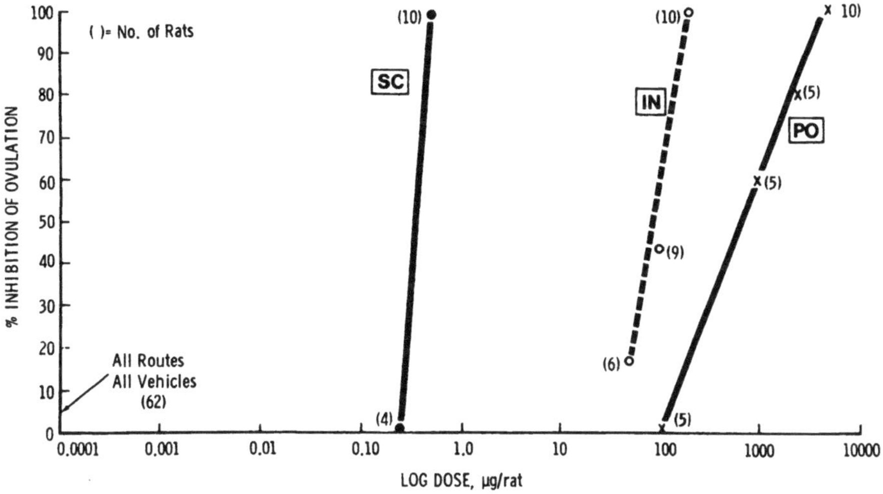

Fig. 2 Ovulation inhibition in unanesthetized, cycling rats treated with Ac-D-Nal(2)^1-pF-D-Phe^2-D-Trp^3-D-Arg^6-LHRH (Salk) at 1200 hr on proestrus: comparison of subcutaneous (sc), oral (po) and intranasal (in) routes.

characteristics of the antagonist. It is noteworthy that acute (proestrous) administration of the antagonist only delays ovulation; the ova that would normally be detected the next morning (estrus) are found one day later (metestrus) intact, with the characteristic cumulus shroud of a fresh ovulation.

Post-coital contraception in rat

Daily subcutaneous administration of either the agonist or antagonist can inhibit pregnancy either pre-(days 1–7) or post-(day 7–12) implantationally (fig. 6). However, under either dosing regimen, the agonist is considerably more potent (by a factor of 100) (tab. 1).

Effect on the rat estrous cycle (fig. 7)

Subcutaneous administration of either analog for 8 days produces a disruption of the estrous cycle, as evidenced by vaginal cytologic dysynchrony. On the afternoon of day 3 (expected proestrous LH surge) evaluation of serum samples revealed a significant inhibition of both LH and progesterone in animals receiving either compound. At autopsy (day after final injection) the uterine weight of agonist recipients were reduced; no such inhibition was seen in antagonist-treated animals. It was determined that approximately 3 days of treatment was sufficient to disrupt the cycle with either agent. Again, a larger dose of the antagonist was required (tab. 1).

	PRIMARY SCREEN[†]				PREGNANCY TERMINATION		Estrous Cycle Disruption	Anti-Fertility Male	Anti-Prostatic Carcinoma●	Anti-Endometriosis●●	Anti-Puberty (µg/rat/day)	
	Ovulation Induction	LH Release	Ovulation Inhibition	LH Inhibition	D1 - 7♦	D7 - 12#						
	(µg/rat▲) (a)		(µg/rat▲) (b)		(µg/rat/day▲)		(µg/rat/day▲)	(µg/rat/day▲)	(µg/rat/day)	(µg/rat/day▲)	♀■	♂♦
AGONIST*	0.1-1.0 sc 10 IN· 10 po;	<1.0 sc	Inactive at 6000 sc	Inactive at 10 sc	1.0 sc	1.0 sc	1-10 x 3 days sc	>10<100 x 7 days ~25 x 14 days, sc	≤500x21 days sc	1.0 x 14 days sc	10 x 11 days	≤10 x 28 days
ANTAGONIST**	Inactive at 100 sc	--	0.50 sc; 200 IN; 2500-5000 po	--	100 sc	100 sc	~50 x 3 days sc	>100x>7 days 100 x 14-28 days, sc	≤500 x 21 days sc	>250 x 21 days sc	100 x 11 days	≤100 x 28 days

† - Proestrous rat
(a) - Nembutal blocked
(b) - Unanesthetized
▲ Estimated MED 100
♦ Preimplantation
Postimplantation
● Transplanted Dunning R-3327 Spontaneous Prostatic Adenocarcinoma
●● Endometrial Homoexplant into Body Wall
■ Inhibition of Vaginal Opening
♦ Inhibition of Sex Accessories

*WY-40972 = D-Trp^6-$N^{\alpha}MeLeu^7$-$DesGly^{10}$-Pro^9-NHEt-LHRH
**SALK = AC-D-$NAL(2)^1$-pF-D-PHE^2-D-TRP^3-D-ARG^6-LHRH

Tab. 1 Comparison of reproductive pharmacologic profile of an LHRH agonist and antagonist in the rat.

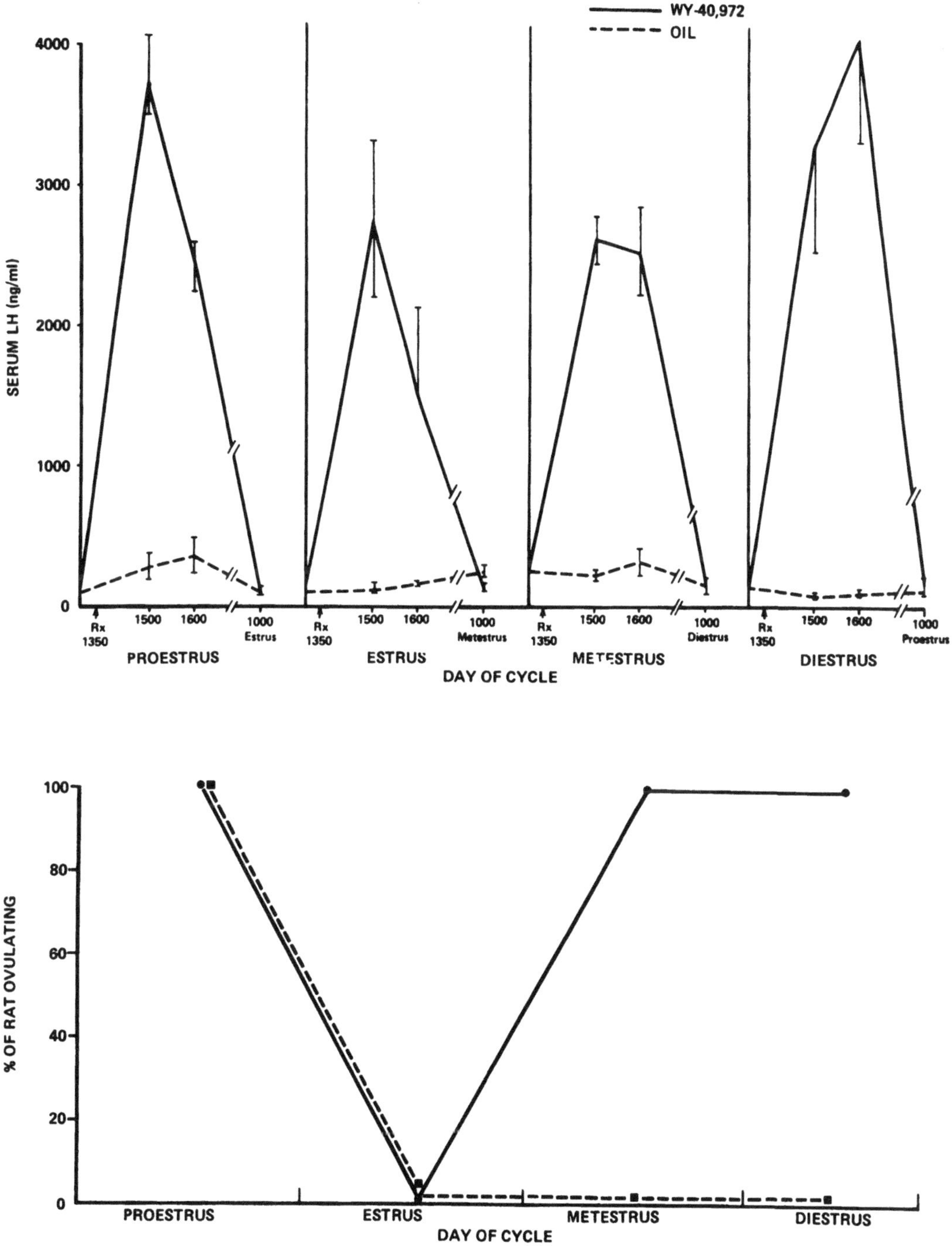

Fig. 3 Serum LH and ovulatory response to Wy-40,972 (10 μg/rat, sc) administered on individual days of the rat estrous cycle.

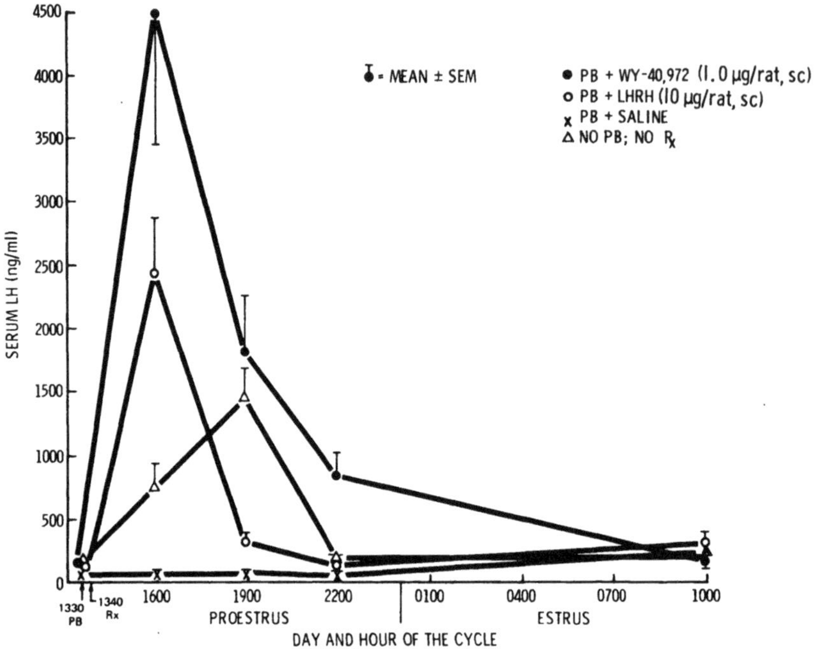

Fig. 4 Effect of a single proestrous administration of Wy-40,972 or LHRH on the pattern of serum LH in pentobarbital (PB)-blocked rats.

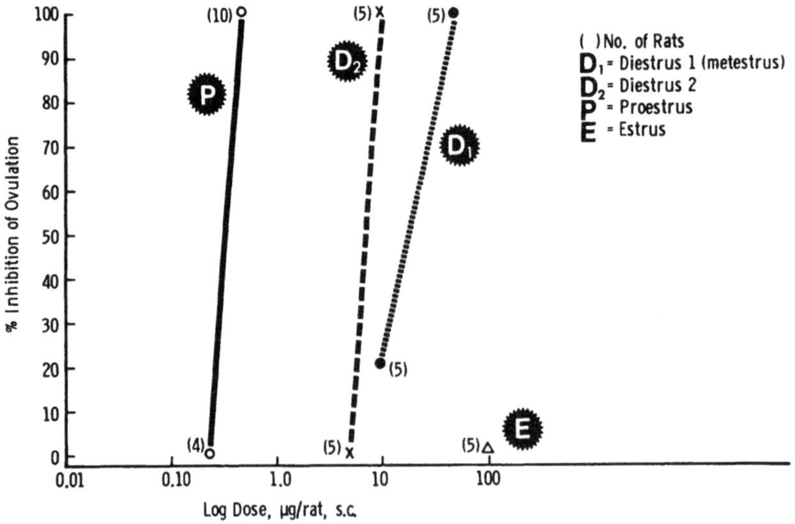

Fig. 5 Ovulation inhibition in unanesthetized, cycling rats treated with Ac-D-Nal(2)[1]-pF-D-Phe[2]-D-Trp[3]-D-Arg[6]-LHRH at 1200 hr on individual days of the estrous cycle.

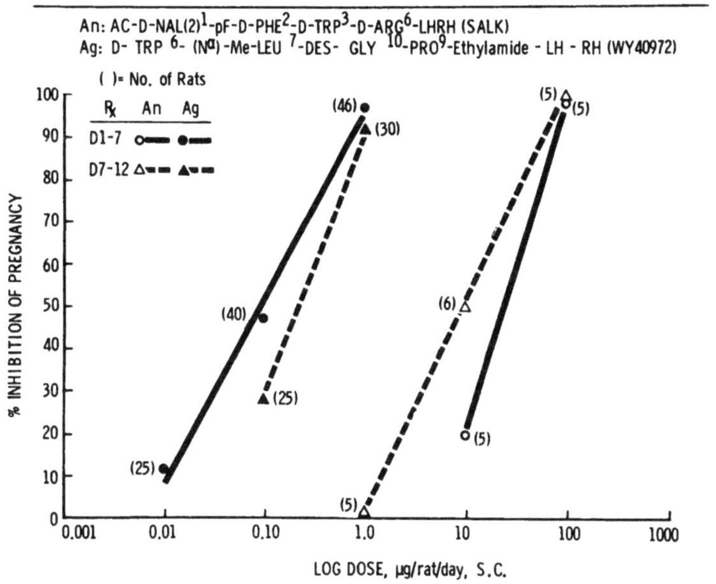

Fig. 6 Pregnancy termination in rat with LHRH analogs: comparison of antagonist (An) and agonist (Ag).

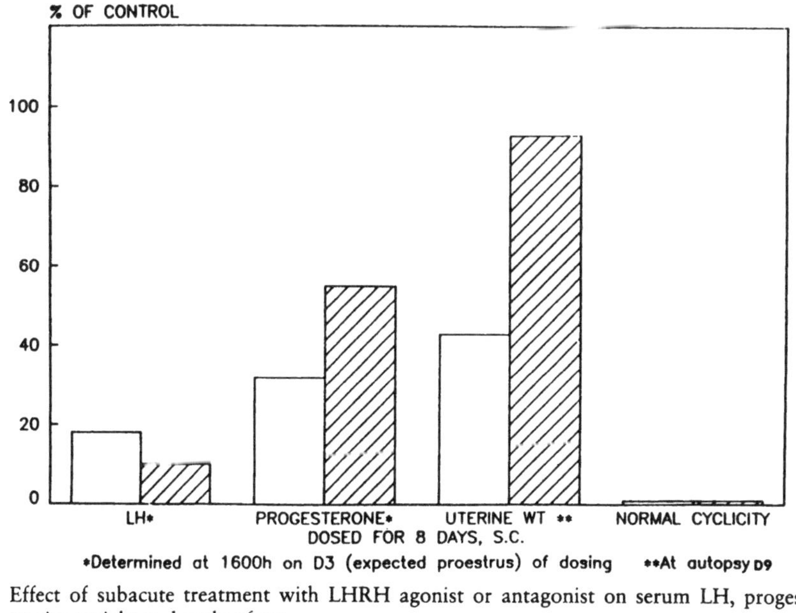

Fig. 7 Effect of subacute treatment with LHRH agonist or antagonist on serum LH, progesterone, uterine weight and cycle of rat.

Effect on male rat

These studies represent not only the contraceptive evaluation of these compounds in the male [1, 7, 9] but also provide a dose-range finding regimen for eventual utility in the prostate carcinoma animal model *(vide infra)*.

Various doses of the agonist and antagonist were administered subcutaneously to mature male rats on a daily basis for up to 35 days. Seven days of treatment with the agonist produces a significant inhibition of serum LH (fig. 8), FSH (fig. 9) and testosterone (fig. 10); significant depression of these parameters occurred with the antagonist at higher doses and over longer (14–28 days) treatment schedules (figs. 8, 9, 10; tab. 1). Important changes in the weight of the testes (fig. 11) and target organs, the ventral prostate (fig. 12), the seminal vesicles (fig. 13), the epididymis (fig. 14) and levator ani (fig. 15), generally occurred with both agents after 14 days of dosing. Again, the agonist proved to be more active and potent than the antagonist, and required a shorter time span, in inhibiting the hormonal and gravimetric components of the pituitary-testicular-androgen dependent organ axis. The very high dose of the agonist (i.e. 500 µg/rat/day) was employed to determine the limits of the dose-response effect in relation to time; notably, the testosterone levels and the weights of the testes and the ventral prostate were severely depressed.

Histologic evaluation of representative testicular sections from agonist- and antagonist-treated animals are visualized in figures 16, and 17 and 18, respectively. In this particular comparison, the agonist used was D-Ala^6-DesGly^{10}-Pro^9-NHEt-LH-RH (Wy18481) [12], which is about 10 times less potent than Wy40972. Chronic (35 days) high-dose (1.0 mg/rat/day, SC) treatment of the rat with the agonist produced the characteristic disarray of testicular cytoarchitecture [9]: progressive disorganization of the seminiferous tubules, loss of sperm in the tubular lumina, and loss of staining characteristics of spermatogonia and interstitial cells. Additionally, a mixture of inflammatory, degenerative (recoverable) and necrotic (non-reversible mineralization) processes were observed. In many instances, these events were focal, and were associated with tubular calcification. Such effects have been reported by others [26, 28, 31, 34, 43], and they may be characteristic of the rat.

In contrast, subcutaneous administration of the antagonist (50 and 100 µg/rat/day), or of a less potent one [Wy-44,599; Ac-dehydro-Pro^1-pF-D-Phe^2-D-Trp^{3,6}-LH-RH (Salk Inst.)] but at 500 µg/rat/day, for up to 28 days, produced no discernible effects on the total histologic character of the testes of the majority of animals (fig. 17). However, in some of the rats receiving Wy-45,760 or Wy-44,599 daily for either 14 or 28 days, the following changes were observed: at 14 days, slight, multifocal (few sites) decrease in spermatocytes; and at 28 days, diffuse, moderate to marked seminiferous tubular atrophy characterized by a reduction in mature sperm and spermatocytes. The spermatogonia and sertoli cells were unaffected (fig. 18). It is noteworthy that the only dosed rats showing such degenerative testicular changes were those

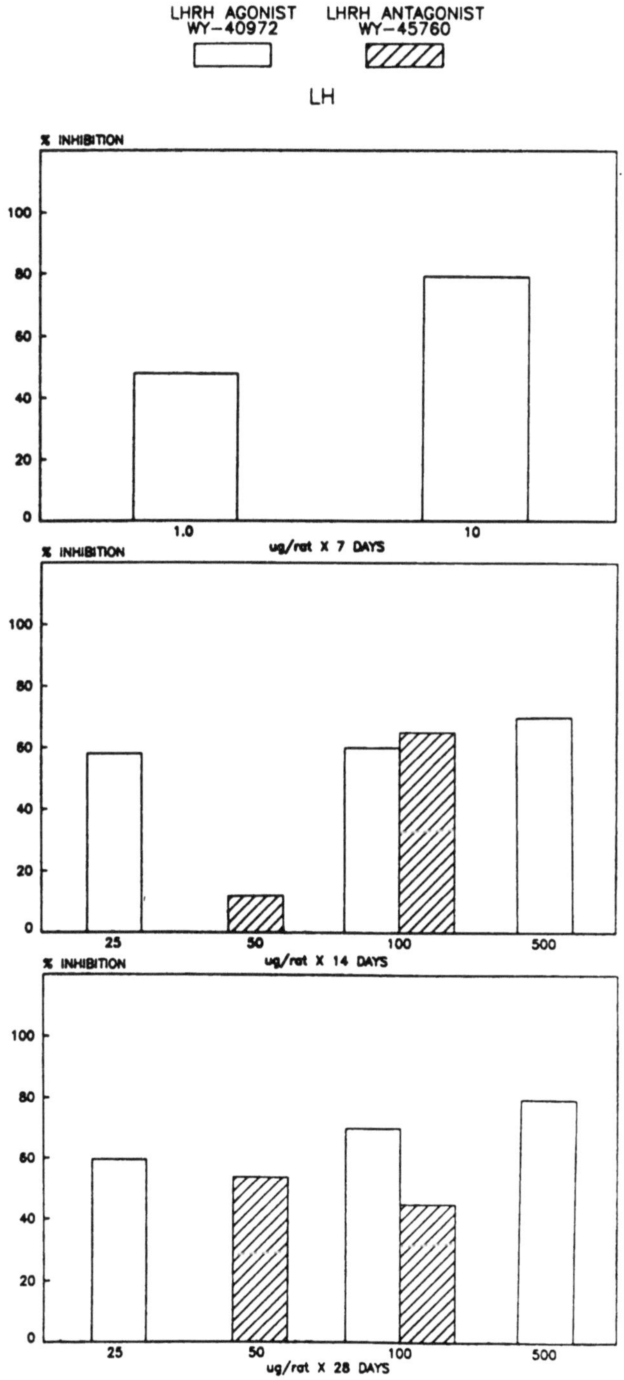

Fig. 8 Effect of an LHRH agonist (Wy-40,972) and antagonist (Wy-45,760) on serum hormone levels in the male rat: LH.

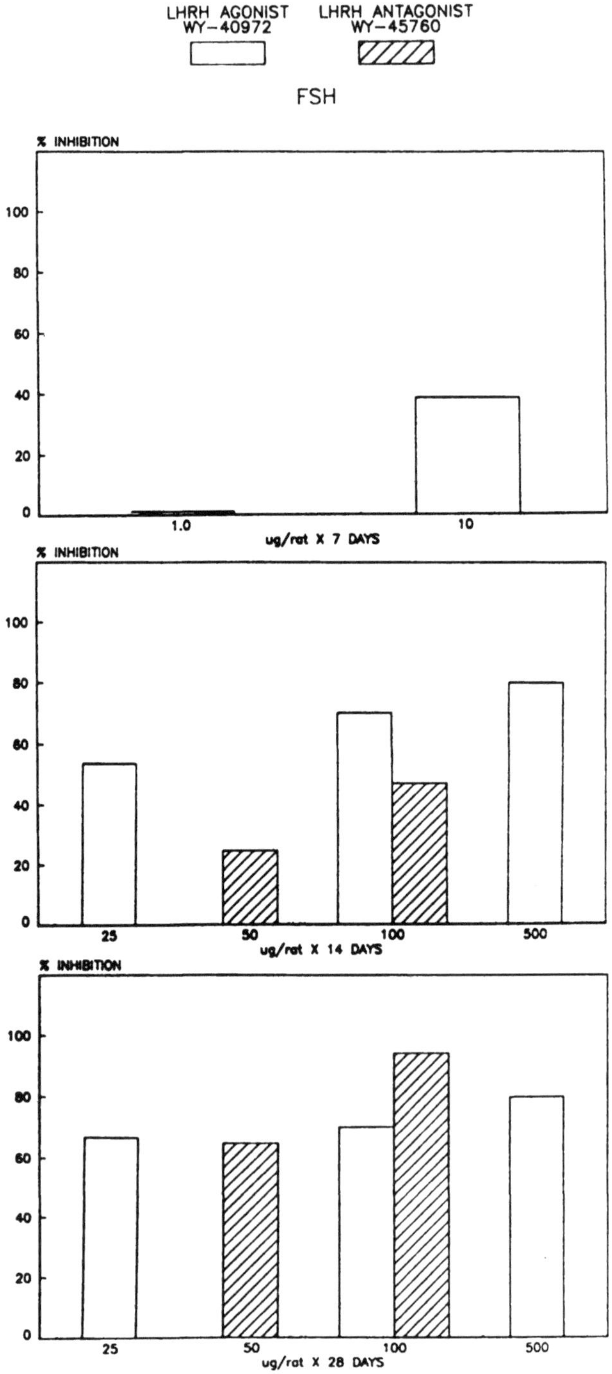

Fig. 9 Effect of an LHRH agonist (Wy-40,972) and antagonist (Wy-45,760) on serum hormone levels in the male rat: FSH.

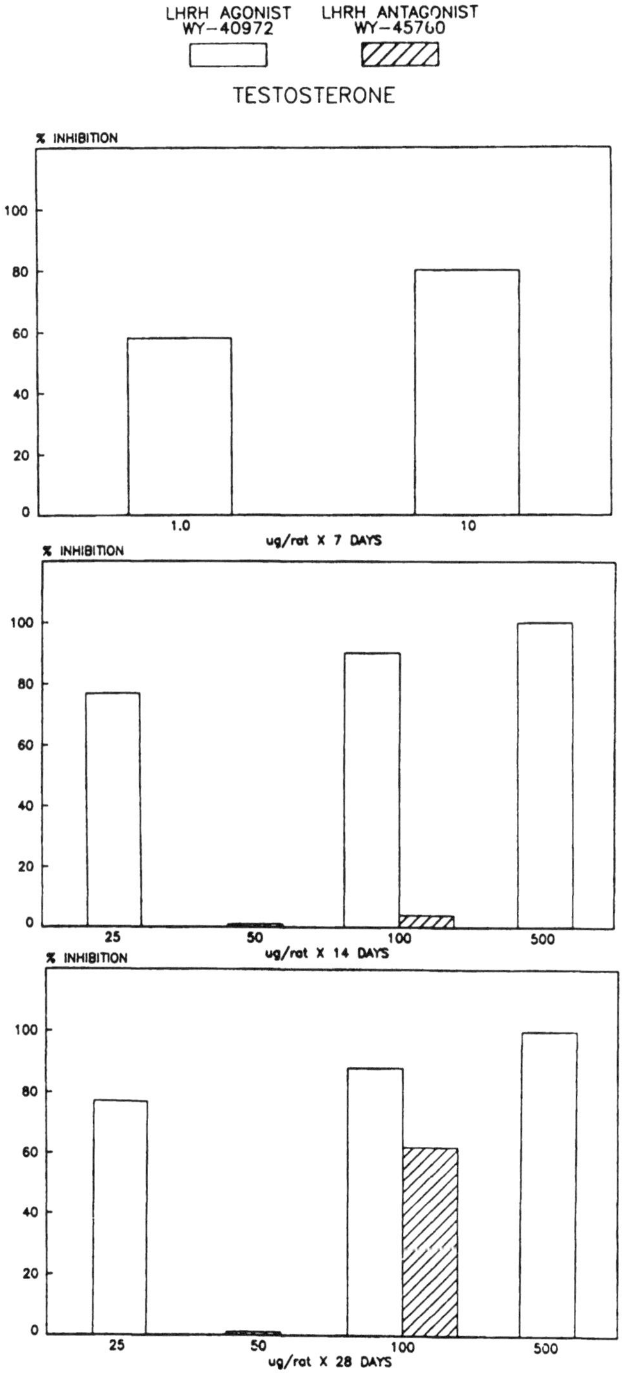

Fig. 10 Effect of an LHRH agonist (Wy-40,972) and antagonist (Wy-45,760) on serum hormone levels in the male rat: testosterone.

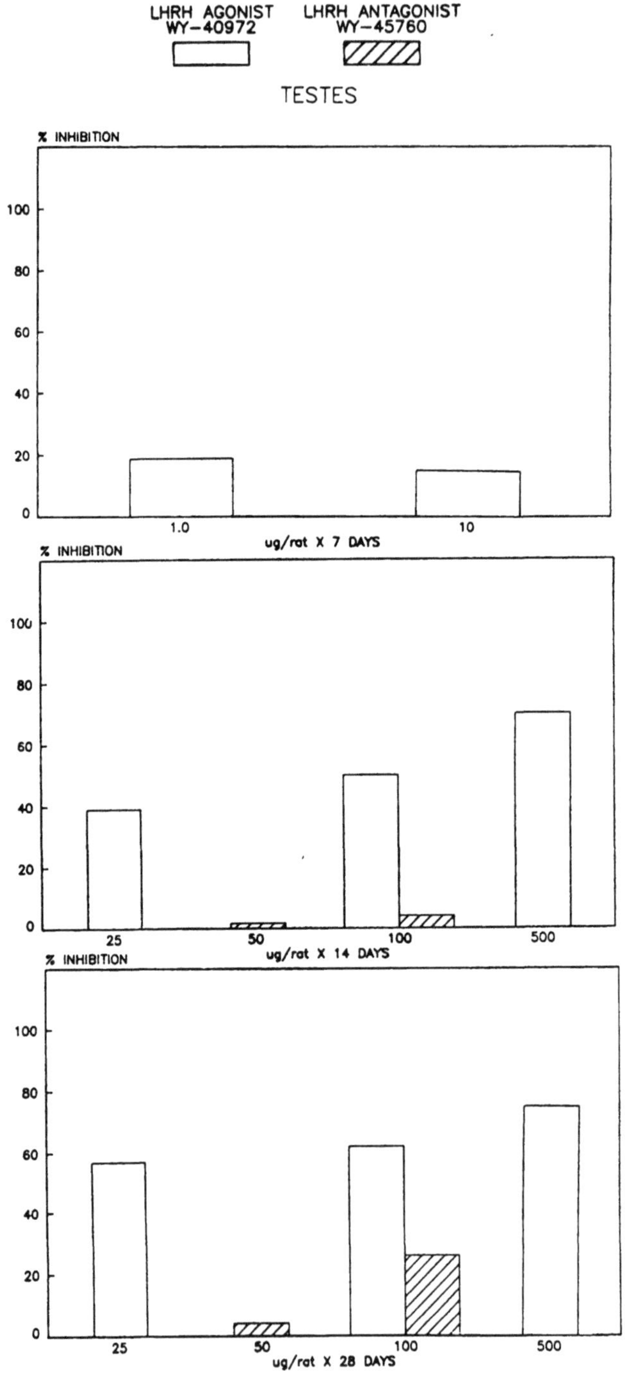

Fig. 11 Effect of LHRH agonist (Wy-40,972) and antagonist (Wy-45,760) on organ weights in the male rat: testes.

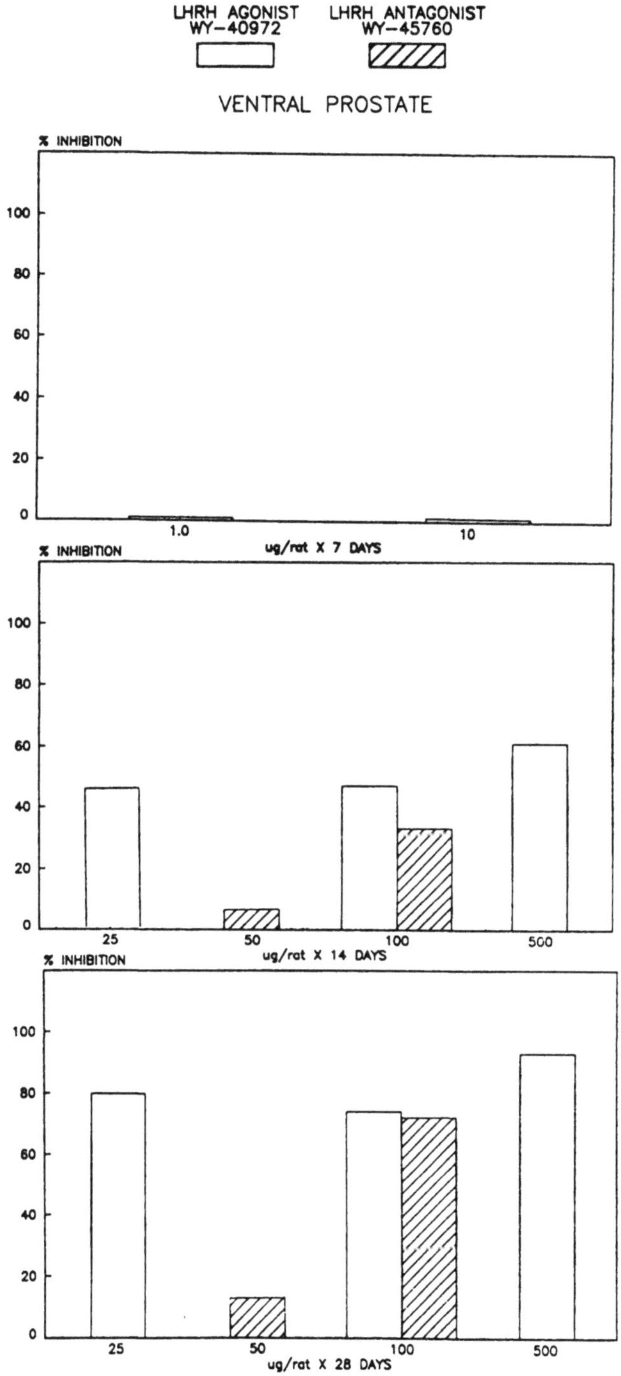

Fig. 12 Effect of LHRH agonist (Wy-40,972) and antagonist (Wy-45,760) on organ weights in the male rat: ventral prostate.

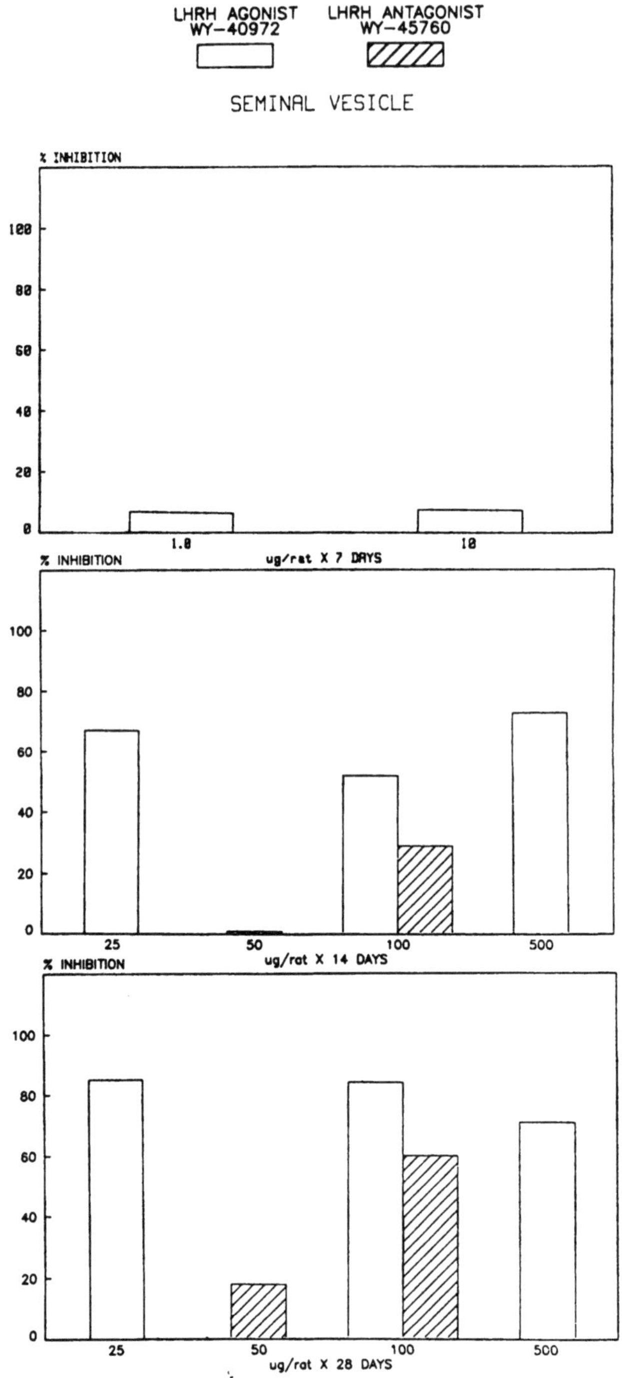

Fig. 13 Effect of LHRH agonist (Wy-40,972) and antagonist (Wy-45,760) on organ weights in the male rat: seminal vesicle.

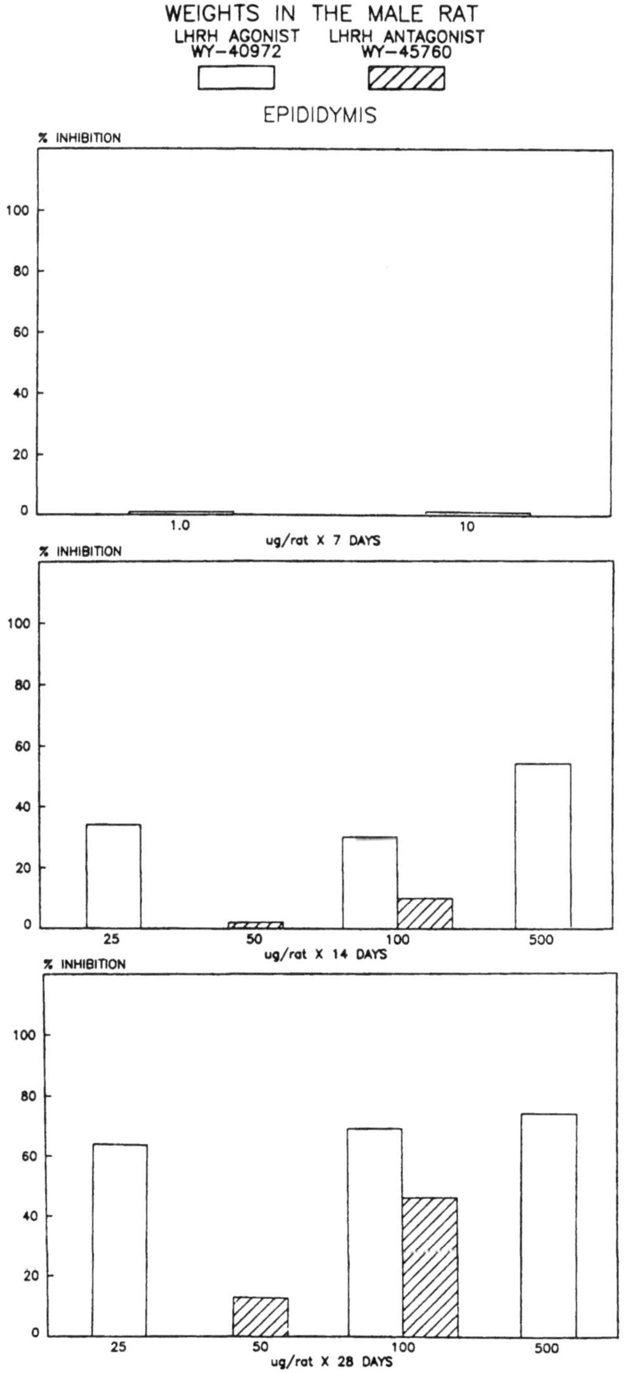

Fig. 14 Effect of LHRH agonist (Wy-40,972) and antagonist (Wy-45,760) on organ weights in the male rat: epididymis.

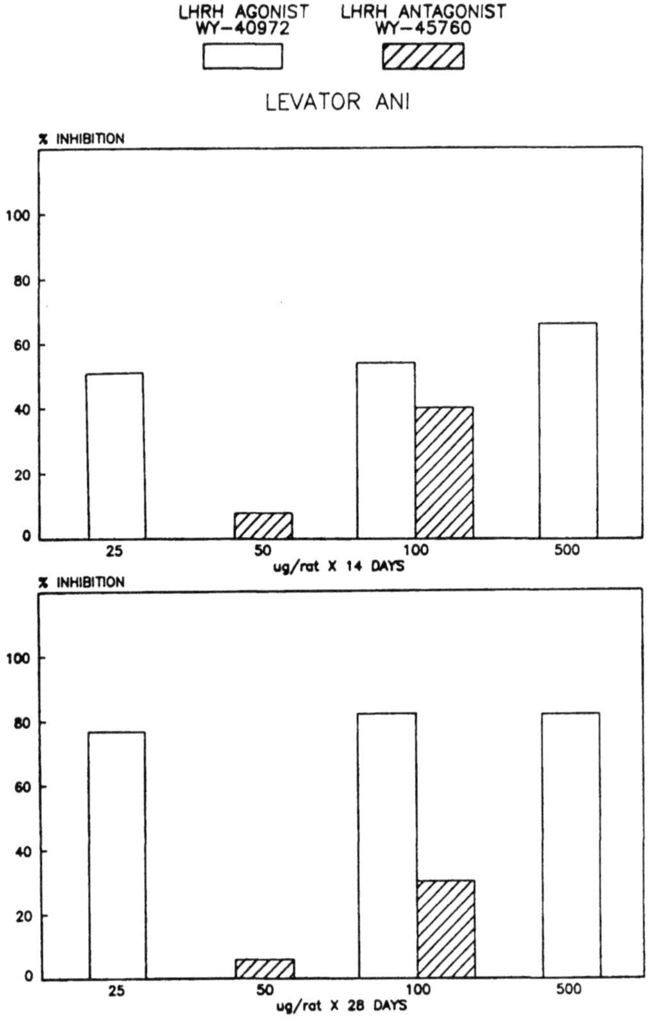

Fig. 15 Effect of LHRH agonist (Wy-40,972) and antagonist (Wy-45,760) on organ weights in the male rat: levator ani.

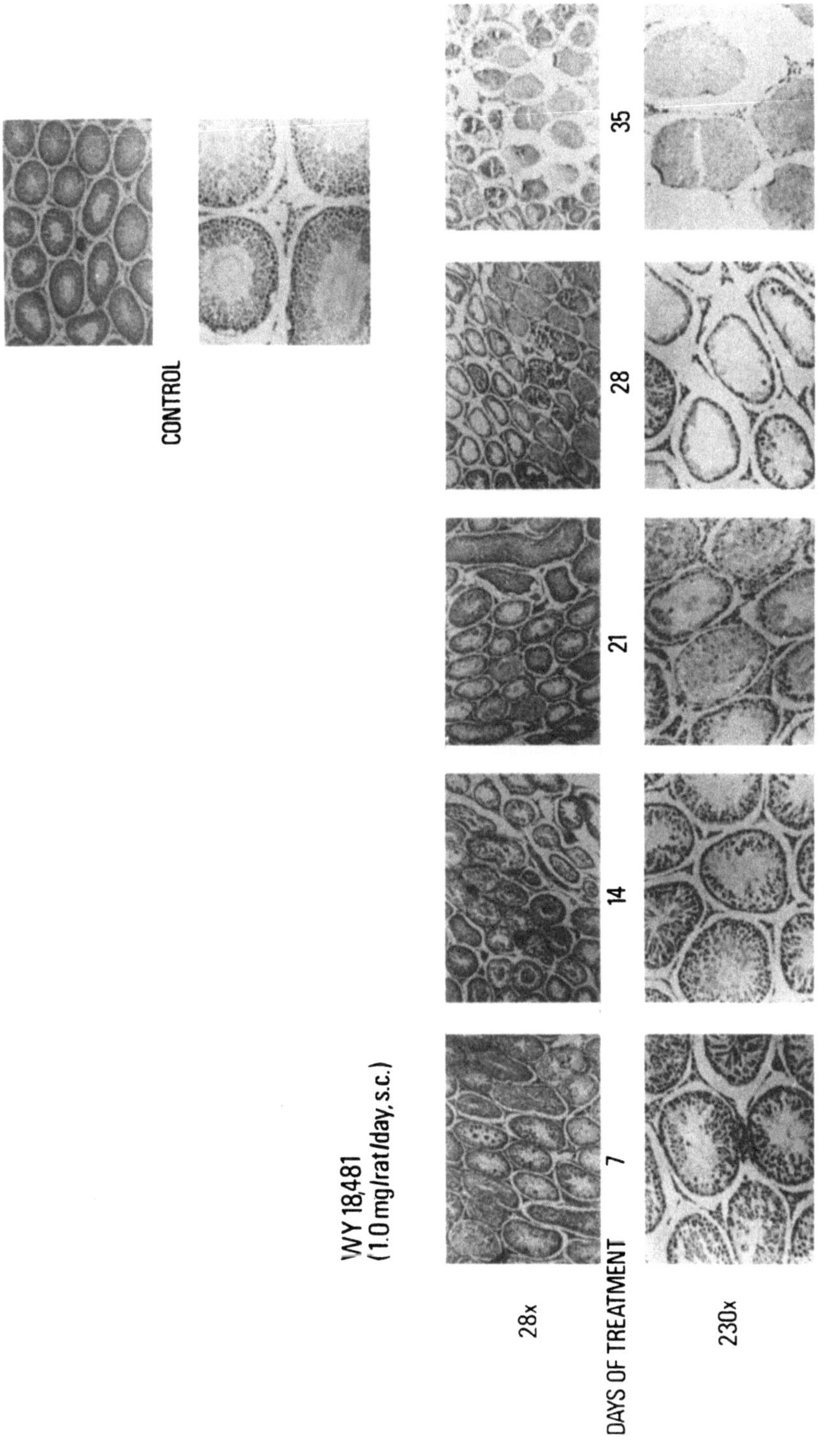

Fig. 16 Effect of chronic treatment with Wy-18,481 on testicular histology of mature male rats.

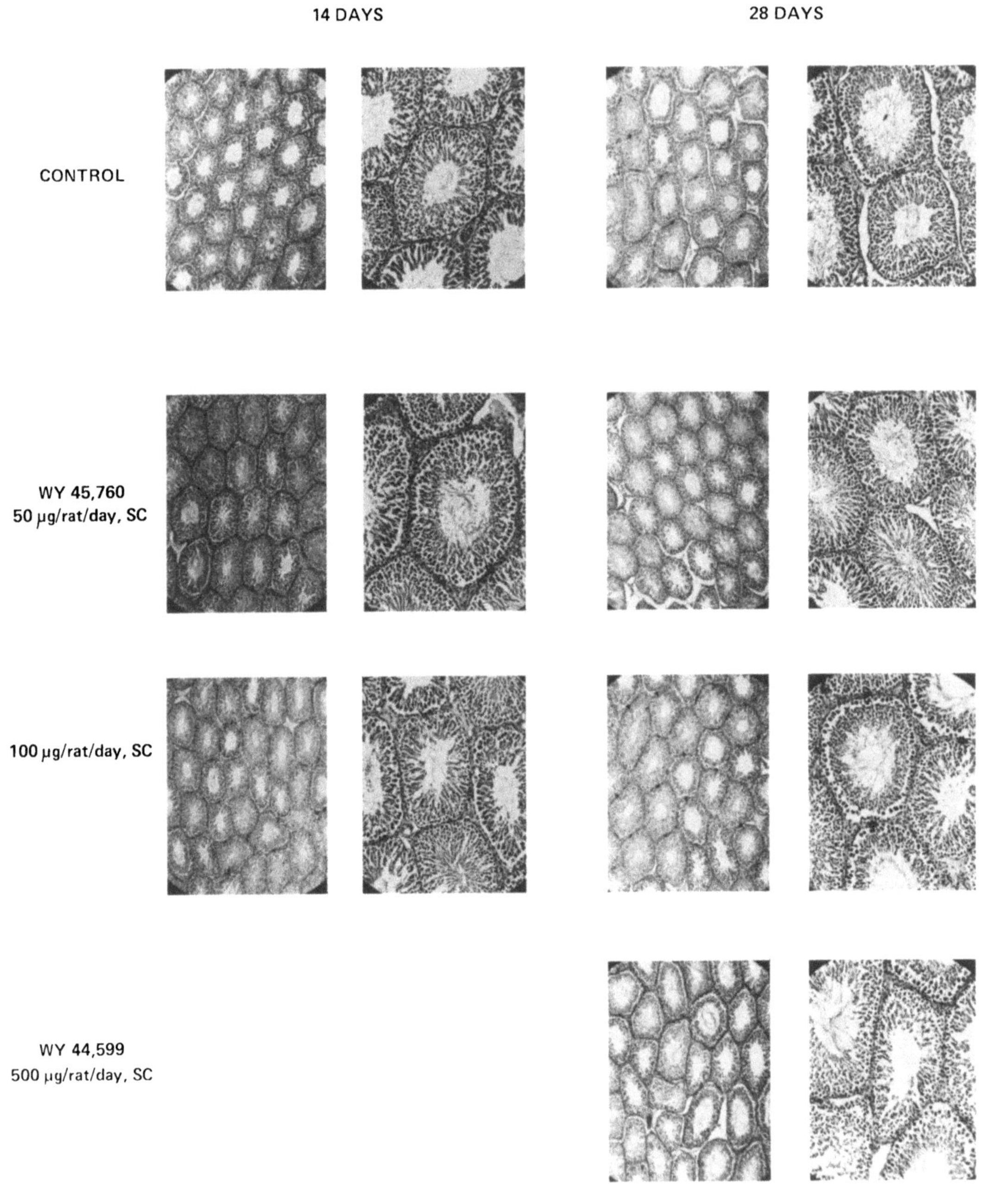

Fig. 17 Effect of chronic treatment with LHRH antagonists on testicular histology on mature male rats: no alteration.

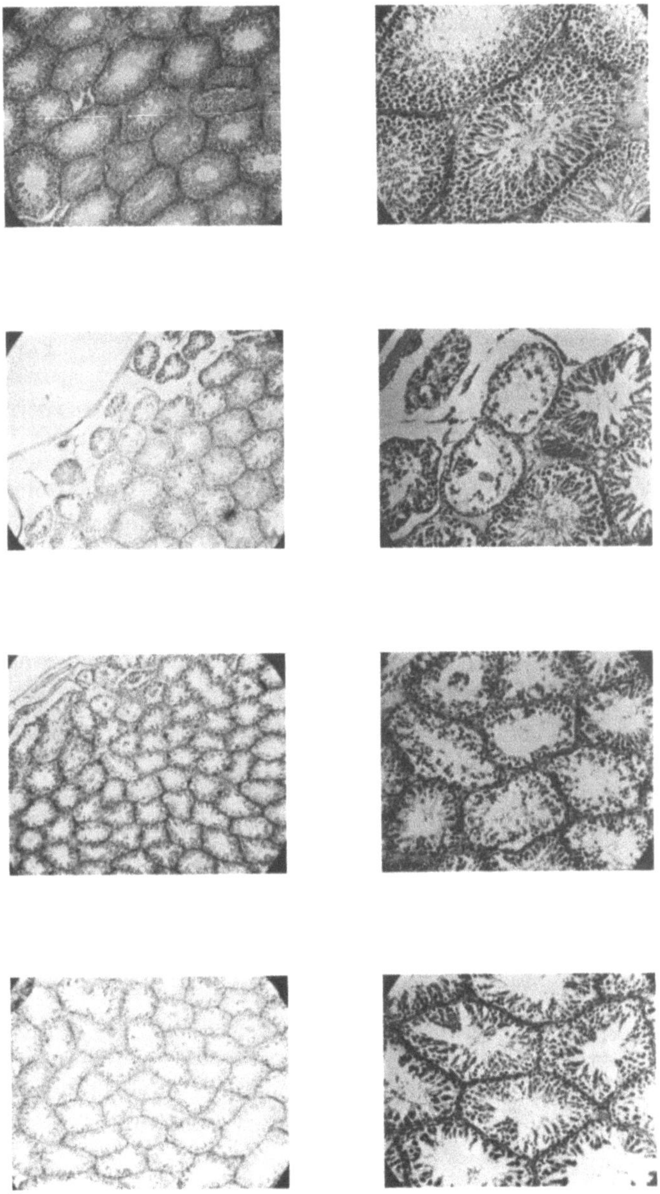

CONTROL 28 DAYS

WY 45,760
100 μg/rat/day, SC X 14 DAYS

WY 45,760
100 μg/rat/day, SC X 28 DAYS

WY 44,599
500 μg/rat/day, SC X 28 DAYS

Fig. 18 Effect of chronic treatment with LHRH antagonist on testicular histology of mature male rats: alteration.

whose gonadal and androgen-dependent organ weights were severely depressed, well below those of their similarly-treated group mates. Thus, a definite chronological progression of testicular disruption emerges, especially in terms of tubular size. One would anticipate, therefore, based on the overall reproductive inhibition observed that either of the aforementioned antagonists, at higher doses and/or longer treatment periods, would produce a greater frequency and extent of histologic evidence of depression of testicular morphology.

In a study using a related antagonist, Ac-dehydro-Pro^{1}-pCl-D-Phe^{2}-D-Trp^{3,6}-N$^{\alpha}$Me-Leu^{7}-LH-RH), Rivier at al. [33], reported that 14-day treatment with 1.0 mg/rat/day significantly lowered the weights of the testes, prostate and seminal vesicles. Furthermore, testicular morphology was altered: atrophy of Leydig cells, reduced tubular diameters, depletion of germinal epithelium, spermatogonial arrest and inhibition of spermatogenesis.

The histomorphologic findings of these studies point to definite differences between the morphological effects of an agonist and an antagonist on the testicular compartments; namely, that the antagonist produces a more quantitatively consistent and structurally uniform change with no evidence of calcification. These differences in biologic effect within the gonad may be attributed to the different mechanisms of action of the two classes of analog: a complex one with the agonist that includes down regulation and desensitization of the pituitary-testicular axis, including the possibility of a direct agonist-gonadal interaction, and, with the antagonist, a simpler, unidirectional inhibition of LH-RH receptors at the pituitary level, with no evidence that the antagonist possesses any intrinsic pharmacologic activity of its own.

Therapeutic evaluation

The curative or palliative utility of the LH-RH analogs lies in their ability to dramatically reduce the levels of gonadal steroids required to support several pathologic reproductive states. In particular, the lowering of blood androgen and estrogen levels by the LH-RH agonists to oophorectomy and orchiectomy ranges, is tantamount to pharmacologic or "medical" castration.

Endometriosis

The inhibition of gonadal steroidogenesis in the female and the resultant regression of uterine function provides the basis for the potential anti-endometriotic utility of the LH-RH analogs.

Several animal models (i.e. rat, rabbit, monkey) for the study of this endocrine distortion have been documented in which uterine tissue, for the sake of practicality and expedience, either has been ectopically implanted or seeded onto peritoneal surfaces [14, 48]. In our hands [25], a uterine segment of a rat is stripped of its myometrium and homologously explanted into the body wall of the peritoneal cavity (fig. 19). Figure 20 demonstrates that 3 weeks of treatment with 30 μg Wy-40,972/rat/day sc causes regression of the explant similar to that produced by ovariectomy; a daily dose as low as 1.0 μg also is effective (fig. 21). It is noteworthy that upon cessation of treatment, the explant shows a slow growth resurgence. This might indicate the need for continuous, but perhaps intermittent treatment in the clinical condition. In comparison studies using levonorgestrel and danazol [25], the anti-endometriotic effects were less pronounced and consistent; in fact, such effects of these steroids became apparent many weeks after treatment was terminated, underscoring the qualitative, quantitative and chronologic superiority of the agonist over the steroids.

A comparison between Wy-40,972 and the antagonist, Wy-45,760, is depicted in figure 22. The anti-endometriotic property of the agonist is clearly far superior to that of the antagonist, both in terms of efficacy and of potency.

The study of Werlin and Hodgen [48] demonstrated the effectiveness of the agonist, D-Leu^{6}-DesGly^{10}-Pro^{9}-NHEt-LH-RH (Leuprorelin®, Abbott), in inhibiting and resolving the growth of surgically-induced ectopic endometrial tissue in monkeys when administered on an intermittent basis. Several preliminary clinical studies employing the agonist, D-Ser(TBU)^{6}-DesGly^{10}-Pro^{9}-NHEt-LH-RH (Buserelin, Hoechst AG) or D-Trp^{6}-DesGly^{10}-Pro^{9}-NHEt-LH-RH (Salk Institute) have provided encouraging results in relieving the subjective symptoms and objective signs of endometriosis [3, 5, 24, 25].

Prostatic carcinoma

The therapeutic value of the LH-RH analogs in hormone-dependent cancer has been the subject of many animal and clinical investigations. Numerous reports are available [3, 5, 17, 23, 27, 32, 39, 45, 47, 49] that discuss this new approach in both males and females.

The dramatic anti-reproductive effects, particularly of the agonists, in causing amerlioration of prostatic carcinoma has provided a novel, non-toxic treatment of this disease. In laboratory studies, the spontaneous androgen-dependent rat prostatic adenocarcinoma, R-3327, has been employed as the model most relevant to the human condition [41]. Figure 23 demonstrates the growth of this tumor and the respective serum testosterone values in vehicle control, Wy-40,972-treated, and surgically castrated rats after 16 weeks. The LH-RH agonist proves to be approximately as effective as surgical castration in rapidly inhibiting the growth of the tumor and eliminating the associated supportive androgen. Such results confirm those reported by other investigators [39]. Representative *in situ* tumors after 14 weeks are visual-

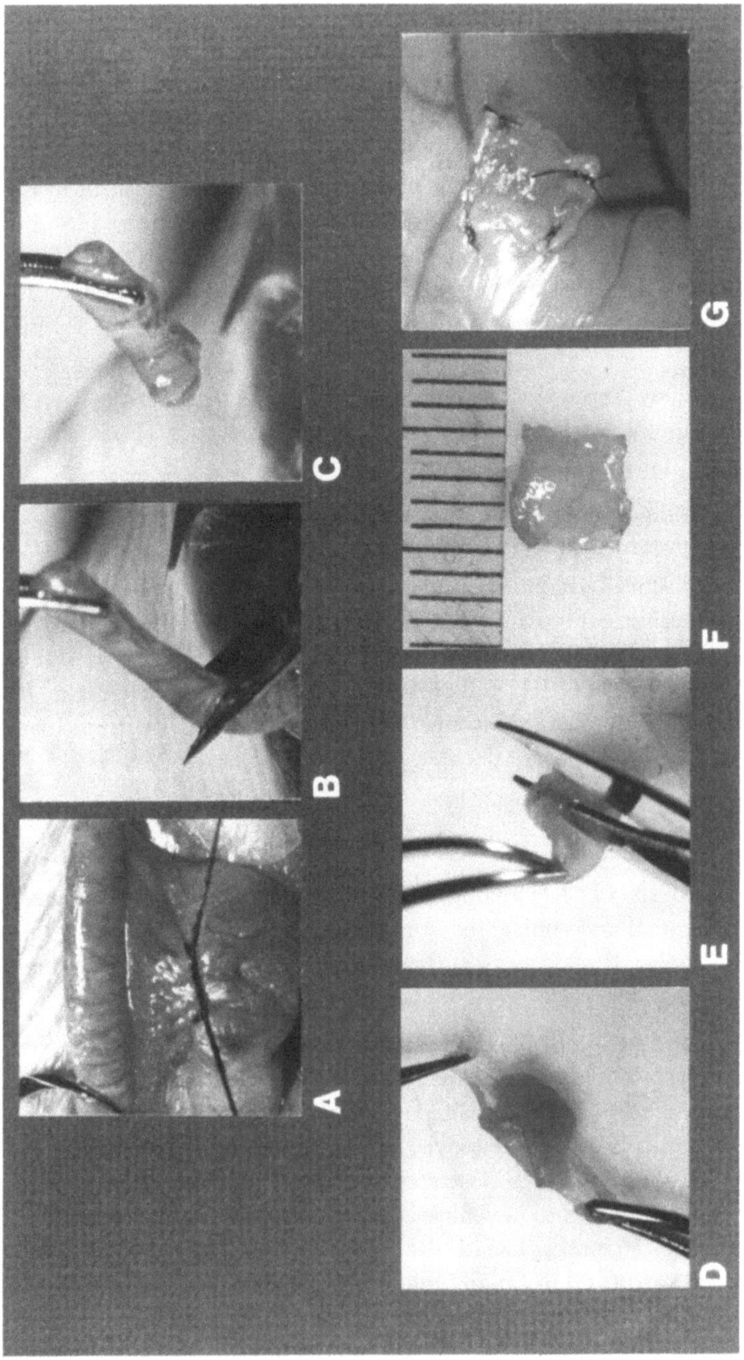

Fig. 19 Procedure for inducing endometriosis in the rat. A) ligation of uterine blood vessels; B–C) uterine segment excised and removed from peritoneal cavity; D) myometrium separated from endometrium; E–F) endometrial segment cut longitudinally and laid open; G) 5×5 mm endometrial segment sutured to body wall of peritoneal cavity.

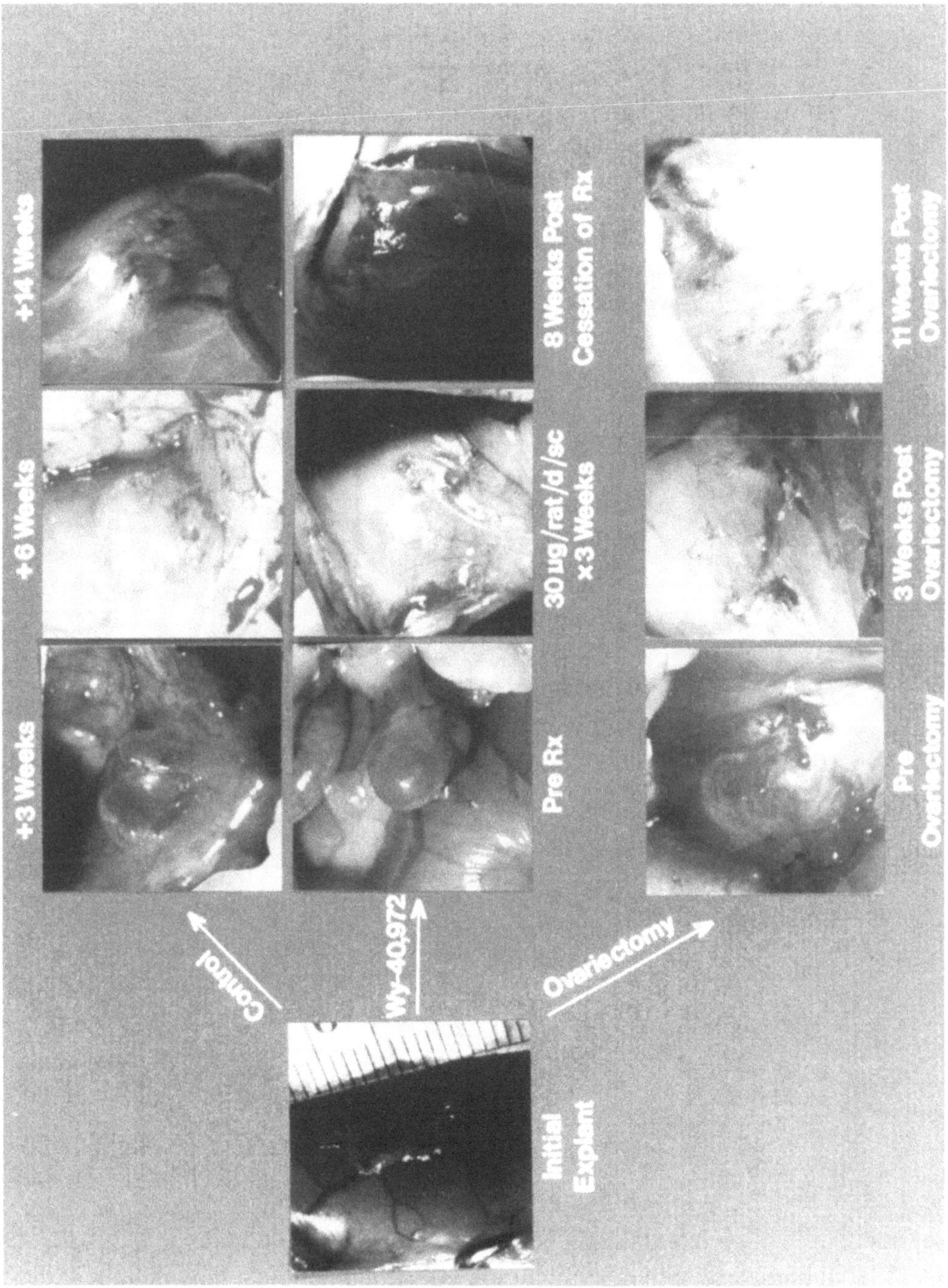

Fig. 20 Effect of treatment with Wy-40,972 or ovariectomy on growth of endometrial explant in the rat. + 3 weeks: explant prior to treatment; + 6 weeks: explant after 3 weeks of treatment; + 14 weeks; explant 8 weeks after cessation of treatment.

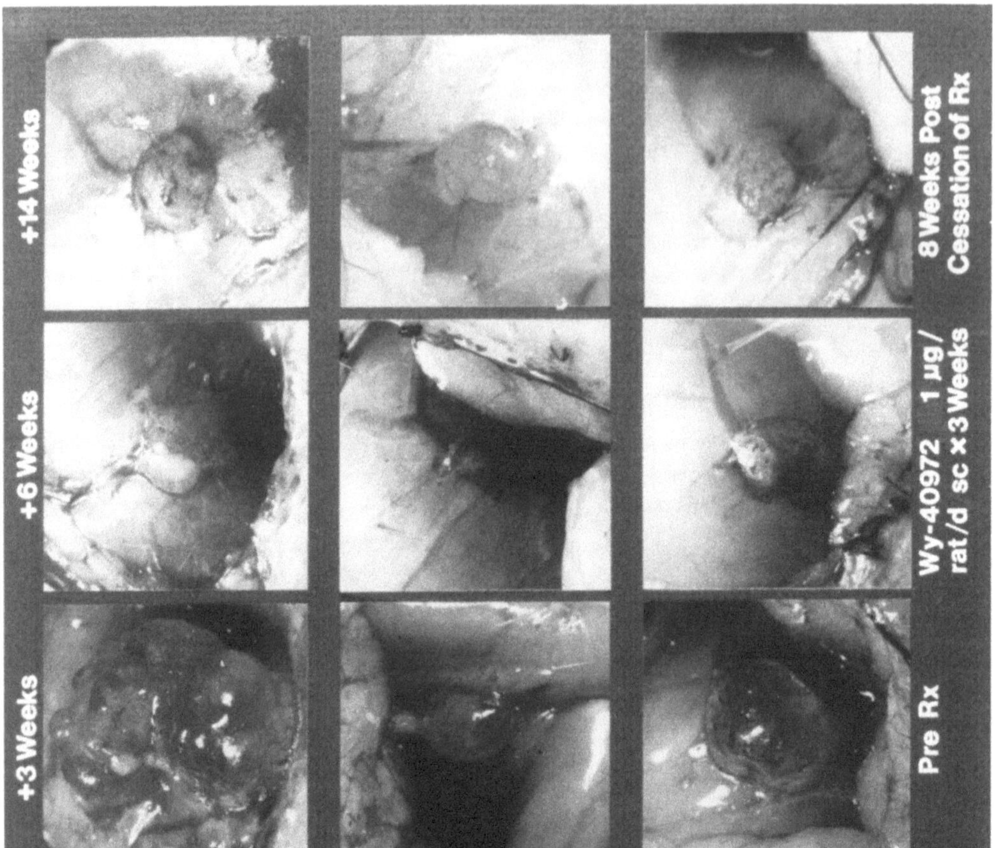

Fig. 21 Effect of treatment with Wy-40,972 on growth of endometrial explant in 3 rats. + 3 weeks: explant prior to treatment; + 6 weeks: explant after 3 weeks of treatment; + 14 weeks; explant 8 weeks after cessation of treatment.

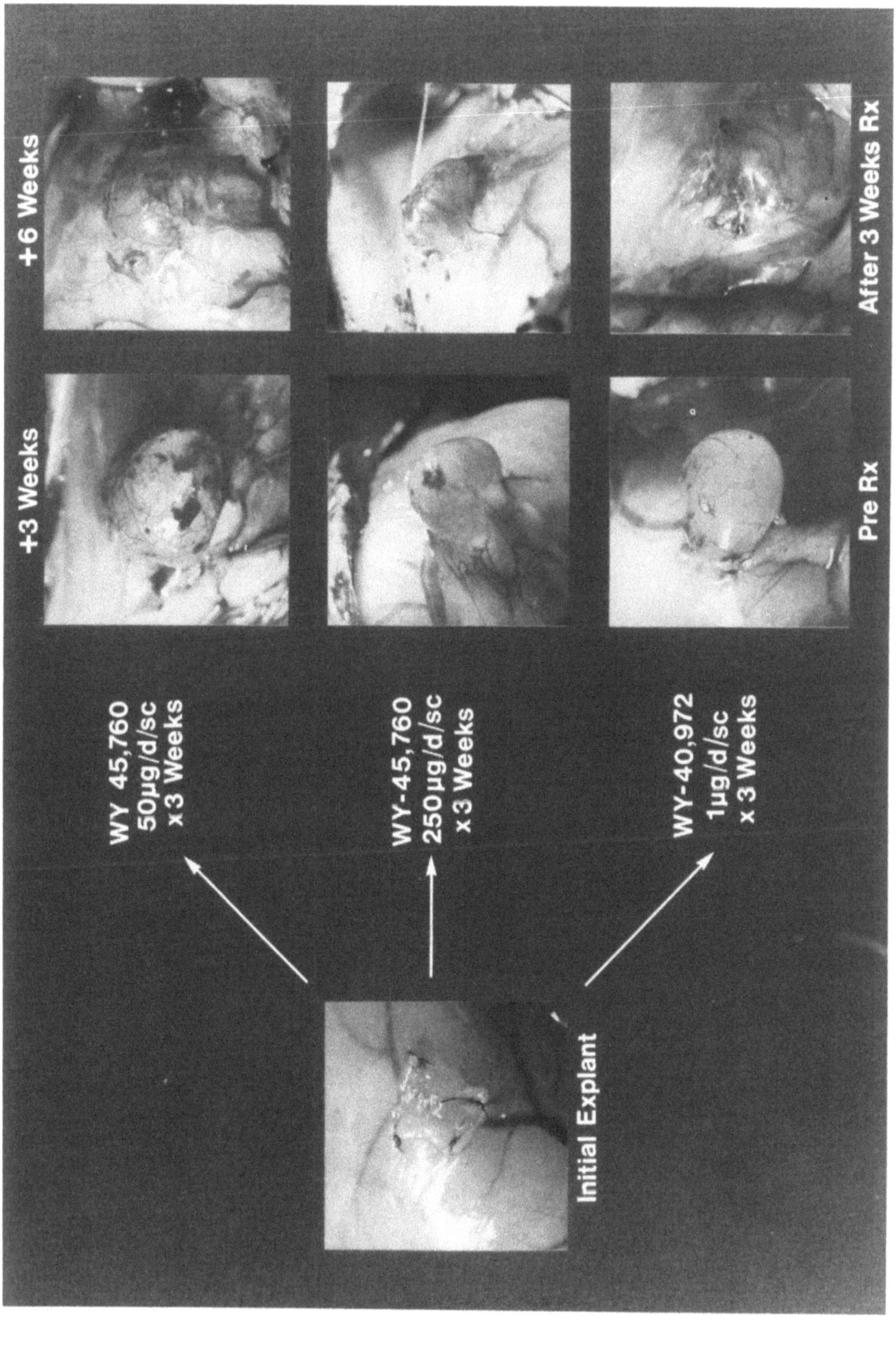

Fig. 22 Experimental endometriosis in the rat: comparison of LHRH agonist and antagonist.

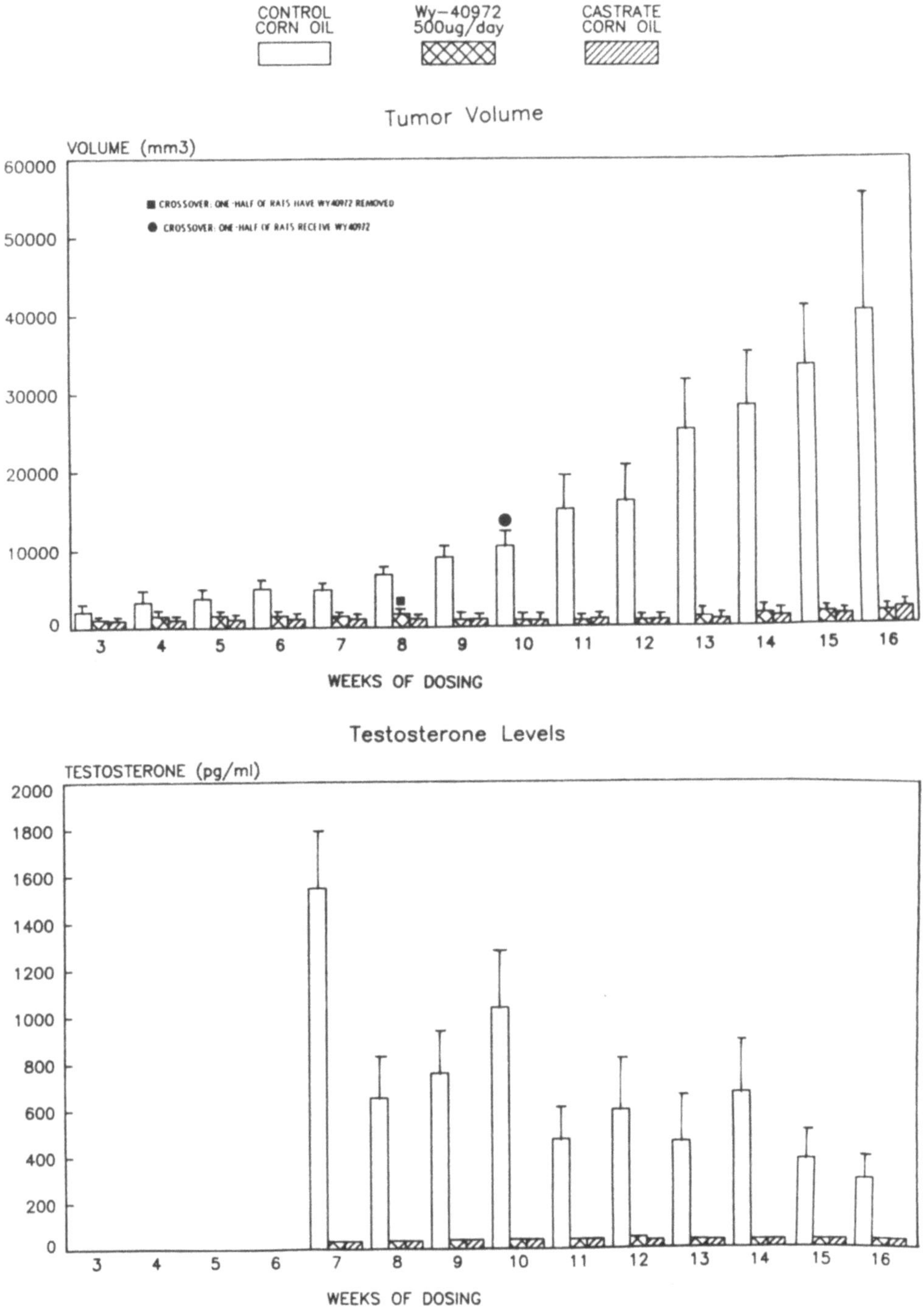

Fig. 23 Effect of Wy-40,972 on androgen-dependent prostatic tumor (Dunning R-3327) growth in male rats: tumor volume and serum testosterone.

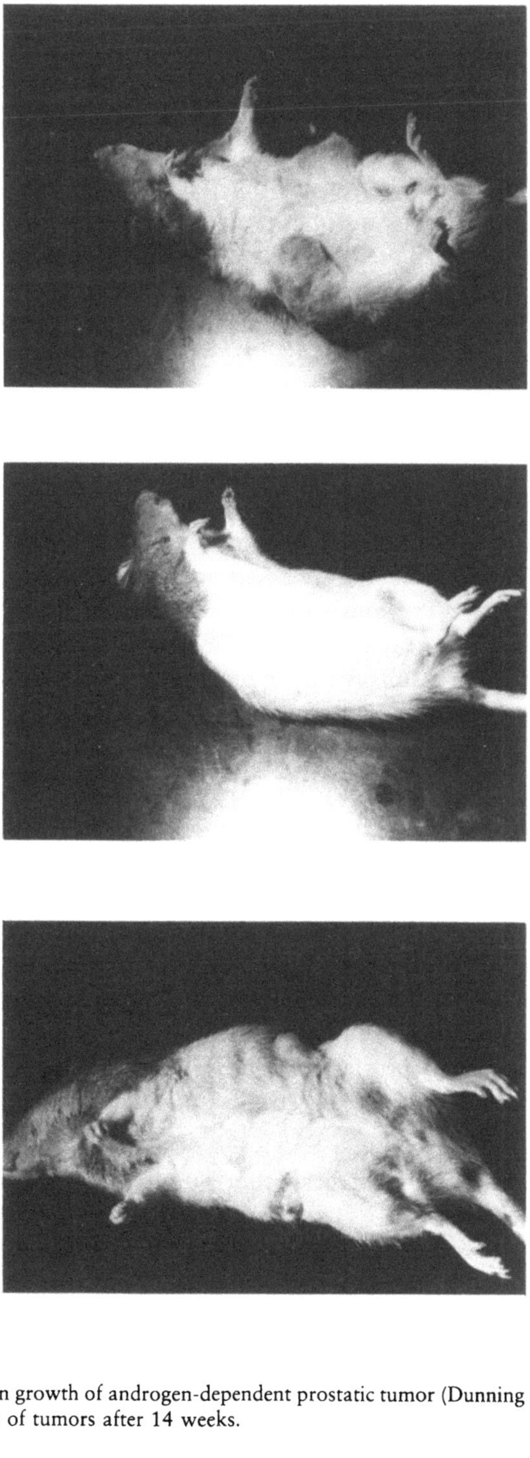

CONTROL

SURGICAL
CASTRATION

WY 40,972
500 μg/rat/day, SC

Fig. 24 Effect of LHRH agonist on growth of androgen-dependent prostatic tumor (Dunning R-3327) in rat. *In situ* representation of tumors after 14 weeks.

ized in figure 24. Crossover studies (fig. 25) further demonstrate that the compound is effective in causing regression of the tumor in control animals subsequently placed on treatment which had borne this tumor for 10 weeks without drug. Additionally, animals that originally were receiving the agonist (for 8 weeks), which was then withdrawn, show a slow resurgence of tumor growth; this attenuated tumor re-growth pattern may reflect the time required for regeneration of the hypophysial LH-RH/gonadal gonadotropin receptor milieu that had been continually desensitized and downregulated by the agonist. This would indicate that chronic (but perhaps intermittent) treatment might be required to ensure tumor inhibition. Figure 25 also shows the time-related changes in serum levels of testosterone consonant with these crossover groups. In these 2 particular cases, the former group (i.e. new Wy-40,972 recipients) reveals a decline in testosterone values, whereas in the latter group (i.e. Wy-40, 972 removed), the testosterone levels rise. Once again, the testosterone levels are directly associated with the changes in the growth patterns of the tumor.

With regard to the LH-RH antagonist, figure 26 depicts the suppression of serum testosterone levels and the attendant restraint of tumor growth following 7 weeks of daily treatment. Previously, it had been shown that the antagonist, Wy-44,599, could inhibit the growth of a mouse mammary tumor (MMT) in neonatal hamsters [5]. The present results reinforce previous reports on the anti-tumor efficacy of the antagonists [39].

While both classes of LH-RH analogs indirectly inhibit steroidogenesis and consequently the androgen-dependent target organs, via pituitary involvement, the possibility of a direct, extrapituitary, extragonadal effect on the tumor exists. In an earlier preliminary study [7], the *in vitro* growth of MMT cells was inhibited by Wy-40,972 in an apparent dose-related fashion. Recently, Hierowski et al. [20] reported that an LH-RH agonist and antagonist can bind to Dunning R3327H prostatic tumors, thus presupposing the presence of LH-RH-like receptors. Interestingly, normal rat prostatic tissues showed no such binding capacities. These authors suggest that the process of carcinogenesis produces structural and compositional membrane alterations which give rise to prostatic LH-RH-like binding sites. Thus, perhaps an LH-RH analog can influence the growth of a prostatic tumor directly, as an ancillary mechanism.

The plethora of recent clinical reports underscores the enthusiasm generated by the application of the LH-RH agonists as a first-line management of hormone-responsive prostatic cancer [5, 23, 45, 46, 47]. Whether the LH-RH analogs have clinical application to the treatment of benign prostatic hypertrophy must await the results of future investigations.

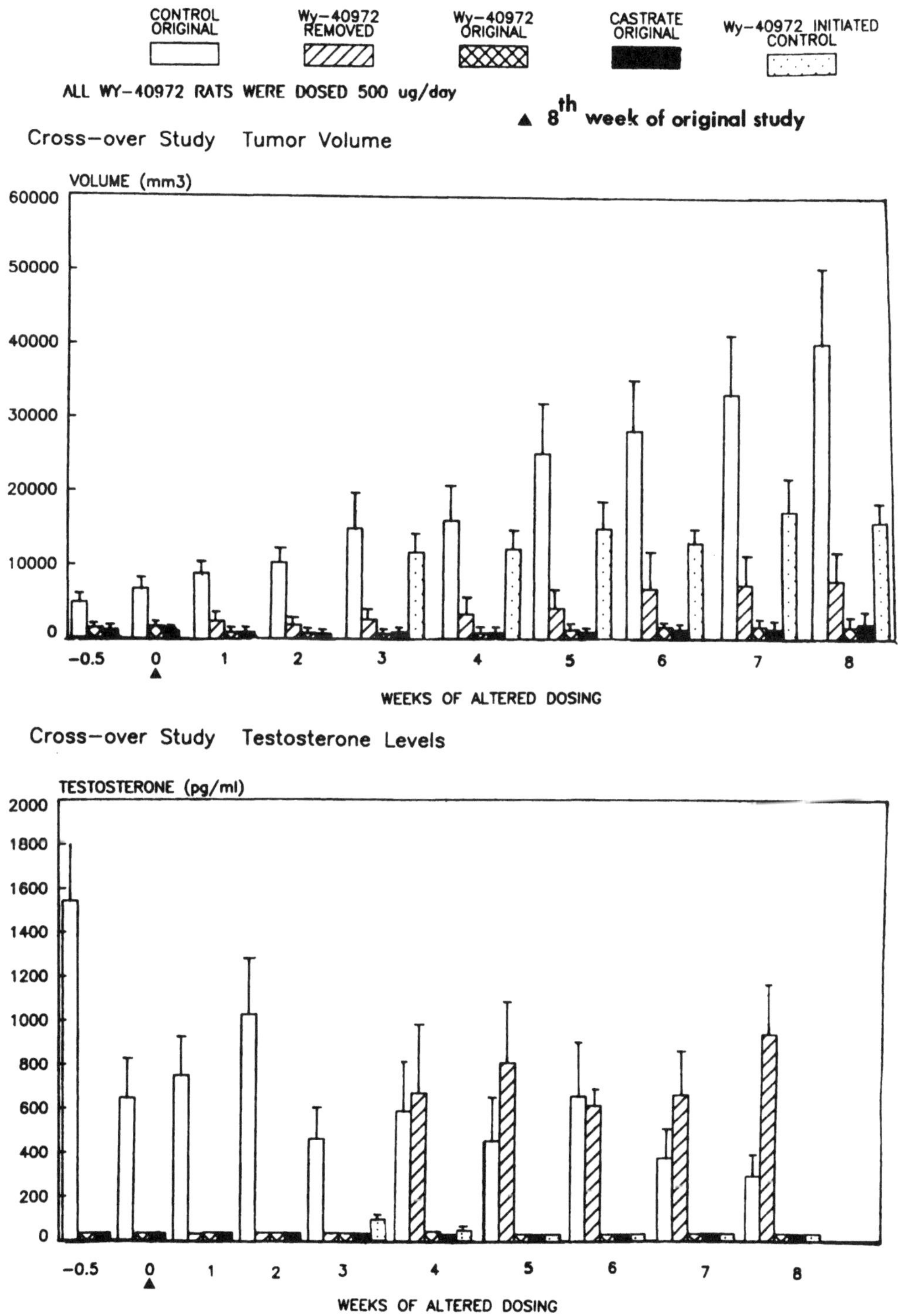

Fig. 25 Effect of Wy-40,972 on androgen-dependent prostatic tumor (Dunning R-3327) growth in male rats: cross-over study. Tumor volume and serum testosterone.

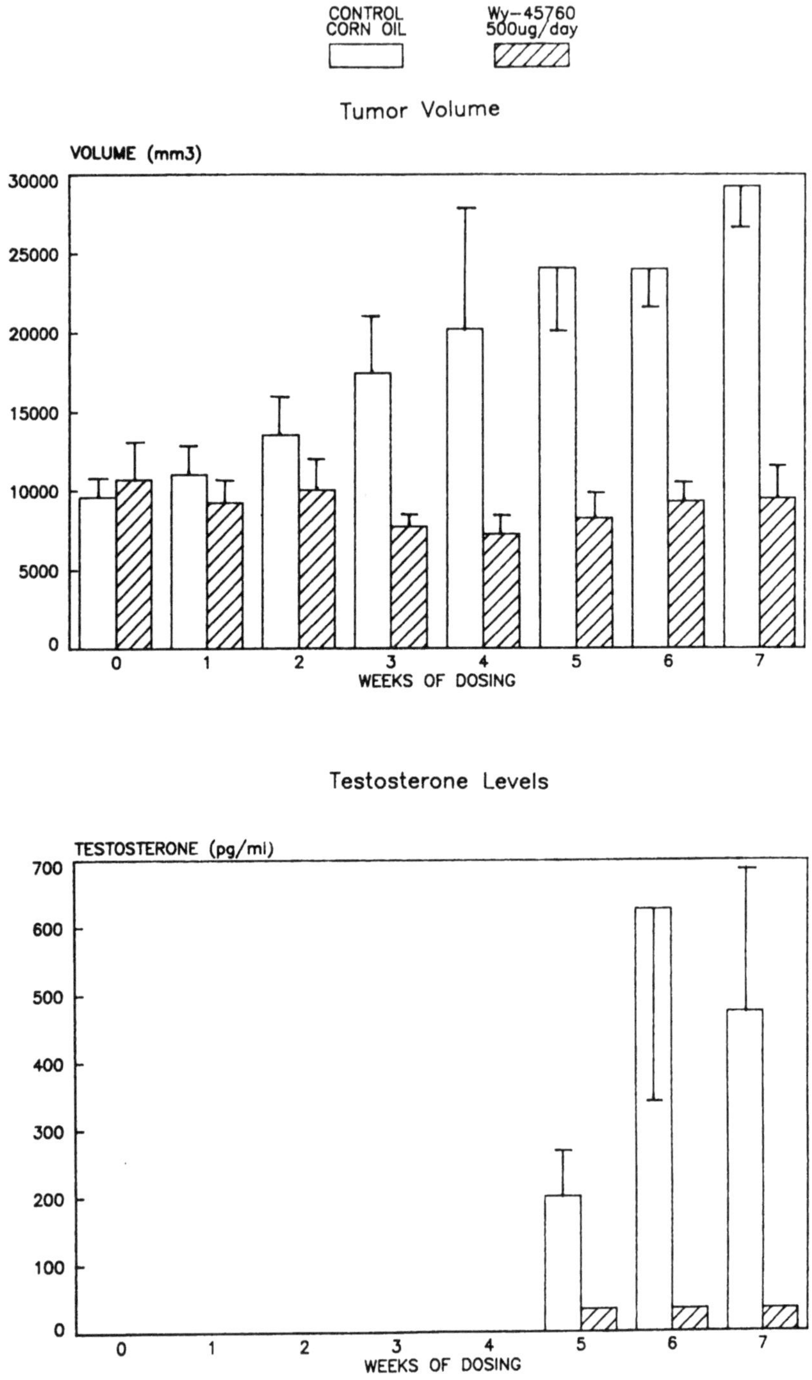

Fig. 26 Effect of Wy-45;760 on prostatic tumor (Dunning R-3327) growth in rat: tumor volume and serum testosterone.

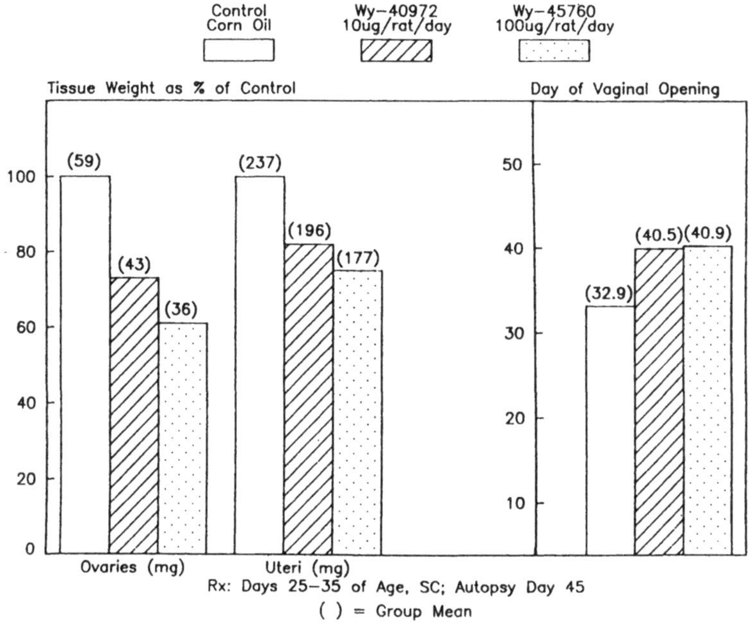

Fig. 27 Effect of LHRH agonist and antagonist on puberty in immature female rats.

Pubertal Inhibition

Several studies have demonstrated that the LH-RH agonists can retard the advent of puberty in female and male rats [3, 7–9, 24, 40, 44]. The chronic non-pulsatile treatment of prepubertal animals retards the functional gonadotropic capacity of the pituitary, leading to maintained gonadal-target organ immaturity. Such anti-reproductive effects in the very young animal have had far-reaching application in the treatment of human idiopathic precocious puberty [13, 15].

In the female rat, vaginal canalization is a sensitive index of pubertal onset. Figure 27 shows that sub-acute treatment with either an agonist (Wy-40,972) or an antagonist (Wy-45,760) from days 25–35 of age delays vaginal opening, and retards the normal gravimetric progression of the ovaries and uteri as determined on age day 45, ten days after treatment had ceased. The antagonist appeared to be more effective than the agonist regarding the organ weights. In fact, as long as the animal is exposed to an agonist, for example, reproductive retardation remains; as soon as treatment is halted, reproductive organ weight and function rebound rapidly, and estrous cyclic patterns are established within 8–10 days (approximately 2 cycle lengths).

In the male rat, both the agonist and antagonist were quite effective in retarding sexual development (fig. 28). In fact, the reproductive-retarding effect of the antagonist far exceeded that of the agonist. Of particular note is that the agonist, in spite of

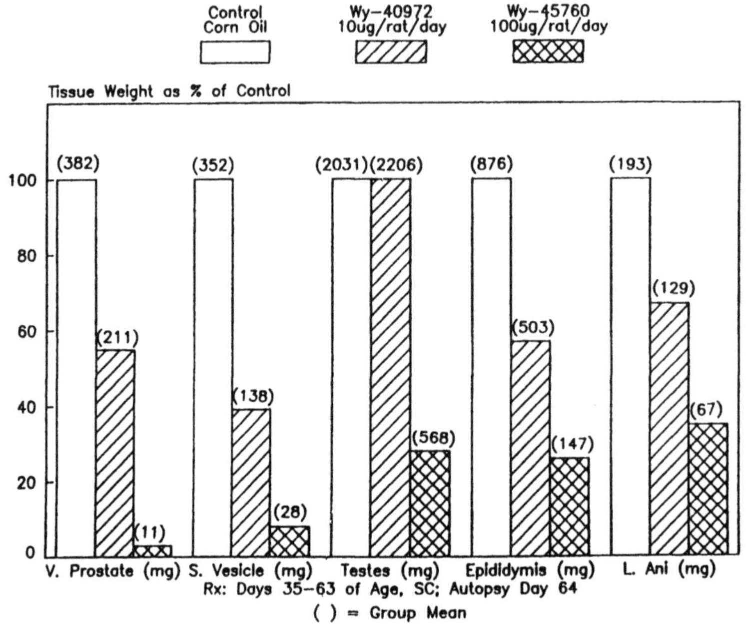

Fig. 28 Effect of LHRH agonist and antagonist on puberty in immature male rats.

having no effect on testicular weight, still produced inhibition of the androgen-dependent organs.

The fact that the antagonist produced a more pronounced suppression of the reproductive axis than did the agonist in these immature animals may be a reflection of the differing mechanisms of action: the antagonist may cause an immediate inhibition of LH/testosterone secretion by virtue of its competitive blockade of pituitary LH-RH receptors (and perhaps of the hypothalamic gonadostat), whereas the agonist required a longer period to induce pituitary and testicular down-regulation/desensitization during a less sensitive (prepubertal) phase of the animal's reproductive continuum [42].

Safety evaluation

Toxicology, ancillary pharmacology, reversibility, metabolism

LH-RH and numerous agonistic analogs have been subjected to a wide array of tests in several female and male animal species (rat, mouse, rabbit, dog, primate). These tests have been performed acutely and chronically using various routes of administration (e.g., iv, im, sc, intranasally) at doses in considerable excess of those producing the primary and therapeutically desired reproductive effects [10, 11, 18, 36].

Aside from the traditional and predictable effects observed on the reproductive tract, no deleterious, overt, toxic and biologically important effects have been noted on non-reproductive endocrine endpoints or on the central nervous system, gastrointestinal tract, cardiovascular and pulmonary systems, immunologic system, or the hepatic and renal systems. There is no teratogenic liability, and reversibility and recovery from the chronic antireproductive effects (in both sexes, including humans) of these compounds are relatively rapid and complete.

The development of new methodologies including specific radioimmunoassay systems as well as sophisticated extraction and chromatographic procedures have contributed much to our understanding of the metabolic fate of LH-RH and its agonists [35]. Although potencies depend on both binding characteristics and resistance to enzymatic degradation, these peptides are relatively rapidly inactivated and appear in the periphery shortly after administration as biologically inactive fragments. In particular, the processes that the agonists initiate (LH-release, antigonadal effects) persist far longer than their detectable blood levels. Resistance to degradation may be a more important factor for antagonist activity. Due to rapid inactivation and clearance of the LH-releasing peptides there is no evidence for accumulation or antibody formation [16] upon chronic administration that can account for the rapid reversal of their effects upon discontinuance of treatment.

The information regarding the safety of the LH-RH antagonists is relatively limited. Daily subcutaneous doses of approximately 1500 μg/kg of the aforementioned antagonists, under the conditions of the above experiments, to male and female rats for 28 days produces no apparent effects outside the reproductive tract; no compromise to other organ systems is evident. In clinical studies employing several different antagonists, single intramuscular doses as high as 90 mg in both men and women, er 80 μg/kg intravenously, produced no untoward side effects [4, 37].

Collectively, the LH-RH analogs, as a specific and selectively-acting chemical class, are well-tolerated, safe and do not compromise non-reproductive endocrine and non-endocrine physiological systems; they provide a wide and outstanding therapeutic margin apparently unprecedented in pharmacologic research, substantiated by a plethora of animal and clinical investigations.

Overview

The chemical identification and synthesis of the hypothalamic hormone, LH-RH, has led to the generation of over 1600 analogs during this past decade. As a result, numerous highly potent peptidic derivatives have become available, either as LH-RH agonists or antagonists, that have received considerable pharmacologic evaluation as potential fertility-regulating agents.

The antagonists, by virtue of their ability to competitively inhibit LH-RH, have received attention as inhibitors of ovulation. Only recently have antagonists of sufficient potency become available to enable their broader pharmacologic evaluation as for the agonists. In contrast, the "super" agonists possess a more complex reproductive pharmacologic profile, and have been studied for their pro-fertility (conceptive) potential in hyporeproductive states, and more extensively, for their paradoxical contraceptive promise. In the latter case, a plethora of animal and clinical studies has demonstrated that these agonists can inhibit reproductive processes in both females and males, as evidenced by gonadotropin hypersecretion, pituitary desensitization, ovulation inhibition, gonadal downregulation, steroidogenic inhibition, luteolysis, interference with estrous and menstrual cycles, early onset of menses, pregnancy termination, retardation of puberty and spermatogenic inhibition.

In animal and clinical safety studies, the agonists (and to a limited extent, the antagonists) have been observed to be well-tolerated and free of untoward side effects at efficacious doses. Any undesirable side effects observed during toxicologic, pathologic and secondary (non-reproductive) pharmacologic testing, in a variety of animal models, associated with varied dosing regimens and routes of administration, have occurred at doses in considerable excess of those required for practical and utilitarian application. Thus, these compounds provide excellent therapeutic margins.

In human males, the agonist-induced testosterone inhibition and resultant loss of libido and potency has discouraged agonist development as a male contraceptive.

Extensive clinical studies, employing chronic nasal delivery of the agonists to females, reinforce continued support of this novel approach to contraception. Trials are in progress to establish practical routes of administration and dosing strategies (e.g. discontinuous treatment in which the agonist is administered for 3 weeks, followed by abbreviated treatment with a progestational agent) [19] to optimize contraceptive efficacy, reliability, predictability, cycle control, and patient compliance.

The original concept that LH-RH and derivatives would be useful as fertility-regulating agents, and moreover provide a novel approach to contraception, now has been extended to include other areas of potential clinical therapeutic utility. The basic animal studies on these molecules have guided us from the conceptive and contraceptive realm into novel and realistic therapeutic applications, including the potential management of an array of reproductive endocrinopathies.

Based on the animal studies herein described, in terms of the various experimental models (tab. 1), both the representative agonist and antagonist were active in the several tests employed. Overall, in terms of dose and time requirements, the agonist would appear to be more effective in producing the various contraceptive and therapeutic responses. Furthermore, the possibility exists that the antagonists might be used in conjunction with the agonist in treating the various gonadal-steroid based

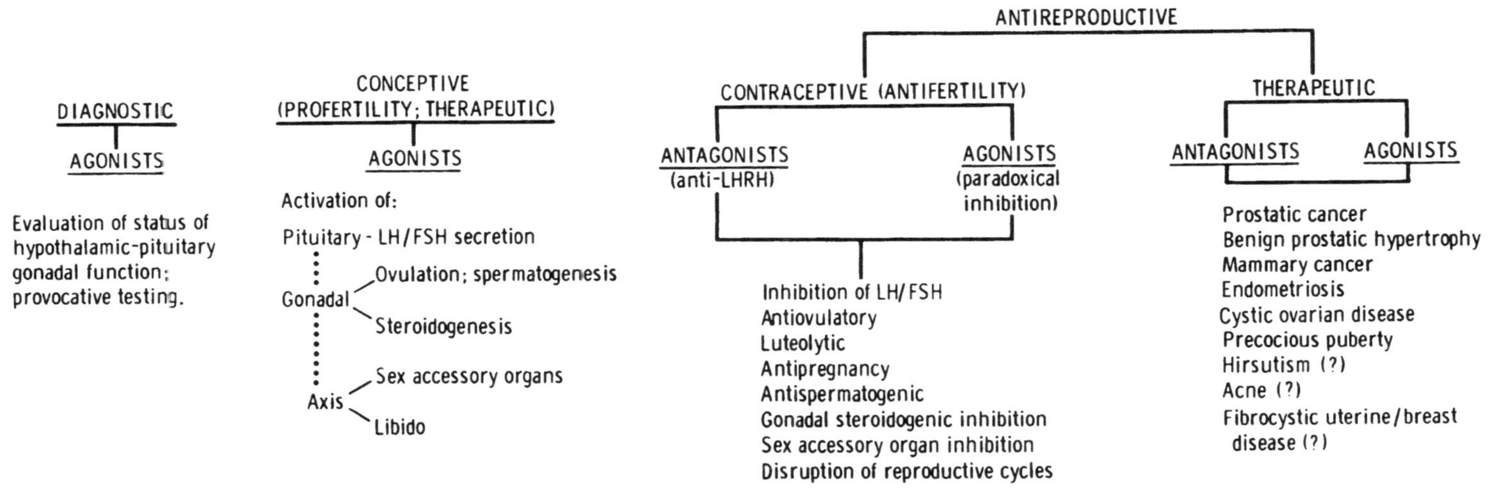

Fig. 29 An overview of the developmental aspects of the reproductive pharmacology of LHRH and analogs.

pathologies: primary treatment with the antagonist will produce an initial decline in the supportive hormones (thereby avoiding the early phase of exacerbation purported to occur with the agonists), followed by continuous administration of the agonist alone to maintain the hyposteroidal state. On the other hand, the introduction of an anti-androgen, for example, co-administered with an agonist [27], during early therapy of prostatic carcinoma, might eliminate the potential need for an antagonist in this disease's management.

Use of the inhibitory (steroid-lowering) properties has been extended to cancer therapy based on the ability of the LH-RH analogs (particularly the agonists) to inhibit the growth of steroid-dependent tumors (e.g., mammary, prostate) similar to that produced by gonadectomy and antisteroid treatments. The use of these peptides for selected hormone-sensitive tumors, as well as for endometriosis, cystic ovarian disease and precocious puberty, presents novel pharmaco-therapeutic applications for this class of drug that are receiving expanded clinical evaluation. Whether the LH-RH antagonists can provide advantages over the agonists in the various clinical settings must await the results of extensive human investigations.

An overview of the application of the LH-RH analogs to the reproductive domain is presented in figure 29.

Acknowledgments

The excellent technical assistance of the following associates is gratefully acknowledged: S. Caltabiano, K. Koch-Michalak, L. Lofton, and C. Marchione. We thank Drs. R. Sharma and E. Carlisle of our Pathology Section for the histomorphologic evaluation of the testicular sections.

References

[1] Bex, F. J., A. Corbin: In "Reproductive Processes and Contraception" (Ed. K. W. McKerns), pp. 109–141. Plenum Publishing Corp., New York 1981.
[2] Bex, F., A. Corbin: In "Hormone Antagonists" (Ed. M. K. Agarwal), pp. 609–622. Walter de Gruyter, Berlin 1982.
[3] Bex, F. J., A. Corbin: In "Frontiers in Neuroendocrinology" (Eds. W. F. Ganong, L. Martini), vol. 8. Raven Press, New York 1984.
[4] Cetal, N. S., J. Rivier, W. Vale et al.: J. Clin. Endocrinol. 57 (1983) 62–62.
[5] Corbin, A.: Yale, J. Biol. Med. 55 (1982) 27–47.
[6] Corbin, A., C. W. Beattie: Endocr. Res. Commun. 2 (1975) 445–458.
[7] Corbin, A., C. W. Beattie, R. Jones et al.: Int. J. Gynaecol. Obstet. 16 (1979) 359–372.
[8] Corbin, A., C. W. Beattie, J. Tracy et al.: Int. J. Fertil. 23 (1978) 81–92.
[9] Corbin, A., F. J. Bex: In "Regulation of Male Fertility" (Eds. G. R. Cunningham, W. B. Schill, E. S. E. Hafez), pp. 55–63. Martinus Nijhoff Publisher bv., The Hague 1980.

[10] Corbin, A., F. J. Bex: In "Progress in Hormone Biochemistry and Pharmacology" (Eds. M. Briggs, A. Corbin), vol. 1, pp. 227–297. Eden Press, Montreal 1980.
[11] Corbin, A., F. J. Bex: In "LH-RH Peptides as Female and Male Contraceptives, PARFR Series in Fertility Regulation" (Eds. G. I. Zatuchni, J. D. Shelton, J. J. Sciarra), pp. 68–84. Harper and Row, Philadelphia 1981.
[12] Corbin, A., F. J. Bex, J. P. Yardley et al.: Endocr. Res. Commun. **6** (1979) 1–14.
[13] Crowley, Jr., W. F., F. Comite, W. Vale et al.: J. Clin. Endocrinol. Metab. **52** (1981) 370–372.
[14] Daniel, Jr., J. C., P. K. William-Boyce: In "Methods in Mammalian Reproduction" (Ed. J. C. Daniel, Jr.), pp. 545–558. Academic Press, New York 1978.
[15] Facts About Precocious Puberty. Office of Research Reporting, NICHD, National Institutes of Health Document, 1983.
[16] Fraser, H. M., J. Sandow, B. Krauss: Acta. Endocrin. **103** (1983) 151–157.
[17] Furr, B. J. A., R. I. Nicholson: J. Reprod. Fert. **64** (1982) 529–539.
[18] Garay, G. L., M. B. Wallach, A. P. Roszkowski et al.: In "LH-RH Peptides as Female and Male Contraceptives. PARFR Series on Fertility Regulation" (Eds. G. I. Zatuchni, J. D. Shelton, J. J. Sciarra), pp. 355–359. Harper and Row, Philadelphia 1981.
[19] Hardt, W., K. Schmidt-Gollwitzer, J. Nevinny-Stickel et al.: Geburtshilfe Frauenheilkd. **42** (1982) 874–877.
[20] Hierowski, M., B. Altamirano, T. W. Redding et al.: Febs. Lett. **154** (1983) 92–96.
[21] Hsueh, A. J. W., P. B. C. Jones: Endocrine Rev. **2** (1981) 437–461.
[22] Hsueh, A. J. W., P. B. C. Jones: Ann. Rev. Physiol. **45** (1983) 83–94.
[23] Jacobi, G. H., U. K. Wenderoth: Eur. Urol. **8** (1982) 129–134.
[24] Johnson. E. S., L. Gendrich, W. F. White: Fertil. Steril. **27** (1976) 853–860.
[25] Jones, R. C.: J. Reprod. Fert. (1984) (submitted for publication).
[26] Labrie, F., A. Bélanger, P. A. Kelly et al.: Prog. Clin. Biol. Res. **74** (1981) 273–291.
[27] Labrie, F., A. Dupont, A. Bélanger et al.: Clin. Invest. Med. **5** (1982) 267–275.
[28] Labrie, F., M. Godbout, A. Bélanger et al.: In "LH-RH Peptides as Female and Male Contraceptives. PARFR Series in Fertility Regulation" (Eds. G. I. Zatuchni, J. D. Shelton, J. J. Sciarra), pp. 246–260. Harper and Row, Philadelphia 1981.
[29] Lemay, A., G. Quesnel: Fertil. Steril. **38** (1982) 376–379.
[30] Meldrum, D. R., R. J. Chang, J. Lu: J. Clin. Endocrinol. Metab. **54** (1982) 1081–1083.
[31] Patanelli, D. J.: In "LH-RH Peptides as Female and Male Contraceptives. PARFR Series in Fertility Regulation" (Eds. G. I. Zatuchni, J. D. Shelton, J. J. Sciarra), pp. 290–292. Harper and Row, Philadelphia 1981.
[32] Redding, T. W., A. V. Schally: Proc. Natl. Acad. Sci. **80** (1983) 1459–1462.
[32a] Rivier, C., J. Rivier, M. Perrin et al.: Biol. Reprod. **29** (1983) 374–378.
[33] Rivier, C., J. Rivier, W. Vale: Science **210** (1980) 93–95.
[34] Sandow, J.: In "Neuroendocrine Perspectives" (Eds. E. E. Muller, R. M. MacLeod), vol. 1, pp. 339–393. Elsevier Biomedical Press, Amsterdam 1982.
[35] Sandow, J., R. N. Clayton: In "Progress in Hormone Biochemistry and Pharmacology" (Eds. M. Briggs, A. Corbin), vol. 2, pp. 63–106. Eden Press, Montreal 1983.
[36] Sandow, J., W. V. Rechenberg, W. Konig et al.: In "Hypothalamic Hormones-Chemistry, Physiology, and Clinical Application" (Eds. D. Gupta, W. Voelter), pp. 307–326. Verlag Chemie, Weinheim 1978.
[37] Schally, A. V.: Res. Front. Fertil. Regul. **2** (1983) 1–16.
[38] Schally, A. V., D. H. Coy: In "Role of Peptides and Proteins in Control of Reproduction" (Eds. S. M. McCann, D. S. Dhindsa), pp. 89–110. Elsevier Biomedical Press, New York 1983.
[39] Schally, A. V., T. W. Redding, A. M. Comaru-Schally: Proceedings of the Prostate Cancer Project Workshop, Buffalo, New York, March 21–23, 1983. The Prostate, 1984 (in press).
[40] Sharpe, R. M., H. M. Fraser: J. Reprod. Fert. **60** (1980) 359–368.

[41] Shessel, F. S., L. Block, B. Stover et al.: Invest. Urol. **17** (1980) 531–533.
[42] Steger, R. W.: Pharmac. Ther. **17** (1982) 1–64.
[43] Vickery, B. H.: In "LH-RH Peptides as Female and Male Contraceptives. PARFR Series in Fertility Regulation" (Eds. G. I. Zatuchni, J. D. Shelton, J. J. Sciarra), pp. 275–290. Harper and Row, Philadelphia 1981.
[44] Vilchez-Martinez, J. A., E. Pedroza, A. Arimura et al.: Fertil. Steril. **31** (1979) 677–682.
[45] Warner, B., T. J. Worgul, J. Drago et al.: J. Clin. Invest. **71** (1983) 1842–1853.
[46] Waxman, J.: Brit. Med. J. **286** (1983) 1899.
[47] Waxman, J. H., J. A. H. Wass, W. F. Hendry et al: Brit. Med. J. **286** (1983) 1309–1312.
[48] Werlin, L. B., G. D. Hodgen: Endocrinology **56** (1983) 844–848.
[49] Yen, S. S. C.: Fertil. Steril. **39** (1983) 257–266.
[50] Zatuchni, G. I., J. D. Shelton, J. J. Sciarra (Eds.): LH-RH Peptides as Female and Male Contraceptives. PARFR Series on Fertility Regulation, pp. 1–146. Harper and Row, Philadelphia 1981.

Comparative non-human primate studies with LH-RH analogues

R. H. Asch, J. P. Balmaceda

Introduction

Luteinizing hormone releasing hormone (LH-RH) antagonists are compounds, chemically related to the original structure of the hypothalamic decapeptide, that bind to LH-RH receptors at the pituitary gonadotrope and, consequently, inhibit both the secretion and release of the gonadotropins, follicle stimulating hormone (FSH) and luteinizing hormone (LH) [1, 2]. Since their original theoretical conception by Kastin et al. in 1971 [3], considerable progress has been accomplished to suggest that these compounds present a promising future in the treatment of clinical conditions in which suppression of gonadotropin secretion is desired.

Unfortunately, most of the research carried out until the present has been performed in small laboratory animals [4–7], and only occassionally in human or non-human primates [8–11].

The objective of this chapter is to present an update of the progress of our research in the study of the effects of LH-RH antagonists in non-human primates during the last four years. For that purpose, we have divided the topic into three sections:

- Basic studies of the effects of LH-RH antagonists on gonadotropins.
- Studies on the effects of LH-RH antagonists in the menstrual cycle.
- Studies on the effects of LH-RH antagonists in the adult male rhesus monkey.

Basic studies of the effects of LH-RH antagonists on gonadotropins

Serum gonadotropins after the administration of an LH-RH antagonist to oophorectomized rhesus monkeys [12]

The purpose of this study was to examine the temporal changes in FSH and LH concentrations induced by the administration to castrated female rhesus monkeys of a potent LH-RH inhibitory analogue and to determine its effect on the pituitary response to LH-RH challenges.

Serum concentrations of FSH and LH decreased significantly in all four animals after the administration of ([N-Ac-D-$Trp^{1,3}$,D-p-Cl-Phe^{2},D-Phe^{6},D-Ala^{10}]-LH-RH). Mean FSH serum concentrations decreased to 70% by 4 h and to 80% by 24 h and remained significantly lower than baseline values for up to 72 h following the administration of the inhibitory analogue of LH-RH.

Serum levels of LH also dropped significantly, but followed a different pattern. Concentrations of LH were significantly lower than the baseline levels as early as 2 h after the injection of the inhibitory analogue of LH-RH (44%) and continued to decrease to 64% by 24 h. However, in three of the four animals, LH serum levels increased to values markedly higher than the baseline 48 h after antagonist administration. The fourth monkey presented a similar elevation 72 h after injection of the LH-RH antagonist.

In the control animals, serum FSH and LH increased to levels significantly higher than baseline ten minutes after LH-RH administration. Maximum mean serum levels for both gonadotropins were reached 20 min after the LH-RH injection and they returned to baseline concentrations at approximately 120 min.

When the monkeys received LH-RH 2 h after the injection of the inhibitory analogue of LH-RH, the increase in serum concentrations of FSH and LH was not significantly different from that observed in the control group. Both gonadotropins were elevated significantly 10 min after the administration of LH-RH and returned to baseline levels by 120 minutes. However, when LH-RH was administered 18 h after the inhibitory analogue of LH-RH, serum concentrations of FSH and LH presented a significantly smaller, as well as delayed, response to the injection of LH-RH, compared to controls. It is interesting to note that, even during the LH-RH challenge test, none of the animals reached FSH or LH levels within the range of baseline (prior to injection of LH-RH inhibitory analogue).

Effects of an inhibitory analogue of LH-RH on the postcastration rise of LH and FSH in female rhesus monkeys [13]

The purpose of this study was to examine the ability of an LH-RH antagonist to affect the post-oophorectomy rise of FSH and LH in rhesus monkeys.

In control animals (vehicle-treated), LH and FSH consistently rose from precastration levels as soon as 3–4 days after surgery ($P < 0.01$). Gonadotropins continued to rise until a plateau was reached, 3–7 times baseline levels, between days 8 and 22 after oophorectomy. A similar trend was observed for both LH and FSH concentrations. The course of gonadotropin increase in this group was identical to that observed previously in non-treated regularly cycling rhesus monkeys after bilateral oophorectomy. In contrast, the release of gonadotropins after castration was profoundly altered by the daily administration of ([N-Ac-D-$Trp^{1,3}$,D-p-Cl-Phe^{2},D-Phe^{6},D-Ala^{10}]-LH-RH). Two to four days following the discontinuation of LH-RH antagonist administration, FSH and LH concentrations were significantly higher than the baseline levels ($P < 0.05$). Gonadotropin levels continued to rise reaching a plateau between 22 and 28 days after castration, (12–18 days after the discontinuation of the LH-RH antagonist administration). This magnitude was similiar to that observed in controls (2–6 times baseline levels).

Administration of an LH-RH inhibitory analogue inhibits the positive feedback of estradiol benzoate on gonadotropin secretion in rhesus monkeys [14]

The purpose of this study was to determine if a potent inhibitory analogue of LH-RH could alter the biphasic action of estradiol on FSH and LH levels in oophorectomized rhesus monkeys.

Estrogens cause a biphasic effect on gonadotropin (FSH and LH) secretion in human and non-human primates. Recent studies suggest that estrogens induce a negative as well as a positive feedback on gonadotropins by a direct action at the pituitary gland. To further investigate the intrinsic mechanism by which estrogens modulate gonadotropin secretion, the following experiments were performed: Oophorectomized rhesus monkeys were injected with estradiol benzoate (EB) at a dose of 40 μg/kg s.c. at 0 time (controls). Three groups of animals received, additionally, an inhibitory analogue of LH-RH, ([N-Ac-D-$Trp^{1,3}$,D-p-Cl-Phe^{2},D-Phe^{6},D-Ala^{10}]-LH-RH) daily at 1. −48 to 48 h, 2. 0 to 48 h and 3. 24 to 48 h from EB, respectively. Blood was collected at −72, −48, −24, and 0 h, every 6 h from 6–84 h and at 96 and 116 h following EB; FSH and LH levels were measured by RIA.

Control animals revealed a 70–80% decrease in baseline FSH and LH levels during the first 24 h after EB injection, followed by a sharp rise to 60–80% above basal levels at 42–48 h post-EB. In contrast, animals that received the inhibitory analogue of LH-RH in different regimes showed a more pronounced and prolonged negative feedback of EB on gonadotropin concentrations. The positive feedback release of FSH and LH was significantly diminished or delayed when compared to controls.

The results of this study indicate that this inhibitory analogue of LH-RH potentiates the negative feedback and suppresses the positive feedback of EB on gonadotropins, suggesting that estrogens induce the secretion of FSH and LH through a mechanism that involves the action of LH-RH at the pituitary gonadotrope.

Inhibition of the pulsatile secretion of LH and FSH in rhesus monkeys by administration of a LH-RH antagonist [15]

The pulsatility of luteinizing hormone (LH) and follicle stimulating hormone (FSH) secretion was evaluated in chronically ovariectomized rhesus monkeys before and after the administration of ([N-Ac-D-$Trp^{1,3}$,D-p-Cl-Phe^{2},D-Phe^{6},D-Ala^{10}]-LH-RH) (IA-LH-RH). Animals were divided into three groups receiving, s.c.: 1. vehicle only (controls); 2. 0.5 mg IA-LH-RH; and 3. 2 mg IA-LH-RH. Twelve hours following drug administration, animals were chair-restrained and blood samples drawn every 10 min over a period of 4 h via indwelling femoral vein catheters. LH and FSH levels were measured by RIA to determine the frequency, amplitude and increment of the pulses. Twelve hours after the administration of 0.5 mg of 2.0 mg of IA-LH-RH, levels of LH were reduced by 30% and 68% (P <0.001) and those of FSG by 34% and 53% (P <0.001 and P <0.002), respectively. Doses of 0.5 mg IA-LH-RH decreased the amplitude (20%; P <0.001), increment (17 ng/ml; P <0.001) and frequency 2 per 4 h; P <0.001) of LH pulses. Administration of 2 mg IA-LH-RH produced a fall of increment (8 ng/ml; P <0.001(, frequency (1 per 4 h; P <0.001) and pulse amplitude (26%; P <0.001). In vehicle-treated animals, FSH pulses occurred at intervals of approximately 60–80 min, with an amplitude of 13% of baseline levels and an increment mean of 3.142 ng/ml. Doses of 0.5 mg IA-LH-RH decreased the increment significantly (1659 ng/ml; P <01001); however, neither the frequency (2.6 per 4 h) nor the amplitude (P <0.5) of FSH pulses was significantly altered following administration of the LH-RH antagonist. Treatment with 2 mg IA-LH-RH markedly decreased the frequency (1.75 per 4 h; P <0.001), the amplitude (9%; P <0.05) and the increment (1058 ng/ml; P <0.001) of LH pulses.

Comparison of intranasal and subcutaneous administration of an LH-RH antagonist on circulating levels of FSH and LH in oophorectomized rhesus monkeys [16]

Even though LH-RH agonists have been successfully administered by other than systemic routes (oral, intranasal and vaginal), there is no evidence that inhibitory analogues may be used in any form other than injectable. In the present study we compared the effects on the gondadotropin levels in oophorectomized monkeys of two forms of administration of the LH-RH antagonist ([N-Ac-D-$Trp^{1,3}$,D-p-Cl-Phe^{2}, D-Arg^{6},D-Ala^{10}]-LH-RH): 1. subcutaneous (0.05, 0.2 and 1 mg) and 2. intranasal (0.2, 1 and 5 mg) in a single dose. After subcutaneous administration of the antagonist, FSG and LS exhibited, as soon as 1 h after the injection, a dose-response decrease which lasted for up to 12 h. The magnitude of the decrease ranged from 23–40% and 42–59% (0.2–1 mg) for FSH and LH, respectively. Intranasal administration of LH-RH antagonist induced a significant fall of serum FSG and LH – 19–39% and 32–52%, respectively (1–5 mg). These decreases were dose-related and lasted for up to 12 h. Analysis of the data revealed that the bioavailability of the intranasal route versus the subcutaneous ranged from 16–26%. This high effectiveness of the intranasal route is markedly greater than that previously reported for LH-RH agonists (1%) and is probably due to a resistance to enzymatic hydrolysis in the nasal mucosa. These results show for the first time that antagonists of LH-RH can be administered by other than injectable routes, increasing their potential clinical use in conditions in which inhibition of gonadotropins is desired, as in contraception and the treatment of endometriosis, precocious puberty, and hormone-dependent neoplasms.

Studies on the effects of LH-RH antagonists in the menstrual cycle

Administration of LH-RH analogues during the early follicular phase of the rhesus monkey menstrual cycle [17]

It has been reported that administration of the LH-RH agonist during the early follicular phase of the menstrual cycle disrupts normal gonadotropin secretion and induces inadequate luteal phases [18]. However, other laboratories have not been able to confirm those observations [19]. To aid in settling the controversy, the present experiment was designed. Regularly cycling rhesus monkeys received the administration of either 1. a potent LH-RH agonist, D-Trp^6-LH-RH 20 μg/day, 2. a potent LH-RH antagonist ([N-Ac-D-Trp^{1,3},D-p-Cl-Phe^2,D-Phe^6,D-Ala^{10}]-LH-RH), 1 mg/day or 3. vehicle, from day 1 to 6 of the menstrual cycle. While controls showed normal cycles by dates of ovulation, length of luteal phases and hormonal profiles, animals treated with either analogue of LH-RH presented disruption of the menstrual cycles. Animals from both groups presented delayed ovulation (LH-RH agonist = 22, 23, 17, 19, 20 of the cycle. LH-RH antagonist = 22, 22, 24, and 20 days of the cycle and one animal remained anovulatory for 65 days) (fig. 1). Monkeys treated with either LH-RH analogue presented normal serum progesterone concentrations and luteal phase lengths (15, 15, 16, 14, 15 days and 15, 16, 16 and 13 days, respectively). In conclusion, the administration of LH-RH analogues during the early follicular phase disrupts gonadotropin secretion and delays ovulation without inducing luteal phase defects.

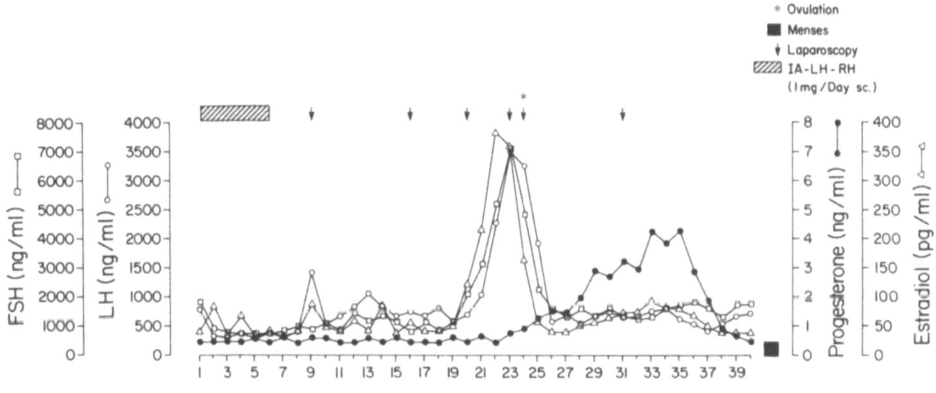

Fig. 1 Serum concentrations of FSH, LH, progesterone and estradiol in a regularly cycling rhesus monkey that received an LHRH antagonist (IA-LHRH) from day 1 to 6 of the menstrual cycle. Note, the delayed ovulation and normal luteal function.

Administration of an LH-RH inhibitory analogue in the preovulatory period of the rhesus monkeys menstrual cycle [20]

The purpose of this study was to determine the effects of a potent LH-RH antagonist ([N-Ac-D-Trp^{1,3},D-p-Cl-Phe^{2},D-Phe^{6},D-Ala^{10}]-LH-RH) during the immediate preovulatory period of regularly cycling rhesus monkeys.

Seven regularly cycling rhesus monkeys were used in this experiment. The animals were followed during two consecutive cycles. During the first cycle (control), the animals did not receive any treatment and the date of ovulation was determined by measuring daily total serum estrogen levels and by serial laparoscopies. In the second cycle, the animals received 1 mg daily of the LH-RH antagonist by intramuscular injection from days 10 to 14. Blood samples were drawn daily from day 8 of the cycle until onset of menses, and the serum was used to measure total estrogens, progesterone and LH. A significant delay of the preovulatory LH peak and ovulation occurred in 5 of the 7 animals resulting in a proportional increase in cycle length as compared to the control cycle. No changes in cycle length or date of LH peak occurred in the other 2 animals. One of them did not present signs of ovulation as determined by laparoscopy (no recognizable stigma or corpus luteum = luteinized unruptured follicle). Progesterone production and length of the luteal phase were not affected by the treatment.

Administration of an LH-RH inhibitory analogue during the luteal phase of the rhesus monkeys menstrual cycle [21]

Controversy exists on the factor(s) that maintain corpus luteum function in the non-pregnant primate. To address the question of whether luteinizing hormone (LH) plays an important role, the following experiment was performed in cycling rhesus monkeys. Ovulation was determined with an accuracy of ± 12 h by serial laparoscopies and daily serum estradiol measurements. Starting on day 1 post-ovulation, animals received either a daily administration of a potent inhibitory analogue of LH-RH ([N-Ac-D-Trp^{1,3},D-p-Cl-Phe^{2},D-Phe^{6},D-Ala^{10}]-LH-RH) (n = 5), or vehicle (propylene glycol 20%, saline 80%) (n = 5) until the onset of menses. Daily measurements of serum FSH, LH, progesterone and estradiol were performed by RIA. Concentrations of FSH and LH diminished to levels ranging on the sensitivity of the assay in animals treated with the inhibitory analogue of LH-RH (concentrations of approximately 50% of controls). However, estradiol and progesterone levels did not differ between the two groups. Luteal phase lengths of animals treated with either vehicle or the LH-RH antagonist were normal (14–16 days and 14–17 days respectively). The results of this study show that the marked decrease of gonadotropin levels during the post-ovulatory period induced by an LH-RH antagonist does not alter the luteal phase in rhesus monkeys. This evidence supports studies [22] indicating that the primate corpus luteum functions independently of the postovulatory influence of LH.

Anovulation after continuous administration of agonistic and antagonistic analogues of LH-RH in *Macaca fascicularis* [23]

This study was designed to compare the effects of [N-Ac-D-Trp^{1,3},D-p-Cl-Phe^{2},D-Phe^{6},D-Ala^{10}]-LH-RH, an inhibitory analogue (IA-LH-RH), and D-Trp^{6}-LH-RH, an agonist of LH-RH, administered to normally cycling cynomologous monkeys. Animals were divided into three groups according to the drug administration: 1. 20 μg of D-Trp^{6}-LH-RH daily, 2. 1 mg of IA-LH-RH daily and 3. vehicle, daily during the first 25 days of the menstrual cycle. Ovulation was established by serial laparoscopies, serum estradiol and progesterone levels.

There was no significant delay or change in the length of the luteal phase in the control group as a result of vehicle administration. However, ovulation was suppressed or delayed markedly in the animals treated with either analogue of LH-RH. All animals treated with the LH-RH agonist or antagonist remained anovulatory during drug administration and ovulated 28, 18, 54, 20, and 28 days (fig. 2) and 7, 8, 15, 13 and 125 days, respectively, following discontinuation of the drugs. Follicular and luteal phase lenghts in the cycles following treatment were not significantly different from those observed in the control cycles.

Even though LH levels tended to be depressed in both groups during administration of LH-RH analogues, individual responses were erratic and variable. Serum levels of estradiol were, in general, below 100 pg/ml during administration of either LH-RH analogue, indicating a lack of follicular development.

The preovulatory estradiol and LH peaks that occurred after discontinuation of both LH-RH analogues were similar in amplitude to those observed in the controls.

Prior to documentation of ovulation by laparoscopic visualization, serum progesterone values remained within preovulatory ranges. When ovulation occurred after discontinuation of analogues, serum progesterone rose to levels similar to those observed in controls and in our non-treated colony.

The effect of LH-RH analogues in the histology and steroid receptors of the rhesus monkey endometrium [24]

Agonistic and antagonistic analogues of LH-RH induce an anovulatory state in several animal species, including human and non-human primates. However, some concern has been expressed regarding these possible new approaches to fertility control due to some reports that showed the occurence of endometrial hyperplasia in humans and non-human primates [25, 26]. In order to study this possibility further the following experiment was performed. We administered either 1. vehicle, 2. LH-RH agonist (D-Trp^{6} LH-RH 20 μg/day) or 3. LH-RH antagonist ([N-Ac-D-Trp^{1,3},D-p-Cl-Phe^{2},D-Phe^{6},D-Ala^{10}]-LH-RH) 200 μg/day s.c. for 90 days. Serum concentrations of FSH, LH, estradiol and progesterone were measured by RIA until 30 days

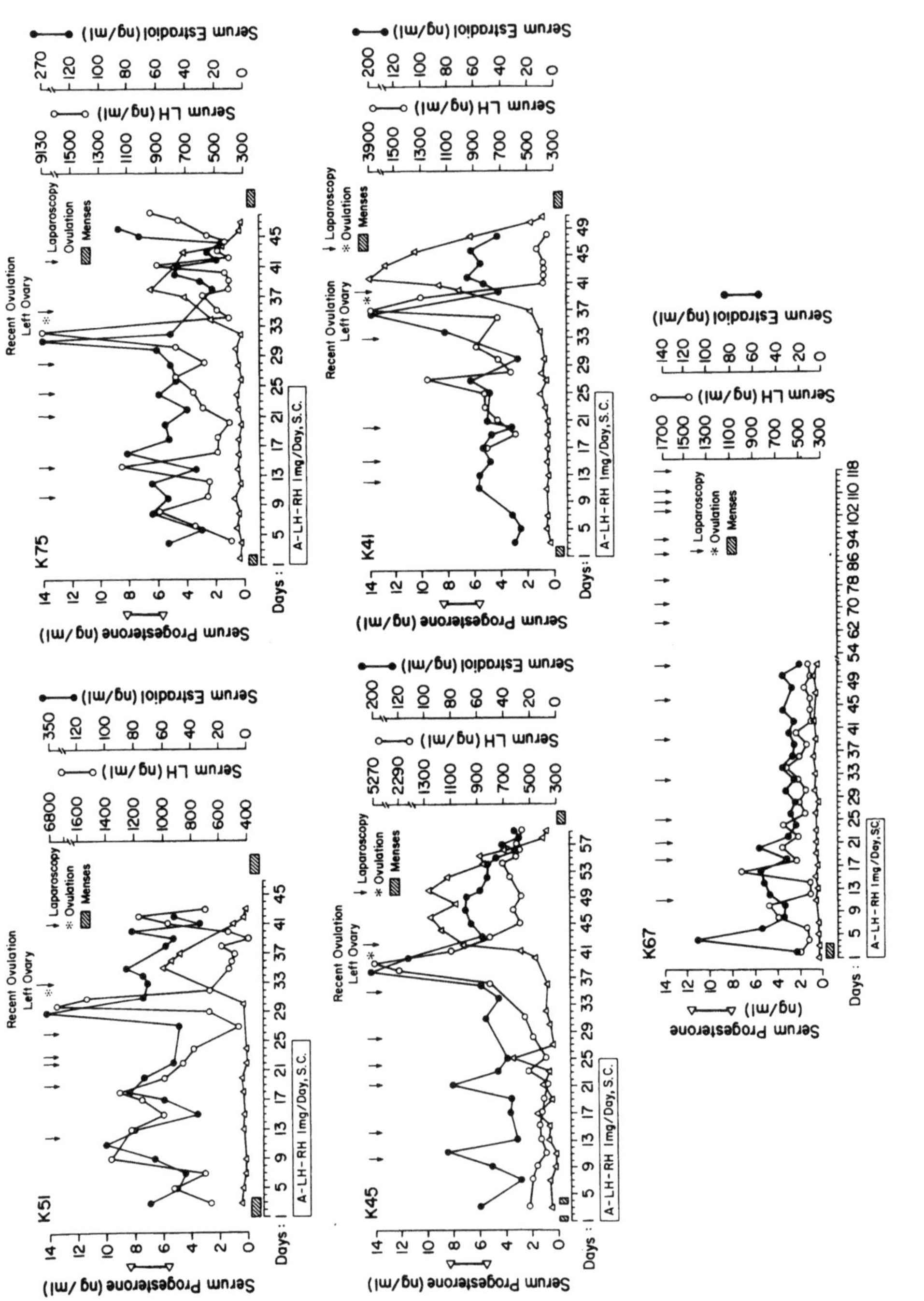

Fig. 2 Serum concentrations of progesterone, luteinizing hormone (LH) and estradiol in cycling *Macaca fascicularis* treated with an antagonist of LHRH (A-LHRH) from day 1 to 25 of the menstrual cycle. Note the consistent delay of ovulation and normal luteal phases, evidence for the postovulatory lenght and progesterone levels.

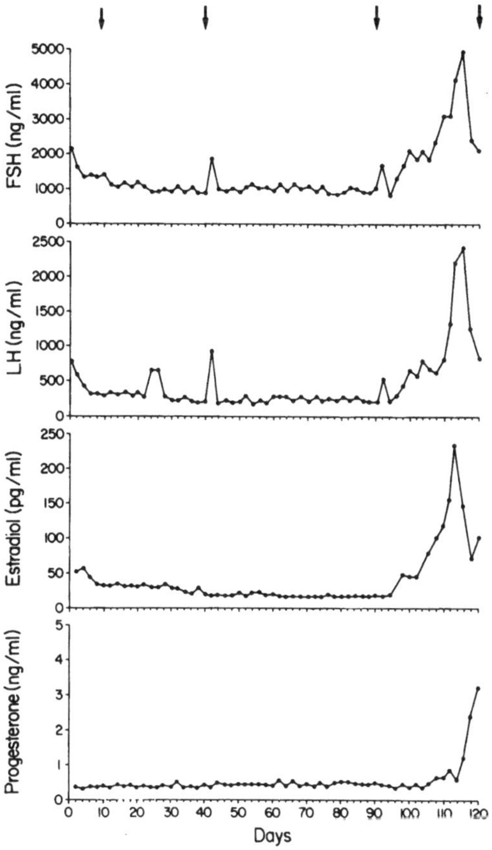

Fig. 3 Serum concentrations of follicle stimulating hormone (FSH), luteinizing hormone (LH), estradiol and progesterone in a regularly cycling animal that received continuous adminstration of an LHRH antagonist from day 1 to 90. Arrows denote when endometrial biopsies were performed. Note the lack of FSH, LH and estradiol surges and low progesterone levels demonstrating anovulation during treatment.

following the discontinuation of drug administration (fig. 3). Endometrial biopsies were obtained at days 1, 40, 90, and 120 and processed for histology (H+E) and determination of estrogen and progesterone cytosol receptors. While LH-RH agonist-treated animals presented different degrees of endometrial hyperplasia during treatment, animals that received the LH-RH antagonist showed either resting or atrophic endometrium (tab. 1). LH-RH agonist administration produced a marked increase in estrogen and progesterone endometrial receptors, while LH-RH antagonist induced a decrease in progesterone receptors (fig. 4). In both instances, reversal of the effects was observed 30 days after discontinuation of drug administration. Animals from both groups remained anovulatory during the course of drug administration.

Table 1 Endometrial histological results before (1), during (2, 3), and after (4) the treatment with vehicle, LH-RH agonist or LH-RH antagonist to rhesus monkeys

	Animal #	1	2	3	4
Group 1	E 01	Proliferative	Proliferative	Proliferative	Secretory (16–17)
(Control)	E 17	Proliferative	Proliferative	Proliferative	Proliferative
	E 21	Proliferative	Proliferative	Proliferative	Proliferative
	E 27	Proliferative	Proliferative	Proliferative	Proliferative
	A 01	Proliferative	Secretory (15–16)	Proliferative	Proliferative
Group 2	137	Proliferative	Proliferative	Hyperplasia	Proliferative
(Agonist)	C 17	Proliferative	Proliferative	Resting	Secretory (19–20)
	E 29	Proliferative	Proliferative	Hyperplasia	Secretory (16)
	J 45	Proliferative	Proliferative	Proliferative	Proliferative
	K 61	Proliferative	Resting	Hyperplasia	Secretory (17)
Group 3	195	Proliferative	Proliferative	Resting	Proliferative
(Antagonist)	312	Proliferative	Proliferative	Proliferative	Secretory (15–16)
	881	Proliferative	Resting	Atrophic	Proliferative
	973	Proliferative	Resting	Resting	Proliferative
	F 09	Proliferative	Proliferative	Resting	Secretory (17)

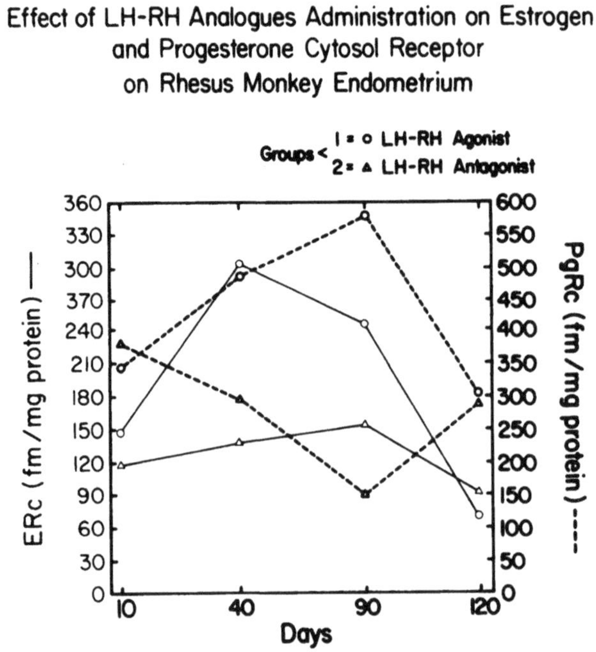

Fig. 4 Self-explanatory.

Studies on the effects of LH-RH antagonist in the adult male rhesus monkey

Inhibition of serum luteinizing hormone and testosterone with an inhibitory analgue of LH-RH in adult male rhesus monkeys [27]

The effects of single and repeated administration of a potent LH-RH inhibitory analogue (antagonist) ([N-acetyl-D-p-chloro-Phe^{1,2},D-Trp^{3},D-Arg^{6},D-Ala^{10}]-LH-RH) on serum concentrations of luteinizing hormone (LH) and testosterone (T) in intact adult rhesus monkeys were studied. In Experiment 1, a single subcutaneous injection of the LH-RH atagonist (400 µg and 50 µg) or vehicle was administered and the temporal changes in serum LH and T were determined. Both LH and T declined markedly in all animals as soon as 30 min following the LH-RH antagonist injection, reaching the nadir (80%) approximately 8 h later and remaining significantly lower than baseline levels for up to 24 h. Control animals showed no marked variations in either LH or T serum levels. In Experiment 2, daily subcutaneous injections of differenct doses of LH-RH antagonist (400 µg, 50 µg and 10 µg) or vehicle were administered during 7 days to 4 animals in each group. The animals in the control group showed no significant changes in LH or T levels, while those treated with the lowest dose of LH-RH antagonist (10 µg) presented decreased T levels in the absence of appreciable changes in LH. The other two doses of LH-RH antagonist (400 µg and 50 µg) induced, as soon as 8 h after the initial injection, dramatic changes in serum levels of both LH and T and these values remained significantly lower than controls for up to 3 and 4 days after discontinuation of drug administration, respectively.

We conclude from this study that LH-RH inhibitory analogues are potent inhibitors of LH and T in intact adult rhesus monkeys. Their potential use in clinical trials for male contraception as well as in cases in which the inhibition of gonadotropins and steroid secretion in males is desired is warranted.

Abstract

The experiments reported here demonstrate that LH-RH antagonists are potent suppressors of pituitary gonadotropins in non-human primates. This antigonadotropic effect of these drugs clearly results in anovulation when they are administered chronically to regularly cycling animals. The blockade of the preovulatory surge of FSH and LH is a consistent, reproducible phenomenon that presents very few side effects. The studies of endometrial histology and steroid receptors showed that the antagonists may be superior to agonists of LH-RH since they do not induce endometrial hyperplasia. LH-RH inhibitory analogues are not effective when used during the luteal phase or early follicular phase of the cycle with regard to inducing luteal phase deficiencies. The suppression of both gonadotropins and testosterone in male monkeys also suggests that the LH-RH antagonists may offer an alternative form of male contraception.

The potent antigonadotropin effect of LH-RH antagonists not only suggests new and interesting non-steroidal hormonal birth control methods, but also opens the possibility for new therapeutic regimes in cases in which the inhibition of FSH and LH is desired, such as precocious puberty, endometriosis, menopause and hormonally dependent tumors.

Acknowledgements

We are grateful to Drs. Andrew V. Schally and David Coy for their kind supply of different LH-RH antagonists and for their continuous intellectual motifation; to Organon, Oss, Holland for the recent supply of ORG30276B; and to Ms. Gretta Small for her excellent preparation of the manuscript. Support for this project was provided by the Ford Foundation (820–1073) and by the Program for Applied Research on Fertility Regulation (PARFR-347), Northwestern University, under a Cooperative Agreement with the United States Agency for International Development (AID) (DPE-0546-A-00-1003-00). The views expressed by the authors do not necessarily reflect the views of AID.

References

[1] Pedroza, E., J. A. Vilchez-Martinez, J. Fishback et al.: Biochem. Biophys. Res. Comm. **79** (1977) 234–238.
[2] Coy, D. H., I. Mezo, E. Pedroza et al.: In "Peptides: Structure and Biological Function" (Eds. E. Gross, J. Meinhofer), pp. 775–779. Pierce Chemical Company, 1979.
[3] Kastin, A. J., A. V. Schally, C. Gual et al.: J. Clin Endocrinol. Metab. **34** (1972) 753–756.
[4] De La Cruz, A., D. H. Coy, J. A. Velchez-Martinze et al.: Science **191** (1976) 195–197.
[5] De La Cruz, A., D. H. Coy, A. V. Schally et al.: Proc. Soc. Exp. Biol. Med. **149** (1975) 576–581.
[6] Phelps, C. P., D. H. Coy, A. V. Schally et al.: Endocrinology **100** (1977) 1525–1532.
[7] Rivier, C., J. Rivier, W. Vale: Endocrinology **108** (1971) 1998–2001.
[8] Hagino. N., D. H. Coy, A. V. Schally et al: Horm. Metab. Res. **9** (1977) 247–248.
[9] Gosselin, R. E., B. G. Fuller, D. H. Coy et al.: Proc. Soc. Exp. Biol. Med. **161** (1979) 21–24.
[10] Gonzales-Barcena, D., A. J. Kastin, D. H. Coy et al.: Lancet ii (1977) 997–998.
[11] Canales, E. S., H. Monvelinsky, A. Zarate et al.: Int. J. Fertil. **25** (1980) 190–192.
[12] Balmaceda, J. P., D. H. Coy, A. V. Schally et al.: Acta Eur. Fertil. **14** (1984) 249–253.
[13] Asch, R. H., J. P. Balmaceda, C. A. Eddy et al.: Fertil. Steril. **36** (1981) 388–391.
[14] Asch, R. H., J. P. Balmaceda, M. R. Borghi et al.: J. Clin. Endocrinol. Metab. **57** (1983) 367–372.

[15] Burgos-Briceno, L. A., C. G. Smith, D. H. Coy et al.: Acta Europaea Fertilitatis **14** (1983) 255–260.
[16] Asch, R. H., J. P. Balmaceda, M. Neves de Castro et al.: Presented at the 31st Annual Meeting of the Society for Gynecologic Investiagion, San Francisco, California, March 20–25, 1984, A#214.
[17] Borghi, M. R., R. Niesvisky, J. P. Balmaceda et al.: Fertil. Steril. **40** (1983) 678–682.
[18] Sheehan, K. L., R. F. Casper, S. S. C. Yen: Science **215** (1982) 170–172.
[19] Sharin, G., S. J. Nillius, L. Wide: Contraception **25** (1982) 31–33.
[20] Balmaceda, J. P., A. V. Schally, D. Coy et al.: Contraception **24** (1981) 275–281.
[21] Balmaceda, J. P., M. R. Borghi, D. H. Coy et al.: J. Clin. Endocrinol. Metab. **57** (1983) 866–868.
[22] Asch, R. H., M. Abou-Samra, G. Braunstein et al.: J. Clin. Endocrinol. Metab. **55** (1982) 154–161.
[23] Borghi, M. R., R. Niesvisky, D. H. Coy: Contraception **27** (1983) 619–626.
[24] Balmaceda, J. P., M. R. Borghi, L. Burgos et al.: Presented at the 30th Annual Meeting of the Society for Gynecologic Investigation, Washington D.C., March 17–20, 1983, A#99, p. 53.
[25] Schmidt-Gollwitzer, M., W. Hardt, K. Schmidt-Gollwitzer et al.: Contraception **23** (1981) 187–195.
[26] Kerr-Wilson, R. H. J., L. MacKenzie, H. M. Fraser: Contraception **24** (1981) 647–655.
[27] Burgos-Briceno, L. A., A. V. Schally, A. Bartke et al.: J. Clin. Endocrinol. Metab., submitted.

Long-term suppression of ovulation in the stumptailes macaque by active immunization against LH-RH or by LH-RH agonist administration

H. M. Fraser, N. C. Laird, M. P. Swaney

Introduction

Of the several ways for suppressing ovulation by manipulation of LH-RH (see chapter 1) we have investigated two approaches; 1. the immunoneutralization of the endogenous decapeptide by actively immunizing animals against synthetic LH-RH, or 2. conversely, to overstimulate the pituitary gland and disrupt normal pituitary-ovarian function by daily administration of LH-RH agonist. These studies have been carried out in stumptailed macaque monkeys in order to study effects of such manipulations on menstrual cycles, ovarian steroid production and the integrity of the hypothalamo-pituitary-ovarian axis in a species with cyclic hormone changes similar to the human female.

Active immunization against LH-RH

There are two important reasons for studying the effects of active immunization against LH-RH in the monkey. Firstly, a safe and effective LH-RH vaccine which produced specific suppression of gonadotropin release could find application in treatment of ovarian and testicular hormone dependent tumors, being a less expensive and simpler approach than continuous administration of LH-RH analogues. Secondly, studies on neutralization of LH-RH by antibodies have, during the last 12 years, contributed much to our understanding of the physiological role of LH-RH in controlling gonadotropins, pituitary LH-RH receptors, sexual behavior, gonadal receptors and steroid production [1–3]. The versatility of this technique has paved the way for investigations on the inhibitions of LH-RH by chemical antagonists which are only now seeing wide application.

Antibody production and effects on menstrual cycle

To investigate the effects of long-term LH-RH immunoneutralization, three stumptailed monkeys (weighing 8–11 kg) with regular menstrual cycles were immunized

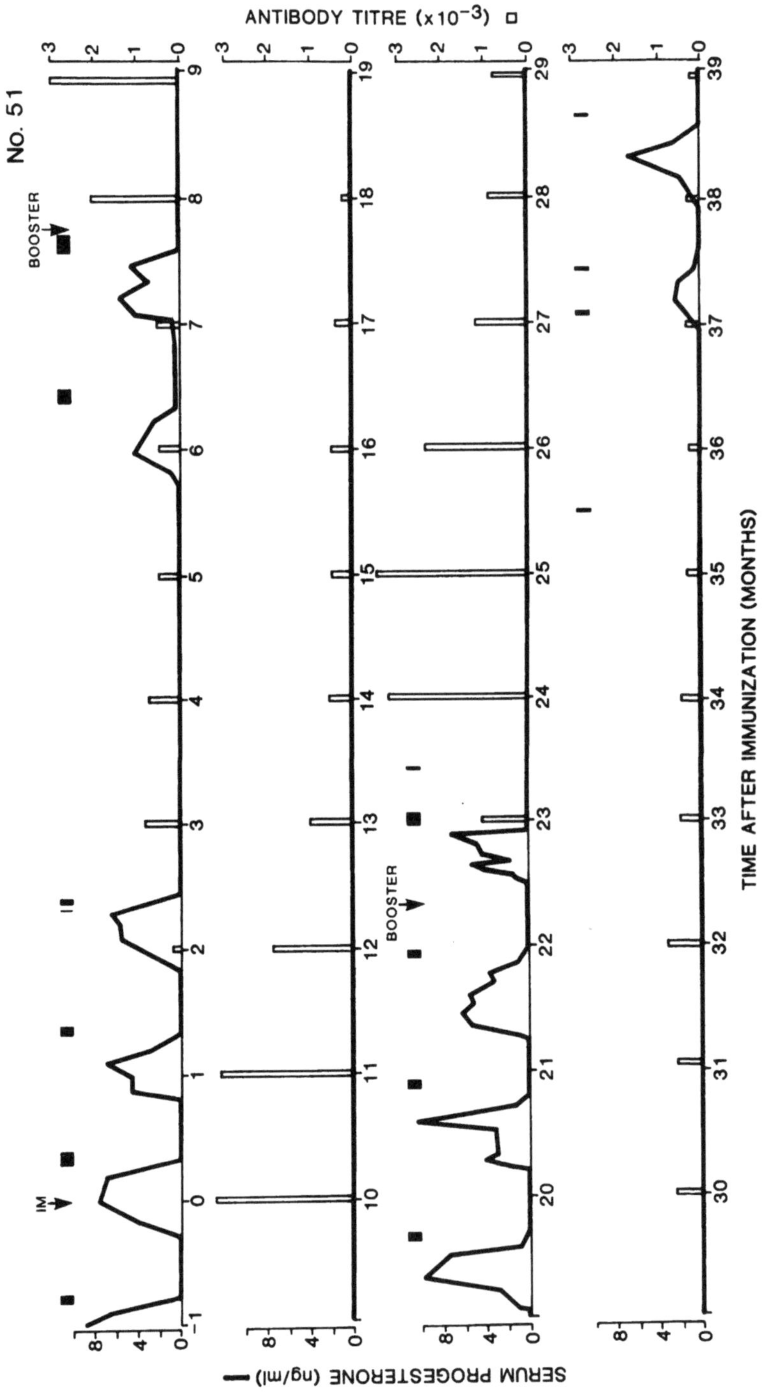

Fig. 1 Effect of active immunization against LHRH (arrow, time 0) on serum concentrations of progesterone (——), menstrual bleeding (■) and LHRH antibody titer (□) in a stumptailed monkey (No. 51). LHRH was conjugted to tetanus toxoid as carrier, and administered, emulsified with Freunds complete adjuvant, at 10 s. c. sites.

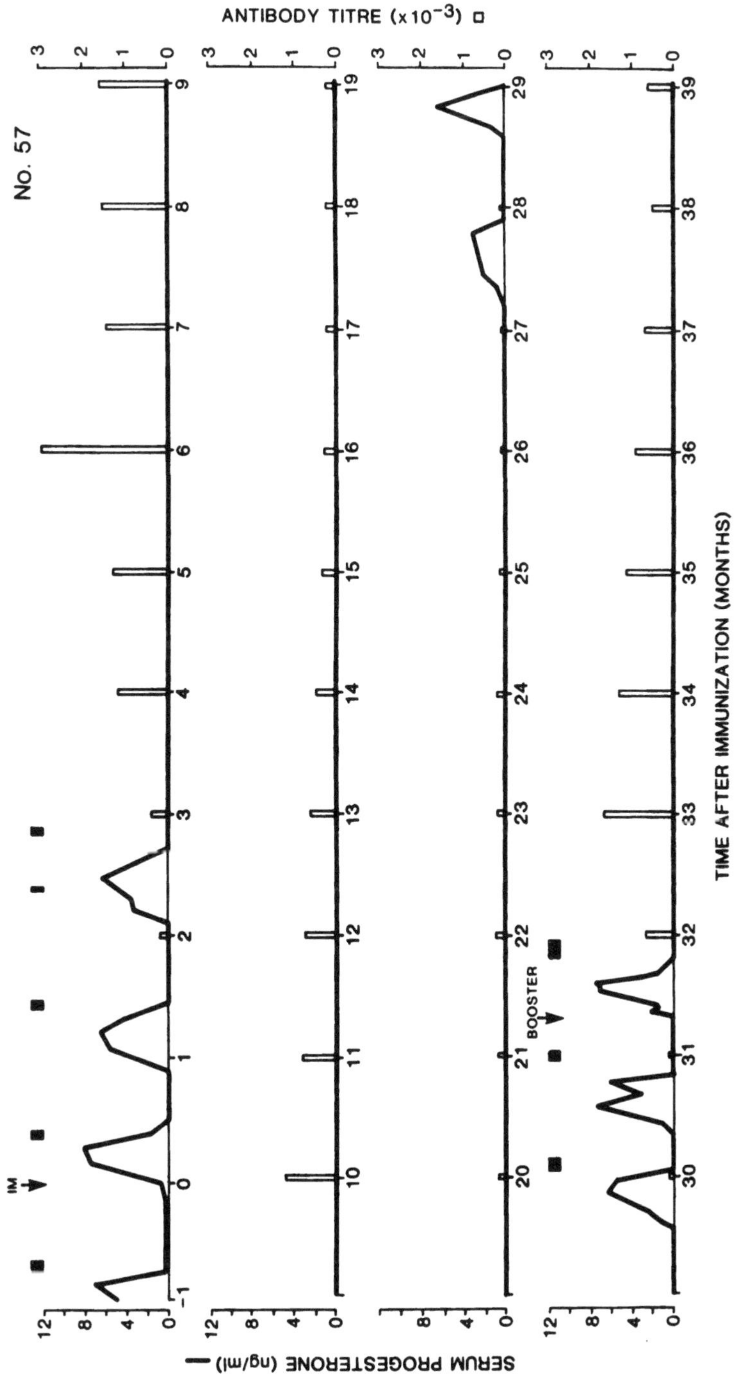

Fig. 2 Effect of immunization against LHRH in stumptailed monkey No. 57. Other details as in figure 1.

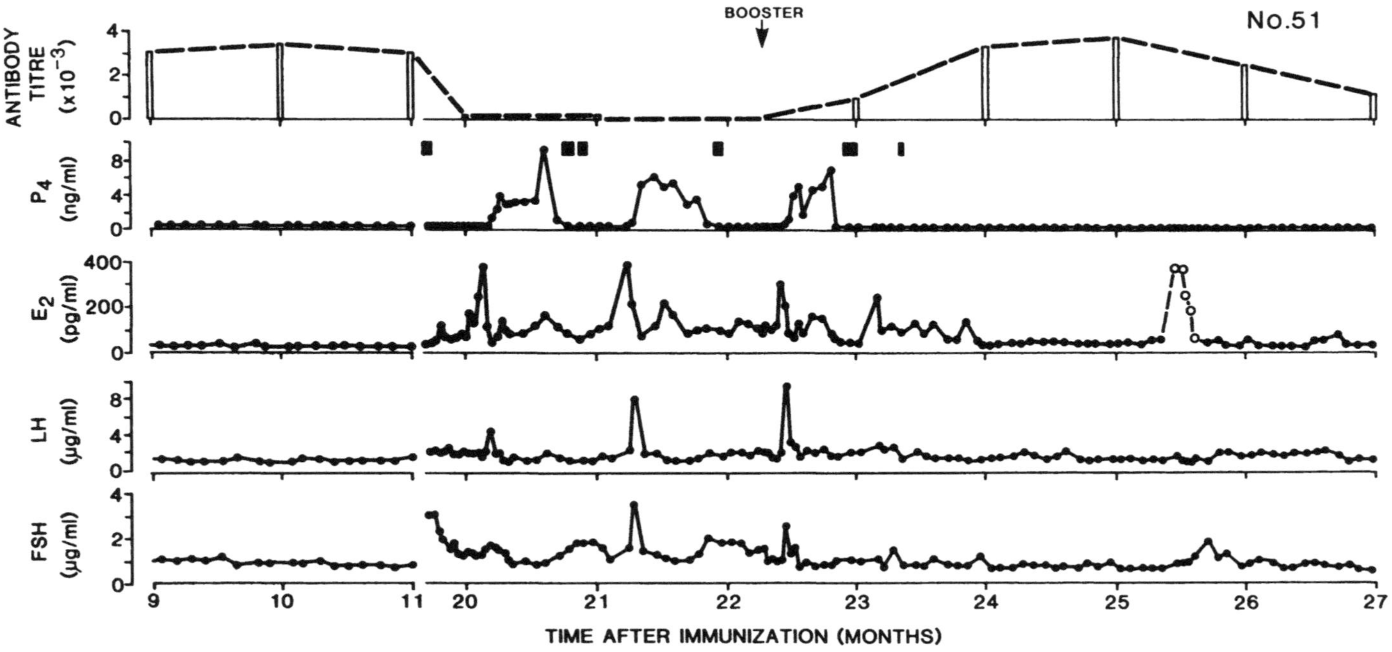

Fig. 3 Effects of active immunization against LHRH on serum concentrations of progesterone (P4), 17β-estradiol (E_2), LH and FSH, and menstrual bleeding in monkey no. 51. The periods shown demonstrate changes during a period when LHRH antibody titers (top panel) are high (Months 9–11 after primary immunization, low antibody levels (months 20–23) and after booster immunization (arrow) to restore antibody titres. Injection of estradiol benzoate (open circles) failed to induce an LH surge.

against LH-RH conjugated to tetanus toxoid and emulsified in Freund's complete adjuvant [4]. Control monkeys immunized with the carrier had normal cycles throughout the study period. The 3 animals immunized against LH-RH all produced antibodies. Antibody titers, assessed by ability of serum to bind ^{125}I-labelled LH-RH, were low during the first 3 months after immunization and cycles continued. Thereafter, antibody titers became established at 1:1000 and there were no longer cyclic rises in serum progesterone and the animals became amenorrheic (e.g. figs. 1 and 2). However, decline in antibody levels led to re-establishment of cycles after 4 months of suppression in monkey 51 and after 22 months suppression in monkey 57 (figs. 1 and 2). This wide variation in biological effectiveness of immunization is one of the problems of hormone immunization. The situation may be aleviated by booster immunization which helps maintain antibody levels. For example, booster immunization in these monkeys resulted in suppression of cycles for a further 14 months in no. 51 and until the end of the 3-year study period in no. 57.

Examples of the detailed hormonal changes during a period of maximal antibody titer, low antibody titer and the response to a booster immunization are shown in Figure 3. No LH surges were detected when LH-RH antibody titers were elevated but the assay is inappropriate for determining changes in basal levels. The cyclical rises in FSH levels in serum were absent when titers were elevated, indicating inhibition of FSH release. Decline in the gonadotropin stimulation of the ovaries was associated with low levels of estradiol-17β in the serum, values most frequently being non-detectable (<25 pg/ml) similar to that observed in serum from ovariectomized macaques.

The third animal demonstrated a similar pattern of antibody production and hormonal response to the primary immunization. Following immunization, two normal cycles occurred but ovulation was suppressed thereafter and antibody levels rose to 1:1000. No ovulations occurred in the following 7 months, but with antibody levels at 1:1000, the animal died suddenly. Post-mortem examination failed to establish the cause of death.

Effect of LH-RH immunization on positive feedback

To determine the effect of active immunization against LH-RH on the ability of the pituitary to respond to the positive feedback effects of estrogen, monkeys 51 and 57 were injected with 50 μg estradiol benzoate per Kg in arachis oil on 2 occassions when cycles were suppressed by LH-RH antibodies.

In three control monkeys treated with estradiol benzoate during the early follicular phase of the cycle, a surge of LH and FSH was observed, with maximal values 48 h after estrogen administration. Results of the first test on LH-RH immunized monkey no. 51 is incorporated into figure 3 and shows an absence of positive feedback. This was also observed on the other tests [4].

Discussion

Active immunization against LH-RH in the female stumptailed monkey led to its neutralization, as indicated by the inhibitory effects on menstrual cycles associated with elevation of serum LH-RH antibody titers. Although the number of monkeys immunized was small, the detailed evaluation of serum hormone values, length of the study period and similarities in the observations made after LH-RH immunization in rats [5–7] ewe [8] and in marmoset monkeys [9], permits a reliable evaluation of the physiological consequences of LH-RH immunizations in the primate.

The occurrence of 2–3 normal cycles after primary immunization was due to the slow rate of production of LH-RH antibodies. Once established, the antibodies produced a decline in serum gonadotropin concentrations. During the periods of anovulation LH surges were not observed, nor could an LH surge be stimulated by exogenous estrogen. Serum fluctuations in FSH observed during normal cycles were absent in the presence of elevated LH-RH antibody titers and were suppressed to basal levels.

The fact that estrogen-induced positive feedback was abolished in these animals is not neccessarily at variance with results in rhesus and stumptailed monkeys showing that passive immunization against LH-RH or pituitary stalk sectioning at the time of estrogen administration failed to inhibit the LH surge [3, 10, 11]. It seems probable that the differences in the ability of the pituitary gland to respond to estrogen depend on whether it has been primed recently by LH-RH, as in the passive immunization and stalk sectioning experiments, or whether this priming effect has been removed by chronic immunoneutralization by active immunization, which may also reduce pituitary gonadotropin stores [5] and a loss of pituitary LH-RH receptors [12].

As far as the prospects for contraceptive and clinical application of LH-RH immunization in women are concerned, the fact that when antibody production reaches certain levels ovulation is inhibited will ensure infertility during this period. The severe reduction in serum estradiol levels produced amenorrhoea, which would probably be acceptable, but might also lead to other unacceptable menopausal symptoms. However, complete suppression of estrogen would be desirable if an "immunological oophorectomy" were required as in the treatment of pre-menopausal women with breast cancer. An LH-RH vaccine would be preferable to the continuous use of LH-RH analogues currently being developed to suppress ovarian function in that it should be inexpensive and administered only infrequently. But, in addition to the possibility of producing undesirebly low estrogen, there is a major problem in individual variability of the immune response and necessity to use a powerful immunological adjuvant. Variability in antibody response leading to variation in time of onset of inhibition of cycles, degree of inhibition of pituitary and gonadal hormones and timing of return to normal cycles are generally observed with methods of LH-RH immunization currently available e.g. rat, sheep [8], marmoset monkey [9] and male rhesus monkey [13]. Also Freund's adjuvant, whilst a powerful stimulator of the immune response, is unacceptable for clinical application. Results using a more acceptable adjuvant (alhydrogel and dipeptide) [14] yielded poor antibody levels. These problems will only be overcome by developing more immunogenic LH-RH conjugates and by advances in ability to control the immune response.

Chronic administration of LH-RH agonist

As discussed in chapter 1, there is a remarkable number of different regimens of LH-RH agonist treatment which will lead to disruption of normal follicular or luteal function. We have investigated the most simple regimen of daily administration of LH-RH agonist beginning during the early follicular phase of the cycle. Administration of 5 μg D-Ser(Bu^t)^6 des $Gly^{10}NH_2$LH-RH ethylamide by s.c. injection for 20 days during the cycle in the stumptailed macaque induced an initial elevation of serum gonadotropins associated with stimulation of estradiol secretion. However, the LH surge failed to occur and there was no rise in serum [15] progesterone concentrations indicating that ovulation had been prevented [15] (fig. 4). Generally, serum estradiol levels fell after about 2 weeks to be followed by endometrial bleeding. However, there were some variations to this pattern. In 2 of 9 monkeys, a higher dose of agonist had to be used to suppress ovulation and in one monkey, it appeared the follicle might have been held in abeyance and ovulated after treatment was stopped, resulting in an inadequate luteal phase (fig. 5). In the other animals, cessation of treatment was followed by pattern of serum estradiol suggesting rapid growth of a new follicle which ovulated 12.1 ± 1 days later (mean ± SEM) resulting in a corpus luteum producing normal amounts of progesterone.

When 9 animals were treated daily for 11–16 months, various degrees of inhibition of ovarian function were observed [16]. These could be divided into 3 types and are illustrated in figures 6, 7, and 8. In the most suppressed state, as represented by 3 of the monkeys (fig. 6), not only was ovulation inhibited, but serum concentrations of estradiol fluctuated between levels associated with the early or mid-follicular phase of the normal cycle, never reaching late follicular phase values. These animals became virtually amenorrhoeic during treatment.

In a further 3 monkeys, while the agonist also inhibited ovulatory cycles, serum concentrations of estradiol occasionally rose to values associated with the late follicular phase, indicating follicular maturation was not fully suppressed on occasional rises in progesterone indicated ovulations or formation of luteinized follicles (fig. 7). These animals demonstrated irregular bleeding patterns.

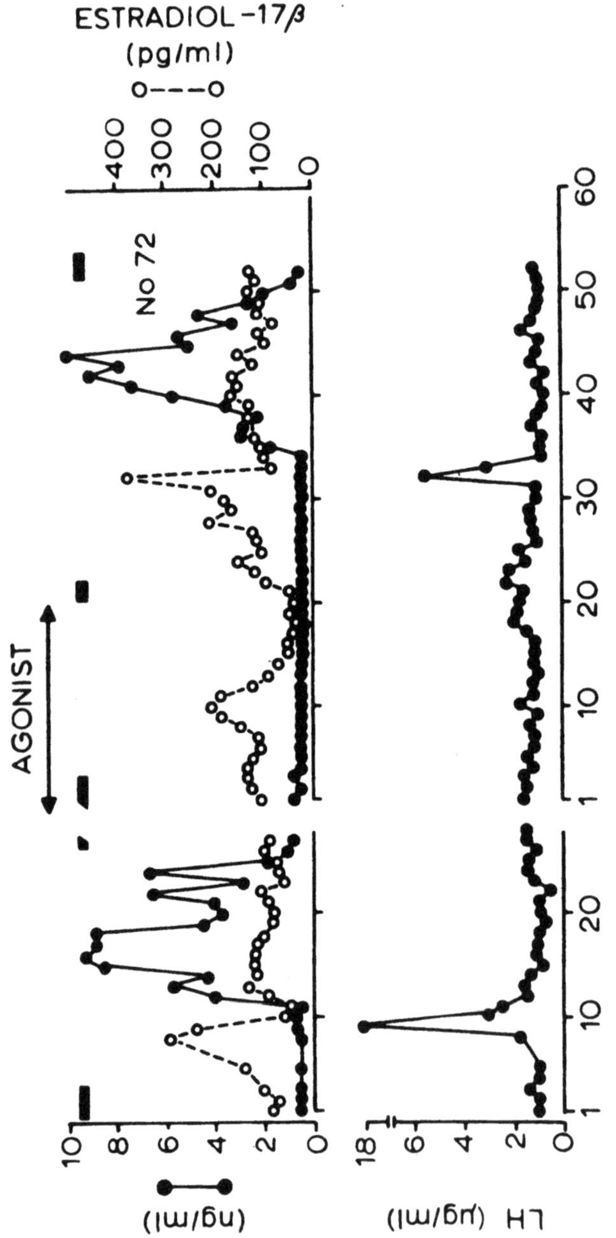

Fig. 4 Plasma progesterone, 17β estradiol, and LH levels during a control cycle and in the following cycle during which the monkey received 5 μg LHRH agonist daily for 20 days beginning on day 1 of the cycle. Note absence of LH surge and ovulation.

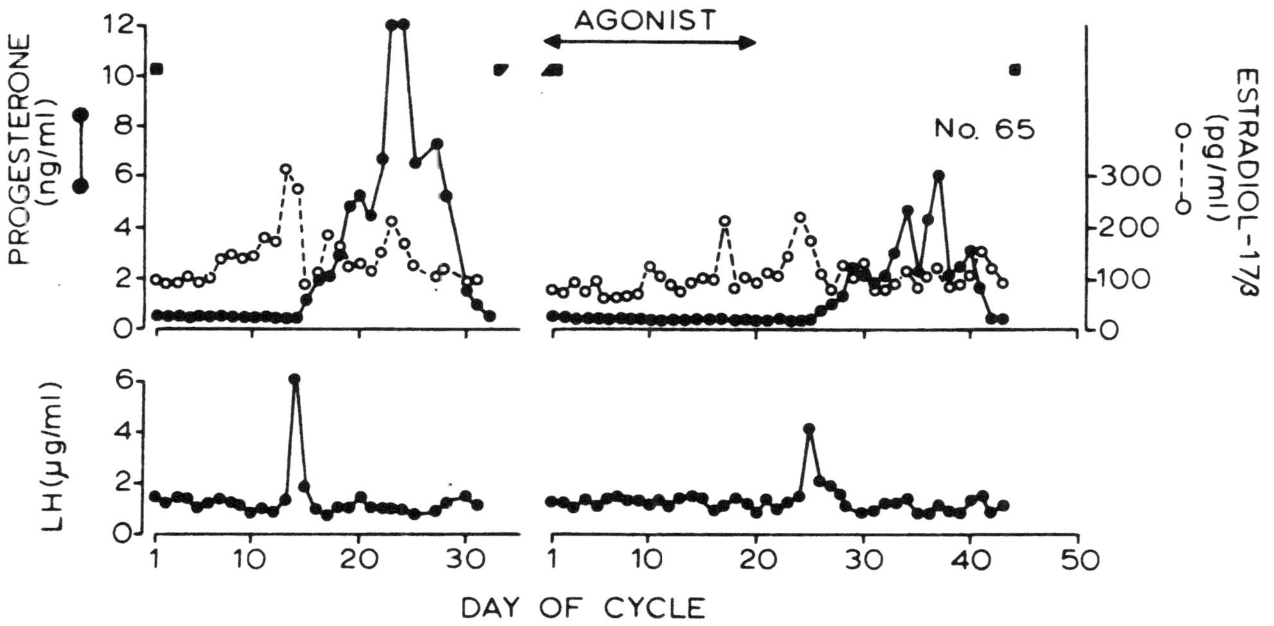

Fig. 5 Monkey receiving same treatment as in figure 4. Expected ovulation is inhibited but follicle appears to persist to ovulate to produce an inadequate luteal phase after cessation of agonist injections.

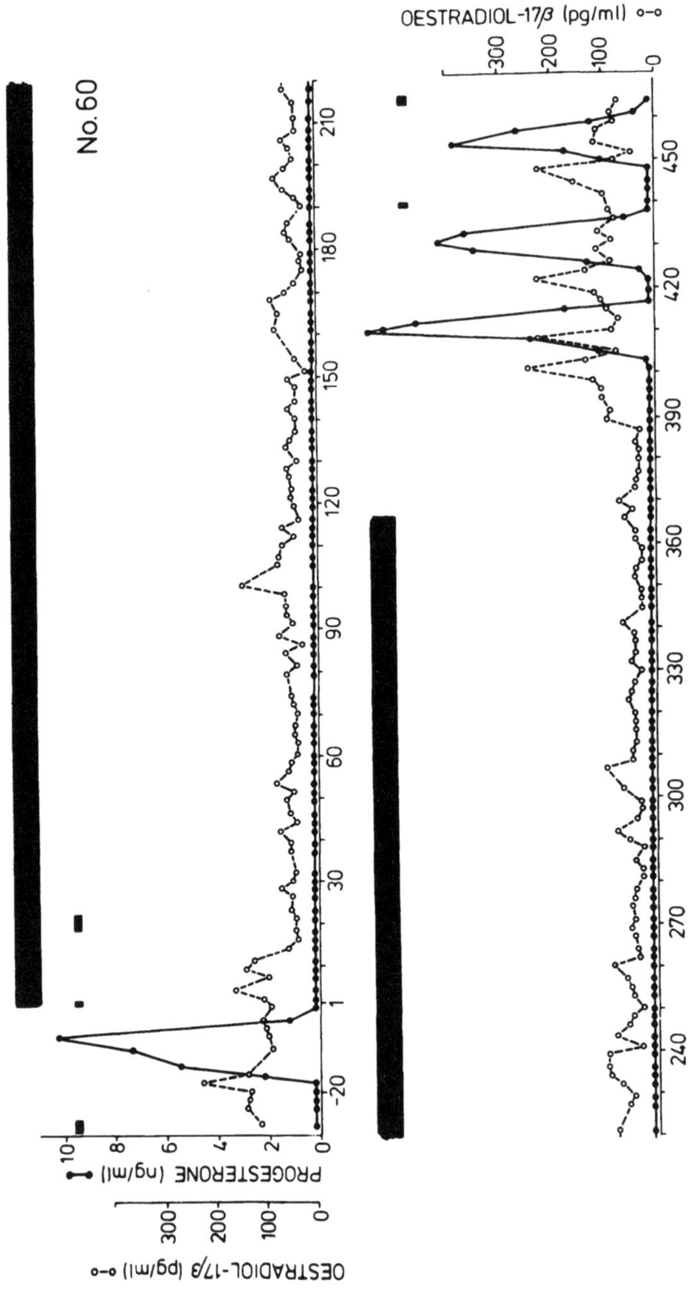

Fig. 6 Effect of daily s. c. injections of 5 μg LHRH agonist on serum concentrations of 17β-estradiol (O–O) and progesterone (●–●) immediately prior to daily agonist administration in one of the monkeys in the most suppressed group. Note fluctuations in oestradiol without levels reaching those observed in a normal late follicular phase and virtual absence of endometrial bleeding during treatment (bars).

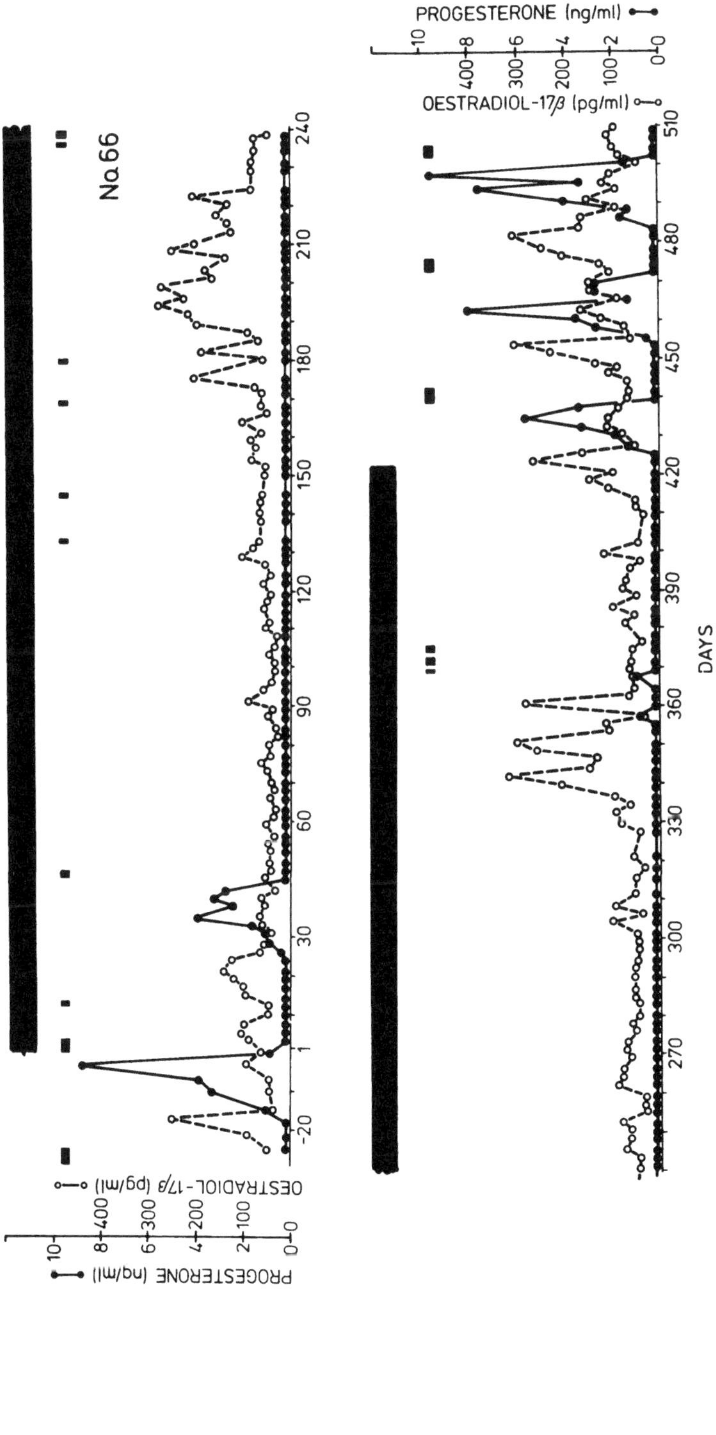

Fig. 7 Effect of daily s. c. injections of 5 µg LHRH agonist on serum concentrations of 17β-estradiol (○–○) and progesterone (●–●) in one of the monkeys showing suppression of ovulation accompanied by irregular phases of follicular development. Note irregular bleeding.

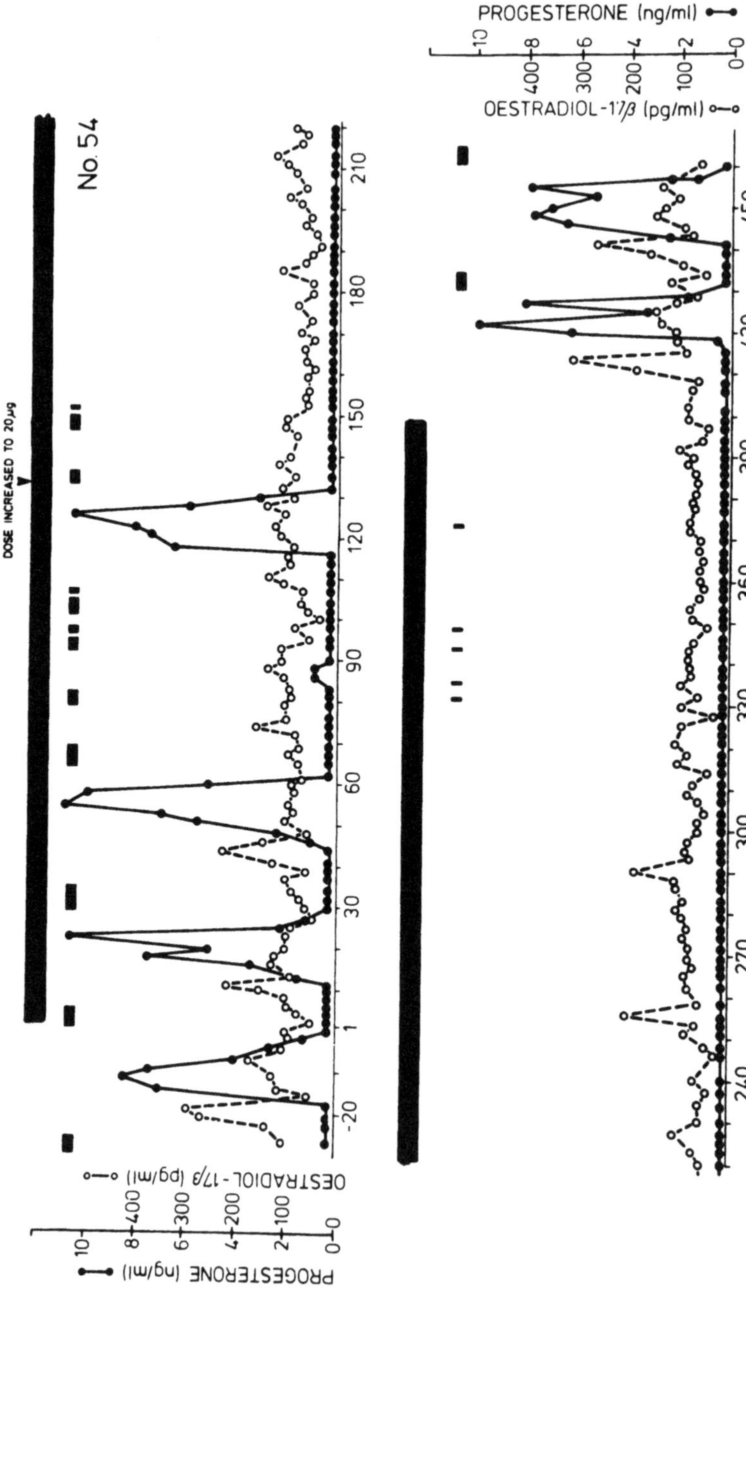

Fig. 8 Effect of daily s. c. injections of 5 μg LHRH agonist on serum concentrations of 17β-estradiol (O–O) and progesterone (●–●) in a monkey representing the non-inhibited group. Note possible luteinized follicle at third ovulation and lengthened follicular phases. When the dose of agonist was increased to 20 μg daily ovulation was inhibited.

In the remaining 3 monkeys, the 5 µg dose failed to suppress ovulation (e.g. fig. 8). Increasing the dose of LH-RH agonist to 20 µg per day suppressed ovulation in two of the animals and reduced the number of cycles in the remaining animal, which was eventually suppressed when the agonist was administered at a dose of 10 µg twice daily.

Serum concentrations of androstenedione remained within the range observed in the normal cycle indicating that cystic follicles had not developed during treatment. When compared to the equivalent pre-treatment control time period, the days of endometrial bleeding were reduced in all monkeys by the agonist treatment [16]. When treatment was stopped, the monkeys ovulated within 2–4 weeks except for one in the most suppressed group whose cycles failed to return.

Effect on endometrium and ovaries

At the end of LH-RH agonist treatment, a laparotomy (17) revealed that the ovaries appeared inactive and were slightly smaller than in control animals. Only one animal had a small ovarian cyst, which was lined with cuboidal cells and considered to be of germinal epithelial origin. The uteri were also smaller than controls. Histological examination showed a range of activity. All the animals with amenorrhea had endometrium with an atrophic or resting proliferative appearence. The glands, some of which were cystic, were lined by flattened epithelium. There was no evidence of mitotic activity in either glands or stroma. The other animals showed a similar or slightly more active appearance with the exception of 2 monkeys (e.g. no. 54, fig. 8) which showed variable degrees of activity. Some of the glands were lined by low cuboidal, inactive cells. Others appeared actively secretory with dilated glands, lined with columnar cells, containing mucinoid material. The epithelium in some areas of the actively secretory glands appeared to show pseudostratification of the nuclei. Gland mitoses were infrequent. The stroma appeared moderately cellular in no. 54 and densely cellular in the other animal. Endometrial polyps were found in no. 54, but were unlikely to be caused by the treatment as polyps were also observed in 2 or 6 control monkeys.

Effect on dysfunctional uterine bleeding

The occurrence of endometrial activity in these two monkeys stressed the possibility that some individuals could be suseptible to the low levels of "unopposed" estrogen during LH-RH agonist treatment and the need for careful assessment in clinical studies. However, the fact that in the majority of monkeys the endometrium was inactive and the days of endometrial blood loss reduced compared to control cycles [16] suggested that this treatment might be of benefit in treating dysfunctional uterine bleeding.

In our colony, 5 animals had had a clear history of dysfunctional uterine bleeding as judged by the high number of days of blood loss over a period of several years as assessed by taking daily vaginal swabs. The number of days of blood loss per month during the 2-year period prior to treatment ranged from a mean of 7.5 to 15.4 days (fig. 9). By comparison, 9 animals with regular menstrual cycles and normal patterns of menstrual bleeding had 2.9±0.8 (mean±S.D., range 2.2–4.5) days per month of bleeding during a 12 month control period.

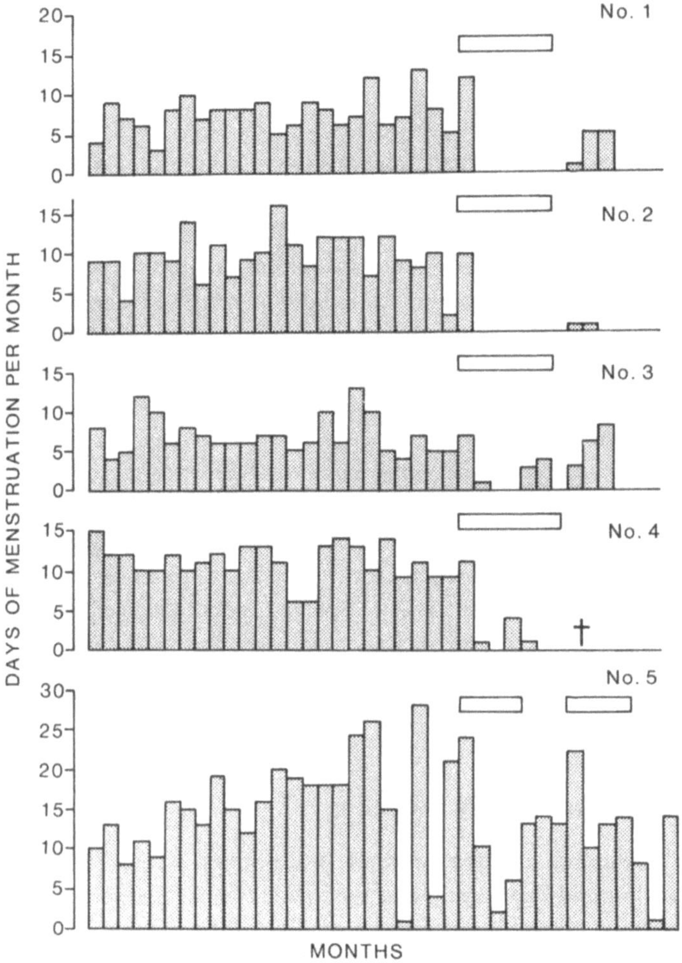

Fig. 9 Days of menstrual bleeding during an 24-month period prior to and during (horizontal bar) treatment with LHRH agonist in stumptailed macaque monkeys. Monkeys 1 and 2 received 50 μg agonist/day for 5 weeks followed by 10 μg injections. Monkeys 3, 4 and 5 received 10 μg/day. Monkey No. 5 received a second course of treatment consisting of 50 μg/day.

Defining the reason for the existence of dysfunctional uterine bleeding in the macaques was difficult, as is found with many women presenting with this disorder. Abnormal ovarian function leading to inadequate secretion of estradiol and progesterone was a possible cause in 3 of the animals with pathological indications of polyps, possible adenomyosis and fibroids being other causative factors.

The pattern of pre-treatment menstruation could be divided into two types. Either prolonged uninterrupted bleeding during the early to mid follicular phase (nos. 1 and 3) or bleeding on two occasions during the early and late follicular phase (nos. 2, 3, 5).

In this study a higher daily dose of LH-RH agonist (10 or 50 μg/day) was employed in an attempt to achieve greater suppression of follicular development and estradiol secretion. Animals were treated for 6 months.

The treatment was successful in suppressing ovarian steroidogenesis in all animals, as indicated by the maintenance of basal serum estradiol levels at <100 pg/ml and serum progesterone at <1 ng/ml. During the first treatment cycle, all monkeys menstruated for their typical time period (fig. 9). The monkeys nos. 1 and 2, receiving the higher dose treatment initially, bleeding stopped completely during the treatment period. In monkeys nos. 3 and 4, days of bleeding was consistently reduced to a few days of irregular bleeding. In monkey no. 5, no significant improvement occurred either when the 10 μg dose was administered nor when the dose of agonist was increased to 50 μg/day.

At the end of treatment, uterine size was reduced in all monkeys. Histological examination indicated decreased endometrial activity. No. 2 had marked reduction in width of the endometrium with only a few inactive glands. The remaining animals, while having a reduction in size of epithelial cells, still showed clear proliferative activity. There was no indication of endometrial hyperplasia, although some dilated inactive glands were observed in no. 4.

After ceasing treatment, cycles with changes in serum concentrations of ovarian steroids similar to pre-treatment profiles resumed promptly. The monkeys resumed menstruation and in the 3 post-treatment cycles observed there were indications of improvement compared with pre-treatment in monkey no. 2 only.

In conclusion, the present results, together with recent preliminary findings on the effects of chronic LH-RH agonist treatment in women and monkeys with endometriosis [19–22] suggest that suppression of ovarian function in this way should have a significant role to play in these disorders of menstruation.

In the interests of clinical application, it should be noted that there was no improvement during the first treatment cycle. In the remaining monkey, no. 5, bleeding continued despite suppression of ovarian steroid secretion. Since monkeys nos. 1 and 2 treated initially with the 50 μg dose of buserelin had made the most dramatic improvement, this dose was employed for a second treatment period in no. 5, but once more had no significant benefit. This monkey was the most severe case of dysfunctional uterine bleeding in the group and had fibroids and exceptionally thick myometrium as well as low steroid profiles prior to treatment. Thus, such a severe condition may not be amenable to the current therapy, although it would be of interest to examine the effects of more frequent agonist administration or infusion in an attempt to gain further ovarian suppression.

Mechanism of inhibitory effect of LH-RH agonist

The mechanisms of the inhibitory effects of agonists on ovulation involve multiple systems and the level of the pituitary gonadotrop and ovary. It is well established for a number of species including the stumptailed macaque that the pituitary response to repeated agonist administration is reduced [15]. Furthermore, we know that administration of estradiol benzoate, which induces an LH surge in normal monkeys, fails to induce a surge or causes only a diminished or delayed rise in LH in macaques treated chronically with the agonist [23] (fig. 10). This is also observed in women given similar treatment [24]. Since the pituitary gland is normally exposed to pulses of LH-RH (see chapter 1), and since the frequency of the pulses is particularly important for the action of estrogen on the anterior pituitary gland to induce an LH surge, then it follows that the LH surge is inhibited primarily because of the prolonged stimulation by the agonist. Important changes must therefore be taking place within the gonadotrops, but these have not been studied in detail in primates. One effect of prolonged agonist treatment may be to decrease the pool of releasable LH or synthesis of factors necessary for gonadotropin release within the gonadotrop. There is some evidence from studies on effect of prolonged agonist treatment in female rats that pituitary gonadotropin content is reduced [25], however we did not observe any marked reduction in rats treated for 3 weeks [36], although the animals had stopped having estrous cycles. We also found there were no obvious changes in pituitary LH-RH receptor numbers during this treatment [36], suggesting the antifertility effects did not involve a simple loss of LH-RH receptors.

Little effect on basal levels of serum LH or FSH were observed after agonist treatment in the stumptailed macaques [16] or in women [27, 28] but it remains to be established whether the pulse rate of gonadotropin release is altered.

From measurement of serum estradiol concentrations it appears that daily injections of agonist in monkeys in women either prevent follicular development or induce follicles to mature but not to ovulate [16, 27, 28]. From studies in rats, we assume that agonist treatment is associated with a loss of LH and FSH receptors on the ovary [29, 30]. While this may also be true for the primate follicle, in our experience the rat responds differently to agonist treatment in that the ovaries contain a predominance of luteal tissue [26, 31] which is not the case in the primate [17]. Little is known

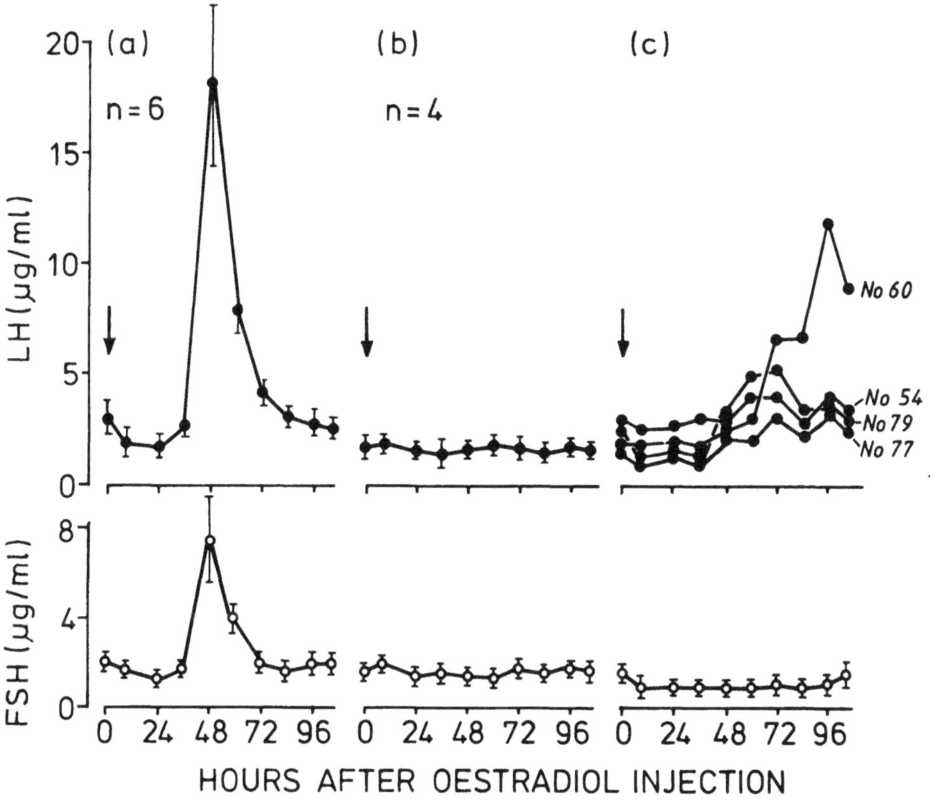

Fig. 10 Effect of estradiol benzoate (50 µg/kg; shown by arrows) on serum concentrations of LH and FSH in (a) six control monkeys on days 1–5 of the cycle, (b) five monkeys treated with LHRH agonist and which showed no LH response and (c) four monkeys treated with the LHRH agonist which did show an LH response. Values are means ± S. E. M. except for the monkeys which showed an LH response.

about ovarian responsiveness during agonist treatment in monkeys and in women, although it has been demonstrated that over-exposure of the follicle to gonadotropin can have a deleterious effect; hCG administration during the follicular phase of the menstrual cycle in women causes an inhibition or postponement of ovulation, apparently by causing luteinization of the theca cells of tertiary follicles and degeneration of the granulosa cells [32]. Since one of the problems of daily agonist administration for contraception is the individual variation in the effect on follicular growth, it seems important that more attention should be given to the mechanism of the inhibitory effect of agonist treatment and to what extent it is due to the pattern of gonadotropin release induced by the agonist or effects on basal gonadotropin release induced by the agonist or effects on basal gonadotropin patterns between agonist administrations.

Finally, LH-RH may have a direct action on the ovarian follicle. However, in this regard, the rat may differ significantly from primates. Rat follicles possess receptors for LH-RH through which its agonists can influence several fundamental functions [33, 34]. Short-term exposure of the preovulatory follicle to LH-RH agonist stimulates prostaglandin production and steroidogenesis [34–37] and promotes oocyte maturation [38]. On the other hand, exposure of preantral follicles to LH-RH agonist for several days inhibits the gonadotropin-induced increase in cAMP, steroidogenesis, LH receptor numbers, and granulosa cell differentiation [39, 40], indicating a dual effect related to both the length of time of exposure and degree of follicular maturation [41]. While it is likely that these direct actions contribute to the antifertility effects of LH-RH agonists in the rat, they are unlikely to occur in monkeys or in the human ovary, since they do not appear to possess the same high affinity LH-RH receptors as the rat [34, 42, 43].

LH-RH agonist treatment and antibody formation

One possible complication of long-term exposure to LH-RH analogues is formation of antibodies against them, since they posses "foreign" amino acid substitutions. LH-RH itself has been reported to have elicited an immune response in at least two individuals being treated by repeated administration of synthetic LH-RH for isolated gonadotropin deficiency [44, 45]. It was suggested that since they had low or absent levels of the endogenous hormone, the exogenous LH-RH may have been seen as "foreign."

In the monkeys receiving LH-RH agonist for prolonged periods in the present study, the sera were tested for the presence of antibodies to the agonist at frequent intervals and at the end of the study, by incubation with ^{125}I-labelled agonist. No antibodies were found. This agrees with experience to date in other species receiving prolonged agonist treatment [46]. While these results suggest a negligible risk of antibody formation, this still merits checking in future clinical trials in which patients receive long-term agonist treatment.

There is also information on the question of whether generation of an immune response to LH-RH agonist would induce antibodies which had the potential to crossreact with endogenous LH-RH. To investigate this, rabbits were actively immunized against D Ser(Bu^t) des Gly^{10}NH$_2$LH-RH ethylamide and the ability of the sera to combine with labelled agonist or LH-RH assessed. All 64 rabbits produced antibodies which bound the agonist, but only 10 of these could also bind LH-RH and this was in very low titer. Thus, LH-RH agonist and endogenous LH-RH seem to have immunochemical differences which would render it unlikely that antibodies induced by agonist treatment would interfer with endogenous LH-RH.

Conclusions

Manipulation of LH-RH, both by active immunization against LH-RH to neutralize the endogenous hormone, or by overstimulation of the pituitary-ovarian axis by chronic LH-RH agonist treatment, resulted in suppression of menstrual cycles. The contraceptive regimes employing LH-RH analogues require daily administration by nasal spray of expensive peptide and as such are not the answer for the population explosion in developing countries. In theory, an LH-RH vaccine would be preferable in that it should be inexpensive and administered only infrequently. However, there is the possibility of producing undersirably low estrogen and there is a major problem in individual variability of the immune response and necessity to use a powerful immunological adjuvant. We have been aware of the potential antifertility effects of LH-RH immunization for many years and it is unfortunate that this approach has not seen sufficient development to overcome these problems. A suitable LH-RH vaccine could at least be of use for "immunological gonadectomy" in cases of hormone dependent tumours. These studies, together with those on passive immunoneutraliziation of LH-RH [1–3], have offered a foresight of the endocrine effets of inhibiting LH-RH action by antagonists. Hopefully, with the latter approach more control will be possible.

The antifertility effects of the LH-RH agonists have been pursued with more vigor and anticipation, but despite their efficacy and lack of metabolic side effects, use of LH-RH agonist for suppression of ovulation has also been criticised because of individual variation, in particular the occurrence of follicular development at unpredictable frequency leading to irregular endometrial bleeding. Further work on use of the agonists to control follicular growth more effectively is required before their contraceptive and therapeutic potential will be realized.

Acknowledgement

H. M. Fraser is grateful to Dr. J. Sandow for helpful discussions and to Hoechst U. K. for supplies of LH-RH agonist.

Reference

[1] Fraser, H. M.: In "Immunological Aspects of Reproduction and Fertility Control" (Ed. J. P. Hearn), pp. 143–171. MTP Press, Lancaster, U. K. 1980.

[2] Fraser, H. M., R. M. Sharpe, G. A. Lincoln et al.: In "Progress Towards a Male Contraceptive" (Eds. S. L. Jeffcoate, M. Sandler), pp. 41–78. John Wiley & Sons Ltd., 1982.

[3] Fraser, H. M., A. S. McNeilly, R. M. Popkin: In "Immunological Aspects of Reproduction in Mammals" (Ed. B. Crighton). Butterworths, 1984.

[4] Fraser, H. M.: J. Reprod. Immuno. **5** (1983) 173–183.
[5] Fraser, H. M., T. G. Baker: J. Endocrinol. 77 (1978) 85–93.
[6] Okon, E., N. Livni, Y. Koch: Br. J. Exp. Path. **61** (1980) 579–589.
[7] Takahashi, M., J. M. Ford, K. Yoshinaga et al.: Biol. Reprod. **17** (1978) 754–761.
[8] Clarke, I. J., H. M. Fraser, A. S. McNeilly: J. Endocrinol. **78** (1978) 39–47.
[9] Hodges, J. K., J. P. Hearn: Nature, Lond. **265** (1977) 746–767.
[10] McCormack, J. T., T. M. Plant, D. L. Hess et al.: Endocrinology **100** (1977) 663–667.
[11] Ferin, M., H. Rosenblatt, P. W. Carmel et al.: Endocrinology **104** (1979) 50–52.
[12] Popkin, R., H. M. Fraser: Unpublished observations.
[13] Chappel, S. C., W. E. Ellinwood, C. Huckins et al.: Biol. Reprod. **22** (1980) 333–342.
[14] Chedid, L., F. Audibert, P. Lefrancier et al.: Proc. Natl. Acad. Sci. U.S.A. **73** (1976) 2472–2475.
[15] Fraser, H. M., N. C. Laird, D. M. Blakeley: Endocrinology **106** (1980) 452–457.
[16] Fraser, H. M.: Endocrinology **112** (1983) 245–253.
[17] Kerr-Wilson, R. H. J., L. MacKenzie, H. M- Fraser: Contraception **24** (1981) 647–654.
[18] Fraser, H. M., R. W. Shaw: Acta Endocrinol. (submitted 1984).
[19] Werlin, L. B., G. D. Hodgen: J. Clin. Endocr. Metab. **56** (1983) 844–848.
[20] Meldrum, D. R., R. J. Chang, J. Lu et al.: J. Clin. Endocrinol. Metab. **54** (1982) 1081–1083.
[21] Lemay, A., G. Quesnel: Fertil. Steril. **38** (1982) 376–379.
[22] Shaw, R. W., H. M. Fraser, H. Boyle: Br. Med. J. **287** (1983) 1667–1669.
[23] Fraser, H. M.: J. Endocrinol. **91** (1981) 525–530.
[24] Bergquist, C., S. J. Nillius, L. Wide: Clin. Endocr. **16** (1982) 147–151.
[25] Cusan, L., C. Auclair, A. Belanger et al.: Endocrinology **104** (1970) 1369–76.
[26] Popkin, R. M., H. M. Fraser, R. G. Gosden: J. Reprod. Fert. **69** (1983) 245–252.
[27] Bergquist, C., S. J. Nillius, L. Wide: Lancet **II** (1979) 215–217.
[28] Schmidt-Gollwitzer, M., W. Hardt, K. Schmidt-Gollwitzer et al.: In "LH-RH Peptides as Male and Female Contraceptives" (Ed. G. Zatuchni), pp. 199–215. Lippincott, U.S.A.
[29] Kledzik, G. S., L. Cusan, C. Auclair et al.: Fertil. Steril **30** (1978) 348–355.
[30] Conti, M., J. P. Harwood, A. J. W. Hsueh et al.: J. Biol. Chem. **251** (1976) 7729–7731.
[31] Sandow, J.: In "Neuroendocrine Prespectives", vol. 1 pp. 339–395. (Eds. E. E. Muller, R. M. MacLeod.) Elsevier Biomedical Press, Amsterdam.
[32] Friedrich, F., P. Kemeter, H. Salzer et al.: Acta Endocrinol. **78** (1975) 332–342.
[33] Clayton, R. N., J. P. Haarwood, K. J. Catt: Nature **282** (1979) 90–92.
[34] Popkin, R., T. A. Bramley, A. Currie et al.: This volume.
[35] Clark, M. R.: Endocrinology **110** (1982) 146–152.
[36] Popkin, R. M., H. M. Fraser, J. Jonassen: Molec Cell Endocr. **29** (1982) 169–159.
[37] Corbin, A., F. J. Bex: Life Sci. **29** (1981) 185–192.
[38] Ekholm, C., T. Hillensjo. O. Isaksson: Endocrinology **108** (1981) 2022–2023.
[39] Hsueh, A. J., P. B. C. Jones: Endocrine Reviews **2**, 437–461.
[40] Knecht, M., A. Amsterdam, K. J. Catt: Endrocinology **110** (1982) 865–872.
[41] Fraser, H. M., R. M. Sharpe, R. M. Popkin: In "LH-RH and Its Analogs – a New Class of Contraceptive and Therapeutic Agents" (Ed. B. H. Vickery, J. J. Nestor, E. S. E. Hafez). M.T.P. Press, Lancaster 1984.
[42] Asch, R. H., M. V. Sickle, V. Rettori et al.: J. Clin. Endocrinol. Metab. 53 (1981) 215–217.
[43] Popkin, R., T. A. Bramley, A. Currie et al.: Biochem. Biophys. Res. Commun. **14** (1983) 750–756.
[44] Brown, G. M., G. R. Van Loon, B. C. W. Hummel et al.: J. Clin. Endocrinol. Metab. **44** (1977) 784–790.
[45] Linder, J., L. W. McNeil, S. Marney et al.: J. Clin. Endocrinol. Metab. **52** (1981) 267–270.
[46] Fraser, H. M., J. Sandow, B. Krauss: Acta Endocrinologica **103** (1983) 151–157.

LH-RH agonists in the male: basic and clinical studies

F. Labrie, A. Bélanger, A. Dupont

Introduction

The availability of LH-RH and its potent agonitic analogues has led to a rapid increase in our knowledge of the pituitary-gonadal axis and has offered new and exciting therapeutic approaches inreproductive endocrinology as well as for the treatment of sex steroid-dependent diseases.

Although, as well described in another part of this symposium, the pulsatile administration of LH-RH itself is highly effective in the treatment of infertility, LH-RH agonists, on the contrary, are potent inhibitors of gonadal functions in both men and women. This presentation will attempt to summarize the data describing the inhibition of testicular functions achieved by LH-RH agonists in the male with special emphasis on the first clinical application of these peptides in the human, namely prostatic cancer.

Inhibition of testicular steroidogenesis

Experimental animals

Stimulated by the unexplained lack of success of LH-RH and its agonists in the treatment of infertility in men [1], we investigated in detail the effect of acute and chronic administration of these peptides on testicular functions in experimental animals. Somewhat unexpectedly, we then made the observation that short-term administration of the LH-RH agonist [D-Leu^6,des-Gly-NH$_2$^{10}]LH-RH ethylamide to adult male rats led to a loss of testicular LH and prolactin receptors, as well as decreased serum testosterone levels accompanied by inhibition of ventral prostate, seminal vesicle and tests weight [2–4].

These inhibitory effects can, at least partly, be explained by LH-RH agonist-induced endogenous LH release cuasing secondary gonadal desensitization [4–8], LH-RH agonists can also exert direct inhibitory effects at the testicular level in hypophysectomized rats *in vivo* as well as in testicular cells *in vitro* [5, 7, 9]. The direct testicular site of action of LH-RH agonists is supported by the finding of high affinity LH-RH binding sites in rat Leydig cells [5, 10, 11].

All *in vivo* studies on the direct gonadal site of action of LH-RH agonists were first performed in hypophysectomized animals. Since hypophysectomy by itself has profound effects on gonadal functions, we have used another approach which minimizes hormonal disturbances, in order to assess the importance of the direct action of LH-RH agonists, namely by using intact animals treated with an excess of equine antibovine LH serum. This study provided, for the first time, an assessment of the importance of the direct testicular site of action of LH-RH agonists in their antifertility activity in intact rats.

It showed that while LH-RH agonists can have direct inhibitory effects on Leydig cell function at high doses, their predominant effect, at least in short-term studies, is mediated by LH-RH agonist-induced LH release rather than by a direct inhibitory action at the esticular level, at least in the rat [7, 12]. Treatment with LH-RH agonists is also known to decrease the gonadotropin responsiveness to LH-RH [6, 13]. However, it is now clear that blockage of the steroidogenic pathway at the level of 17α-hydroxylase and 17,20-desmolase activities is responsible for at east most of the inhibitory effects of LH-RH agonists in the rat [5, 6, 8, 14].

Man

It is of great interest that inhibitory effects on testosterone secretion similar to those first described in the rat [2–4] are exerted in the male hamster [15], rabbit and dog [16]. The only exception so far reported is the monkey where androgen biosynthesis is exceptionally resistant to treatment with LH-RH agonists [17].

Among the species so far studied, man is the most sensitive to the inhibitory effect of treatment with LH-RH agonists on testicular steroidogenesis [5]. In fact, while, in the rat, treatment with LH-RH agonists increases 5α-reductase activity and formation of 3α-androstanedid and 5α-dihydrotestosterone which can partially counteract the inhibitory effect on testosterone production [8, 14], no such effect is seen in man where androgen biosynthesis can be completely inhibited and medical castration is thus achieved relatively easily with no secondary effect other than those related to low circulating androgen levels [5, 18–24].

Following our preliminary study showing that twice daily intrasanal administration of [D-Ser(TBU)^6]LH-RH-EA led to a 75% inhibition of serum testosterone concentration after 16 days [5], we then performed a long-term study of the effect of treatment with the same LH-RH agonist by the intranasal and subcutaneous routes [20, 21]. The effect of chronic treatment with [D-Ser(TBU)^6]LH-RH-EA administered by nasal spray (200 or 500 μg, twice daily) or subcutaneously (50 μg daily) for periods up to 8 months was studied on serum sex steroid and LH levels in 18 patients with cancer of the prostate. Basal serum testosterone concentration decreased to 71.1±18.3 (NS) and 28.6±9.3% ($p < 0.01$) of control in patients receiving the 200 and 500 μg doses by nasal spray, respectively. In patients treated subcutaneously at the 50 µg dose, a more rapid inhibition of serum testosterone levels to 19.6±6.4% of control ($p < 0.01$) was observed [20]. A more complete and rapid inhibition of serum testosterone levels to 5–8% of control (castrated levels) is achieved with the daily 500 µg dose [19, 24]. Elegant studies by Crowley et al. [25] have shown the potent antisteroidogenic activity of another LH-RH agonist in patients with precocious puberty.

Inhibition of spermatogenesis

Since the marked loss of testis weight following treatment with the LH-RH agonist [2–4] was likely due to some defect in spermatogenesis, it seemed important to investigate the cellular changes occurring in rat testis during chronic administration of [D-Ala^6]LH-RH-EA.

When the LH-RH agonist was administrated at the dose of 1 µg every second day, degenerative changes were observed after 4 weeks in almost all seminiferous tubules. In about 20–30% of tubules, both germinal and Sertoli cells were almost completely absent.

Although long-term treatment with LH-RH agonists in male rats causes degeneration changes in a large proportion of the seminiferous tubules with a complete loss of spermatozoa in most the inhibitory effects are never complete. This is probably due to the fact that, in this species, LH-RH agonist treatment increases 5α-reductase activity [8, 26] which, as mentioned earlier, counteracts the inhibitory effect resulting from the almost complete inhibition of testosterone production. Although the rat was the first species where the inhibitory effects of treatment with LH-RH agonist were described on both androgen biosynthesis [2–4] and spermatogenesis [27], and studies in this species have been essential for understanding the mechanisms involved [2–8], it is not the best model for the human. In fact, in man, there is no stimulatory effect of LH-RH agonist treatment on 5α-reductase activity and a parallel inhibitory effect is observed on both testosterone and 5α-dihydrotestosterone formation [5, 18, 19]. Our current studies in the dog indicate that this species is a more appropriate model for studying the antifertility effects of LH-RH agonists. The pattern of serum steroid levels observed after LH-RH agonist treatment in man and in dog is very similar. Histology of the testis after chronic treatment of dogs with [D-Ser(TBU)^6]LH-RH-EA shows a marked atrophy of the tubules and a complete inhibition of sperm formation. That treatment with LH-RH agonists can inhibit spermatogenesis in men has been shown by the study of Linde et al. [28].

So far, the responsibility for fertility control has almost exclusively been limited to women. It is thus important that special efforts be made in order to develop a safe, acceptable, reliable and reversible method of fertility regulation in men. The current approaches in male contraception have serious limitations. While gossypol presents some toxicity problems [29, 30], the combination of gestagens and androgens induces azoospermia in only approximately 70% of men while varying degrees of oligospermia are obtained in the remaining 30% of subjects [31, 32]. Moreover, the development of immunological reactions in vasectomized men is of some concern.

An alternative approach is the combined use of an LH-RH agonist and androgen replacement therapy. Now that reversibility of sperm formation has been observed in an experimental model (Tremblay, Bélanger and Labrie, unpublished observations), clinical studies in adult men receiving androgen replacement therapy should provide the required answers concerning the efficacy and acceptability of this approach.

Cancer of the prostate

Cancer of the prostate is the second cause of death due to cancer in man. The pioneering studies of Huggins and collaborators [33] have demonstrated the role of testicular androgen in prostatic cancer. In fact, significant improvement of the clinical condition follows castration or estrogen administration in 60 to 70% of patients with advanced prostatic carcinoma. Subsequently, during the last 40 years, the principal goal of hormonal therapy in the treatment of prostatic cancer has been the suppression of androgens of testicular origin.

Inhibition of testicular androgen secretion by estrogen administration and removal of the source of testicular androgens by surgical orchiectomy have shown similar palliative effects in advanced prostatic carcinoma. In fact, 60 to 60% of patients with prostatic carcinoma show a positive response to either of these two treatments as evidenced by objective and/or subjective parameters. These hormonal manipulations thus provide remission for various time intervals in a large proportion of patients. However, castration is not always well accepted by the patients while high doses of estrogens have serious cardiovascular side effects [34].

In agreement with all previous endocrine therapies which had shown that a positive response is observed in 60 to 70% of cases of prostatic cancer when serum testosterone levels are reduced to castration levels, it was observed, in a collaborative preliminary study, that a similar rate of response is found following treatment with LH-RH agonists [21]. This has now been confirmed by a study of the Abbott group [22, 23] as well as by ICI studies (unpublished observations).

However, treatment with LH-RH agonists is accompanied, during the first five to fifteen days of treatment, by increased serum androgen levels leading to a disease flare in some patients [22, 23]. Moreover, androgens of adrenal origin could well play a role in the relapse which regularly follows standard hormonal therapy. We thus felt that the next logical step in the hormonal therapy of prostate cancer was the combined use of an LH-RH agonist and a pure antiandrogen.

A major previous limitation to the use of pure antiandrogens in the treatment of prostate cancer has been the escape phenomenon due to the neutralization of the inhibitory feedback action of androgens by the antiandrogen, which led to a progressive increase in gonadotropin and testosterone secretion. This readjustement of androgen secretion at higher levels requires progressively higher doses of the antiandrogen leading to toxicity problems as well as lack of efficient neutralization of the effect of androgens on the growth of the cancer. Since treatment with LH-RH agonists causes a desensitization of the gonadotropin response to LH-RH as well as an inhibition of testicular androgen biosynthesis, a solution is thus available to the previous limitations of pure antiandrogens. We then found that daily administration for five months of a potent LH-RH agonist in combination with a pure antiandrogen, RU 23908, causes an almost complete inhibition of ventral prostate and seminal vesicle weight in the rat [35].

Following these encouraging results, we have performed a preliminary study using combination therapy with the same LH-RH agonist and pure antiandrogen [19] in patients with advanced prostatic cancer. This preliminary study was originally performed in 9 patients at stage D and in 1 patient at stage C of the disease. Objective remission as ascertained by bone scan, acid phosphatase levels and ultrasonography of the prostate was recorded in 9 patients.

The present report is a continuation of this study in 97 patients at stage D of the disease. The combination therapy was used in 44 previously untreated patients as well as in 24 patients previously treated with DES (diethylstilbestrol). In 9 previously untreated patients, complete androgen neutralization was achieved by surgical castration (instead of LH-RH agonist administration) and the antiandrogen. For comparison, in 29 patients showing relapse of the disease after surgical castration, the effect of antiandrogen administration has been studied. In support of our previous suggestion, the present study clearly indicates that drastic changes in the approach to hormonal therapy of prostatic cancer are appropriate.

Serum prostatic acid phosphatase

Serum prostatic acid phosphatase (PAP) measured by radioimmunoassay was elevated in 70 out of 97 patients at initiation of treatment. It can be seen in figure 1 that serum PAP was rapidly reduced to 45% of pretreatment values as early as 5 days after starting the combined antihormonal therapy using the LH-RH agonist and the antiandrogen in previously untreated patients. The serum PAP values progressively decreased and normal values were reached within two months in all except 4 patients who all showed normal serum PAP levels at 4 months. A comparable pattern was seen in the patients previously untreated who were surgically castrated and received the same dose of the antiandrogen (data not shown).

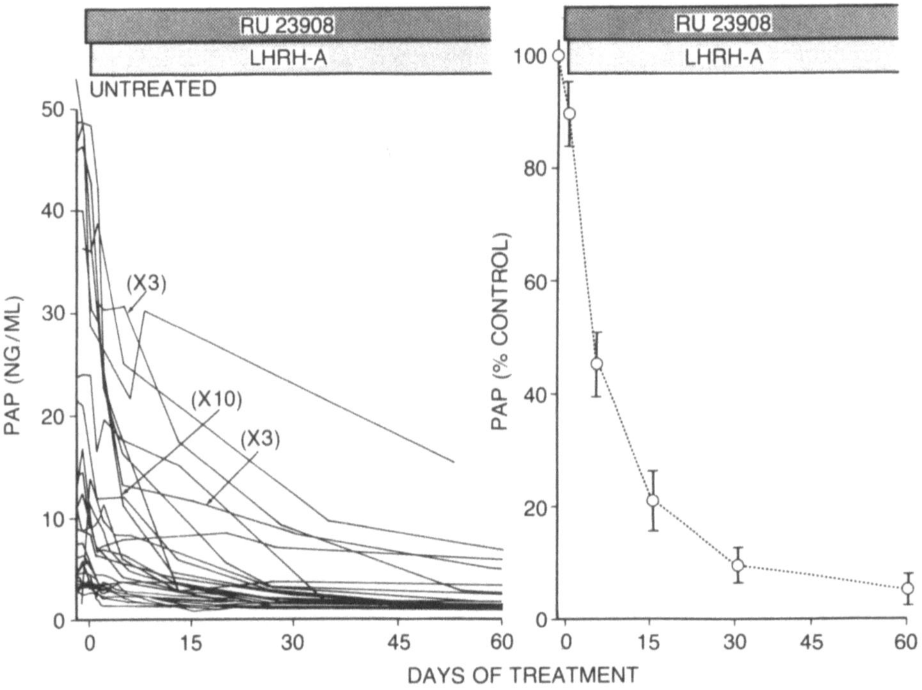

Fig. 1 Effect of combined treatment with an LHRH agonist and a pure antiandrogen on serum PAP levels in previously untreated patients with advanced (stage D2) prostatic cancer. Individual values are shown on the left panel while means ± SEM are illustrated on the right panel (25 patients) [36].

It can be seen in figure 2 that a striking difference is observed when the same treatment is applied to patients previously treated with DES and showing relapse of the disease. In fact, although serum PAP levels decreased to normal values in some patients, the levels of serum PAP continued to increase in 11 out of 24 patients. Similarly, in patients previously castrated, stabilization or an increase of serum PAP levels was seen in 75% of patients (data not shown).

Objective response according to the NPCP criteria to the combined treatment with an LH-RH agonist (or surgical castration) and a pure antiandrogen in previously untreated patients with prostate cancer at stage D or previously treated with DES as well as to treatment with the antiandrogen in stage D patients previously castrated [36].

As already seen in the first adult man treated with a high dose of an LH-RH agonist [5], treatment with LH-RH agonists alone is always accompanied by a rise in serum T and DHT concentration which lasts for 5 to 15 days [5, 19, 22, 23, 24] and is

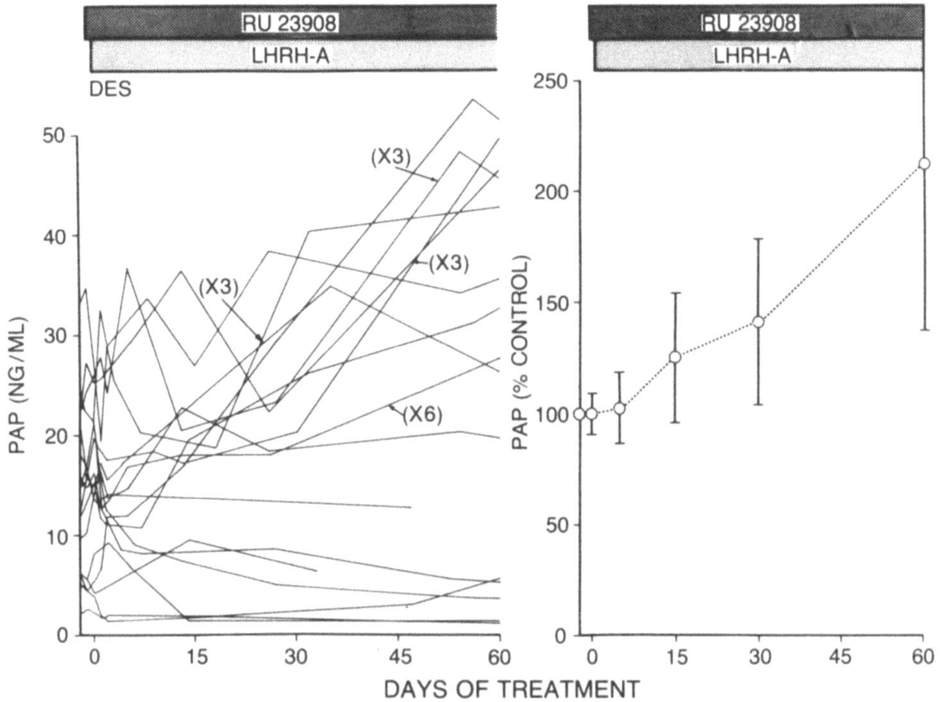

Fig. 2 Effect of combined treatment with an LHRH agonist (HOE-766) and a pure antiandrogen (RU23908) on serum PAP levels in patients with advanced (stage D2) prostatic cancer previously treated with diethylstilbestrol. Individual values are shown on the left panel while means ± SEM are illustrated on the right panel (9 patients) [36].

accompanied in a significant proportion of cases by a flare of the cancer [22, 23]. It is thus of great interest to see in figures 1 and 3 that a 55% decrease in serum PAP is already observed during the first 5 days of treatment with the LH-RH agonist at a time when serum androgens are increased by 100 to 200% ($p < 0.01$, fig. 3).

Hormonal

Before treatment, except in patients treated with high doses of DES, or castrated, serum steroid values were within the normal range. As expected, chronic administration of the LH-RH agonist in combination with RU 23908 led to a marked inhibition of serum T levels to 2.50±0.03% of control. It was also found, somewhat surprisingly, that serum levels of DHEAS and DHEA were also decreased to 45.0±4.7 and 64±5.0% of control, respectively, while serum cortisol levels remained unchanged (fig. 4).

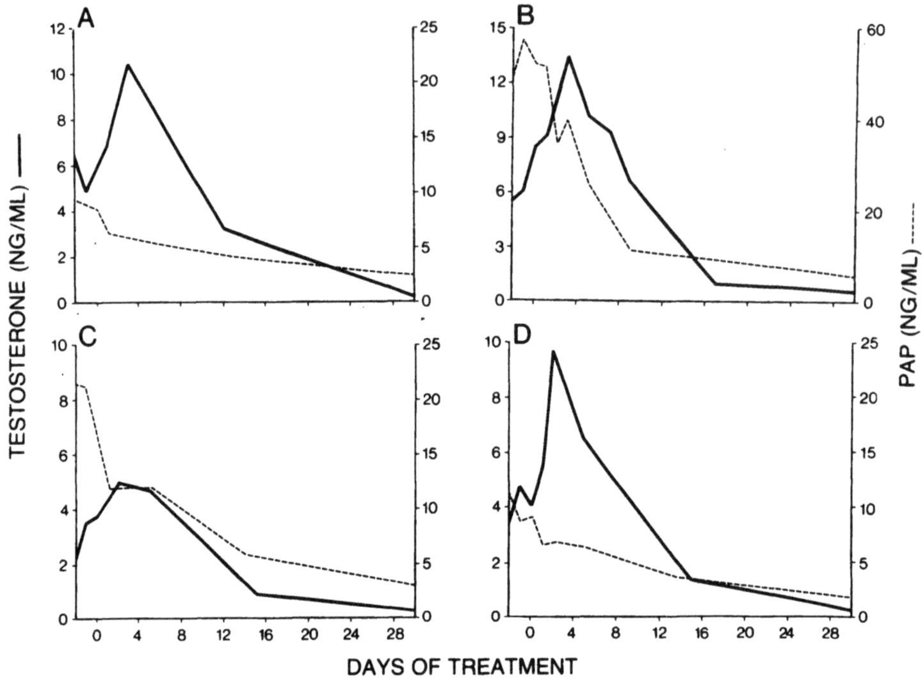

Fig. 3 Changes in serum PAP and testosterone levels during the first month of treatment in four previously untreated patients having advanced prostatic concer and receiving the combined administration of the LHRH agonist HOE-766 and the pure antiandrogen RU23908. Note the rapid and marked decrease in serum PAP concentration in the presence of elevated serum T levels, thus indicating the efficiency of the antiandrogen at the dose used [24].

Bone scanning

In 32 previously untreated patients having metastatic disease, the combined therapy led to at least a 50% decrease in uptake accompanied by a normalization of serum PAP and no appearance of new lesions. A complete disappearance of bone lesions was seen within 5 months in 4 patients, thus indicating complete objective response. In the other 12 patients classified as stable, serum PAP levels are decreasing but have not yet reached normal values. A most important finding is that none of the 44 previously untreated patients receiving the combination therapy showed progression of the diseases (tab. 1).

Clinical signs and symptoms

In the previously untreated patients, a rapid and complete relief of pain was observed in all patients presenting this symptom before treatment. Disappearance of bone pain was seen within a few days. In patients previously treated with DES, complete re-

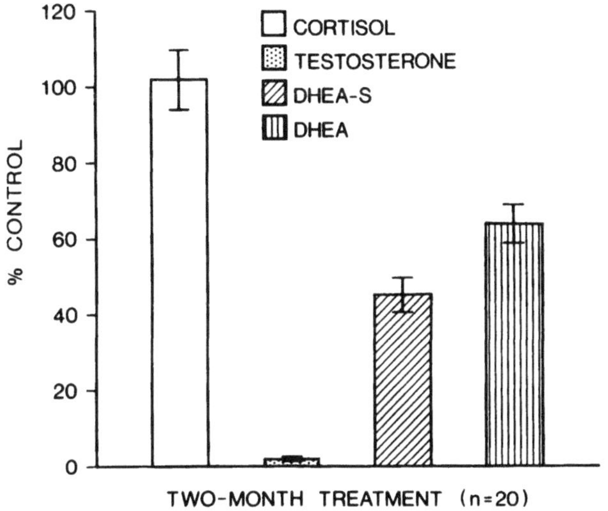

Fig. 4 Effect of 2-month combined treatment with die LHRH agonist (HOE-766) and the antiandrogen RU23908 on serum levels of cortisol (F), testosterone (T), dehydroepiandrosterone (DHEA) and dehydroepiandrosterone sulfate (DHEA-S) in 20 previously untreated patients having prostatic cancer. Control levels of F, T, DHEA-S and DHEA were respectively 156± 6, 5.44 ± 0.44, 834 ± 147 and 1.9 ± 0.3 ng/ml [37].

Table 1 Objective response to the complete removal of androgens

				% Objective response					
Previous treatment	Months of RX	Current RX	No of pts	Complete	Partial	Stable	Progression	Escape	
NIL	9.9 (4–18)	LHRH-A +Anti- Andr.	35	9% (3)	71% (25)	20% (7)	0% 0%	2/35	4.5% 2/44
NIL	7.3 (4–11)	Castr. +Anti- andr.	9	11% (1)	33% (3)	56% (5)	0% 0	0/9	
DES	8.5 (3–14)	LHRH-A +Anti- andr.	24	4% (1)	37% (9)	17% (4)	42% (10)	4/14	25% 6/24
CASTR.	8.1 (4–11)	LHRH-A +Anti- andr.	13	0% 0	8% (1)	31% (4)	61% (8)	2/5	
CASTR. + DES	6.5 (4–10)	Anti- andr.	16	0% 0	19% (3)	12% (2)	69% (11)	0/5	

moval of androgens also led to a disappearance of pain in all patients, while in patients previously castrated, disappearance of pain was seen in 12 out of 16 patients. A partial relief of pain was obtained in the 4 others. Although more diffucult to evaluate due to the frequent concomitant presence of benign prostatic hyperplasia, signs of prostatism were improved in 80 to 100% of patients. The improvement in signs of prostatism was confirmed by rectal examination as well as by transrectal and transabdominal echography in all cases. Improvement in performance and well-being (appetite, sleep, general activity and body weight) was seem in 100% of previously untreated patients while an approximately 60% improvement was seen in the patients previously treated with DES or castrated.

As revealed by a series of standard biochemical and hematological tests, treatment with the LH-RH agonist and the antiandrogen has no detectable effect on any of the following parameters: complete (WBC, RBC, hemoglobin, hematocrit and platelets) and differential blood count, γ-glutamyl transaminase, glutamic oxaloacetic transaminase, glutamic pyruvic transferase, lactic dehydrogenase, creatinine, total bilibu-rin and other parameters of blood biochemistry (SMA-12).

As the duration of treatment and the number of patients included in this study increases, a most consequent conclusion which is clearly seen is that prostate cancer in man is extremely sensitive to androgens. In fact, when complete androgen neutraliziation is achieved in patients previously untreated, a positive objective response assessed according to the criteria of the National Prostatic Cancer Project is observed in more than 95% of patients. In fact, in 44 patients who received the combined therapy with the LH-RH agonist or surgical castration, and the antiandrogen, no progression of the disease was observed in any patient.

Another most important conclusion which can be drawn from the present study is that a large proportion of prostatic cancer cells which continue to grow under the influence of androgens of adrenal origin become insensitive to androgens in this "androgen-poor" milieu. This is clearly demonstrated by the finding that complete androgen neutralization in patients previously treated with estrogens or castrated leads to only 30 to 40% positive/objective responses as compared to more than 95% in previously untreated patients. The much lower rate of response observed in previously treated patients indicates a marked increase in the proportion of androgen-insensitive cancer cells in these patients. The relatively low rate of response observed after removal of adrenal androgens in previously treated patients in our study is in agreement with the data obtained in the same category of patients following surgical or medical adrenalectomy [38–41]. It is thus clear that in these patients, neutralization of testicular androgens left an important proportion of cells growing in an "androgen-poor" milieu.

These two predominant findings, namely extremely high androgen sensitivity of prostatic cancer not previously treated and the transformation into androgen-insensitive cells in the presence of androgens of adrenal origin have major implications for the choice of early versus late hormonal therapy in prostatic cancer as well as complete versus partial neutralization of androgens.

Another important finding in the present study is that concomitant treatment with the pure antiandrogen completely prevents disease flare, a complication unfortunately observed in a significant proportion of patients treated with LH-RH agonists alone [22, 23]. With the present knowledge, there remains no reason to use LH-RH agonists alone since the effect of the initial rise in serum androgens can be so easily prevented, thus eliminating any unnecessary risk to the patient.

Due to its excellent tolerance and lack of secondary effects other than those related to hypoandrogenicity, the present findings strongly suggest that complete androgen neutralization achieved by the present approach should be initiated as early as possible after diagnosis (at least at stage C and D) in order to obtain remission in almost all patients and to minimize the appearance of androgen-insensitive cell clones, thus improving the quality of life and faciliting the possible application of other treatments such as radiotherapy and/or chemotherapy in the cases developing androgen-independent tumors.

References

[1] Krabbe, S., N. E. Shakkeback: Acta Paediatr. Scand. **66** (1977) 361–365.
[2] Auclair, C., P. A. Kelly, F. Labrie et al.: Biochem. Biophys. Res. Commun. **76** (1977a) 855–862.
[3] Auclair, C., P. A. Kelly, D. H. Coy et al.: Endocrinology **101** (1977b) 855–862.
[4] Labrie, F., C. Auclair, L. Cusan et al.: Endocrine Appraoch to Male Contraception. Int. J. Androl. (Suppl. 2) (1978) 303–318.
[5] Labrie, F., A. Bélanger, L. Cusan et al.: J. Androl. **1** (1980) 209–228.
[6] Cusan, L., C. Auclair, A. Bélanger: Endocrinology **104** (1979) 1369–1376.
[7] Séguin, C., A. Bélanger, F. Labrie et al.: Biol. Reprod. **24** (1981) 889–901.
[8] Bélanger, A., L. Cusan, C. Auclair et al.: Biol. Reprod. **22** (1980) 1094–1101.
[9] Hsueh, A. J. W., G. F. Erickson: Nature **281** (1979) 66–68.
[10] Lefebvre, F. A., J. J. Reeves, C. Séguin et al.: Mol. Cell. Endocrinol. **20** (1980) 127–134.
[11] Perrin, M. H., J. M. Vaughan, J. E. Rivier et al.: Life Sci. **26** (1980) 2251–2255.
[12] Séguin, C., A. Bélanger, F. Labrie et al.: Endocrinology **110** (1982) 524–530.
[13] Sandow, J., W. V. von Rechenberg, W. Konig et al.: Hypothalamic Hormones – Chemistry, Physiology and Clinical Applications (Eds. D. Gupta, W. Voelters) pp. 307–326 Verlag Chemie, Weinheim 1978.
[14] Bélanger, A., C. Auclair, L. Ferland et al.: J. Steroid Biochem. **13** (1980) 191–196.
[15] Sandow, J., M. Hahn: Acta Endocrinol. **88** (1978) 601–610.
[16] Vickery, B. H.: In "LH-RH Peptides as Females and Male Contraceptives" (Eds. G. I. Zatuchni, J. D. Shelton, J. J. Sciarra), pp. 109–125, Harper and Row Publ., Philadelphia 1981.
[17] Resko, J., A. Bélanger, F. Labrie: Biol. Reprod. **26** (1982) 378–384.
[18] Bélanger, A., F. Labrie, A. Lemay et al.: J. Steroid Biochem. **13** (1980) 123–126.
[19] Labrie, F., A. Dupont, A. Bélanger et al.: J. Clin. Invest. Med. **5** (1982) 267–275.
[20] Faure, N., F. Labrie, A. Lemay et al.: Fertil. Steril. **37** (1982) 416–424.

[21] Tolis, G., D. Ackman, A. Stellos et al.: Proc. Natl. Acad. Sci. USA, **79** (1982) 1658–1662.
[22] Santen, R. J., B. Warner, L. M. Demers et al.: In "LH-RH and Its Analogs – A New Class of Contraceptive and Therapeutic Agents" (edited by B. Vickery, J. J. Nestor, Jr., E. S. E. Hafez). MTP Press, Lancaster-Boston 1983, in press.
[23] Trachtenberg, J.: J. Urol. **129** (1983) 1149–1152.
[24] Labrie, F., A. Dupont, A. Bélanger: The Prostate (1983), in press.
[25] Crowley, W. F. Jr., F. Comite, W. Vale: J. Clin. Endocrinol. **52** (1981) 370–372.
[26] Carmichael. R., A. Bélanger, L. Cusan et al.: Steroids **36** (1980) 383–391.
[27] Pelletier, G., L. Cusan, C. Auclair et al.: Endocrinology **103** (1978) 641–643.
[28] Linde, R., G. Doelle, N. Alexander: New Engl. J. Med. **305** (1981) 663–667.
[29] National Coordinating Group on Male Antifertility Agents: Clin. Med. J. (Engl.) **4** (1978) 417–423.
[30] Djerasi, C.: The Politics of Contraception (Ed. W. W. Norton), pp. 183–213. New York 1980.
[31] Schearer, S. B., F. Alvarez-Sanchez, J. Anselmo et al.: Int. J. Androl., suppl. **2** (1978) 680–689.
[32] Lee, H. Y., S. I. Kim, E. H. Kwon: Scand. J. Med. **20** (1979) 1–8.
[33] Huggins, C., C. V. Hodges: Cancer Res. **1** (1941) 293–297.
[34] Bailar, J. C., D. P. Byar, Vet. Adm. Coop. Urol. Res. Group: Cancer **26** (1970) 257–259.
[35] Lefebvre, F. A., C. Séguin, A. Bélanger et al.: The Prostate **3** (1982) 569–578.
[36] Labrie, F., A. Dupont, A. Bélanger et al.: In "Hormones and Cancer". Raven Press, in press.
[37] Bélanger, A., A. Dupont, F. Labrie: J. Androl., in press.
[38] Bhanalaph, T., M. J. Varkarakis, G. P. Murphy: Ann. Surg. **179** (1974) 17–23.
[39] Harrison, J. H., G. W. Thorn, D. Jenkins: N. Engl. J. Med. **248** (1953) 86–92.
[40] Huggins, C., C. V. Hodges: Cancer Res. **1** (1941) 293–297.
[41] MacFarlane, D. A., L. P. Thomas, J. H. Harrisson: Amer. J. Surg. **99** (1960) 562–572.

A new approach to male contraception using combined androgen and GnRH analog treatment

R. S. Swerdloff, S. Bhasin, D. Heber

Introduction

The ideal male contraceptive agent would be easily available, immediately effective completely reliable, free of toxic effects and rapidly and assuredly reversible. The only presently available form of male contraception that approaches these goals is the condom. Its widespread usage is limited by complaints that it interferes with the spontaneous and pleasurable aspects of sexual intercourse.

Despite the diversity of effective available female contraceptive approaches, investigations have continued to be directed toward finding new male contraceptives. The incentives for such studies include the recognition of adverse reactions from female agents, the increasing social attitude of shared responsibility for family planning between spouses and the desire of some men with multiple or transient relationships to be free of concerns of possible paternity.

We have been involved for some time in the search for an effective system male contraceptive agent that would result in reversible inhibition of spermatogenesis (azoospermia) without accompanying impairment of sexual function or other undue adverse effects. In these studies, we and others have examined the effects of synthetic androgens, progestational agents and GnRH analogs on the reproductive hormonal system and on spermatogenesis, and their potential role as contraceptive agents.

Since the end point of these studies would be the inhibition of spermatogenesis, a brief description of the regulators of sperm maturation will be presented.

Spermatogenesis in the human results in the progressive maturation of germ cells from spermatgonia to mature spermatozoa. This process requires at least 14 intermediate stanges and takes approximately 70 days [1]. The process requires an intact hypothalamic-pituitary axis resulting in the normal pattern of secretion of the two gonadotropic hormones, luteinizing hormone (LH) and follicle stimulating hormone (FSH). LH effects on spermatogenesis are mediated by its stimulation of secretion of testosterone which diffuses from the interstitial space into the spermatogenic tubule, where it affects spermatogenesis either directly or through effects on Sertoli cell function. FSH acts directly on Sertoli cells to stimulate the production and release of a number of factors which act in concert with testosterone in an incompletely understood fashion to stimulate the spermatogenic process [2, 3].

From this background information, it is apparent that spermatogenesis is dependent on gonadotropic hormones. This is confirmed by observations that hypophysectomized and LH and FSH deficient men demonstrate predictable azoospermia. These observations have led to attempts so suppress gonadotropin secretion which drugs for contraceptive purposes. To this end, several types of agents have been tested. Because of their success as female contraceptives, steroids were a logical first approach.

In our studies with depot forms of testosterone, we utilized testosterone enanthate in doses as high as 200 mg each week. This proved to be relatively effective, resulting in decreased blood levels of LH and FSH (approximately 50% of baseline), testosterone concentrations that were only moderately elevated compared to baseline, and a mean inhibition of sperm concentration of 97% in the semen of our subjects [11]. Almost all subjects (35 of 39) attained sperm counts of less than 5 million/cc and 60% were azoospermia. Other investigators have reported similar results with androgens alone and androgens plus progestogens [4–11]. No regimen has produced azoospermia in all subjects tested. In the short term studies reported (up to 6 months of treatment), very few adverse effects have been observed.

GnRH agonistic analogs were originally developed as longer acting therapeutic agents to treat GnRH deficient patients. After early trials, it became apparent that they were poor therapeutic substitutes for authentic short-acting GnRH and that, when given chronically, they had paradoxical inhibitory actions on LH and FSG secretion [13]. Subsequent studies demonstrated additional direct inhibitory actions on LH and FSH secretion [13]. Subsequent studies demonstrated additional direct inhibitory effects of GnRH agonists on rat testes [13]. Reports of these antigonadal effects raised hopes of their potential application as male contraceptive and clinical trials were begun in several laboratories. Bergquist et al. [12] treated men for 17 weeks with 5 mcg daily of DSer(TBU)^{6}GnRH ethylamide with little effect on spermatogenesis, while LH, FSG and testosterone fell. Linde et al administered 50 μg of (DTrp^6, Pro^9-N-ethylamide) GnRH daily and observed a fall in serum testosterone with a mean nadir of 60 ng/dl by the fourth week of teratment [14, 15]. Agonist treatment was discontinued after 6 or 7 weeks in five of eight subjects because of impotence. Libido and potency returned two weeks after stopping agonist therapy, but the occurence of these symptoms represented a significant drawback to the application of GnRH agonists alone as male contraceptive agents. Of three subjects who completed 10 weeks of therapy, one was azoospermic. Recovery of spermatogenesis occurred within 10 weeks of cessation of therapy in all but the one azoospermic subject, who recovered after 14 weeks. In this regard, studies from our labratory suggsted that combined androgen and agonist treatment might lead to the development of an effective, practical male contraceptive agent. We argued that their combined use was theoretically attractive for two reasons. First, testosterone treatment would prevent the undesirable side effects of impotence and diminished libido; and second, androgens alone are potent inhibitors of spermatogenesis in man, the addition of a second gonadotropin inhibitor might have additive or synergistic effects on the testis.

Our initial studies on combined GnRH agonist and testosterone treatment were performed in laboratory rats. Adult male Wistar rats were treated for 60 days with daily injections of GnRH analog alone, a subcutaneous testosterone implant, or analog and testosterone in combination [16, 17]. The resulting intratesticular sperm counts are shown in table 1. These data confirmed other observations that GnRH agonist would significantly inhibit spermatogenesis and demonstrated a synergistic effect of combined androgen and GnRH agonist therapy. These data were encouraging, but emerging information indicated that the prime site of inhibitory action of GnRH agonists on the reproductive system in the rat was at testicular level, while the human was affected primarily at the pituitary gland [18].

Clinical studies in our laboratories have utilized the GnRH agonist $D(Nal_2)^6$ GnRH (Syntex Research). Preliminary studies assessed two doses of this potent agonist on testosterone, LH and FSH secretion [19]. Daily administration resulted in an early phase of stimulation followed by a progressive decline in LH, FSH and testosterone to serum levels below baseline by day 10 of treatment. The higher dose (100 μg) was more potent in both the stimulatory and down regulatory phases. Combined treatment of a single 200 mg dose of testosterone enanthate with daily subcutaneous injections of 100 μg of GnRH agonist did not blunt the peak LH and FSH responses on day 2, but resulted in significantly lower LH (187±30 vs. 234s±42 mIU-day/ml) and FSH (20.6±3.3 vs. 32.8±4.2 mIU-day/ml) responses, as assessed by paired comparisons of the areas under the curve, from days 3–11 [20].These studies suggested that the addition of testosterone to GnRH analog had additive or synergistic inhibitory effects on LH and FSH secretion and encouraged us to test the combination in longer-term studies assessing spermatogenesis.

In the most recent studies, seven men were given daily subcutaneous injections of 200 μg of $D(Nal_2)^6$GnRH in combination with 200 mg of testosterone enanthate every two weeks [21, 22]. The mean sperm count declined to a nadir of 13.8±7 mil-

Table 1 Intratesticular sperm counts (million/testis) in adult male rats after chronic treatment with D-leu^{6}desGly^{10}-GnRH, testosterone implants or both

Group	Day 40	Day 60
Control (10)	145 ± 7	169 ± 13
Testosterone implanted (10)	156 ± 15	122 ± 16
Analog at 200 ng	62 ± 10	44 ± 11
Analog plus testosterone	34 ± 7	9 ± 1.6

lion/cc (fig. 1). However, one subject did not show any significant suppression of sperm count as assessed by regression analysis. If this subject were excluded, the mean sperm count in the remaining six subjects declined by more than 90%. While no patients became azoospermic, one patient had sperm counts below 50,000 per milliliter of semen. Thus, this combined regimen of intermittent agonist injection with bimonthly injections of testosterone did not induce azoospermia. These results are similar to those of Evans et al., who also noted only partial suppression of spermatogenesis with a combined regimen that employed subsuppressive dose of testosterone [23].

Basal serum LH concentrations after an initial phase of stimulation returned to baseline by d28 and progressively fell to 50% of baseline by the end of the treatment period (fig. 2). Basal FSH concentrations declined more rapidly than LH to 40–50% of baseline by the end of second week and stayed decreased thereafter (fig. 3). Following discontinuation of treatment, both LH and FSH returned to baseline within 4–6 weeks without a significant rebound [22].

Detailed LH responses to GnRH agonists on days 0, 1, 28 and 112 were assessed by multiple blood sampling for LH and FSH over 24 h period. On day 1, LH concentrations rise promptly and stay elevated for the entire 24 h period. In contrast, the LH responses on days 28 and 112 are strikingly blunted with no significant rise in LH after agonist injection. indicating significant down-regulation of pituitary LH secretion.

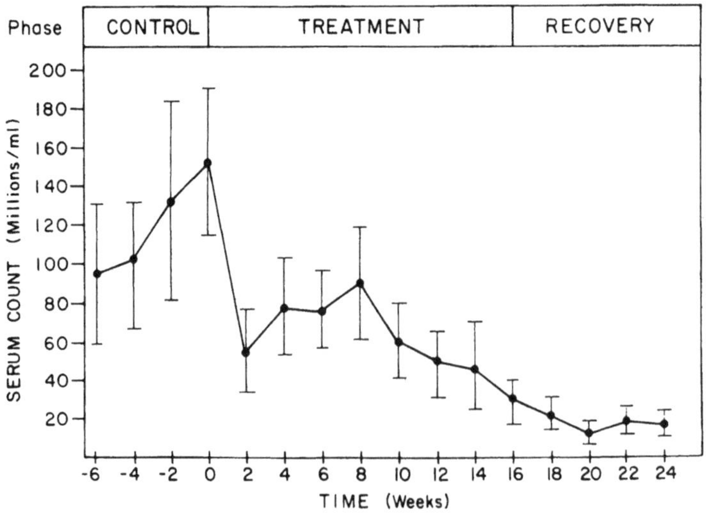

Fig. 1 Effect of combined treatment on sperm count. The data are mean ± S. E. M. n = 7. One subject did not show significant suppression as assessed by regression analysis. No subjects became azoospermic. Reproduced with permission from Bhasin et al. [22].

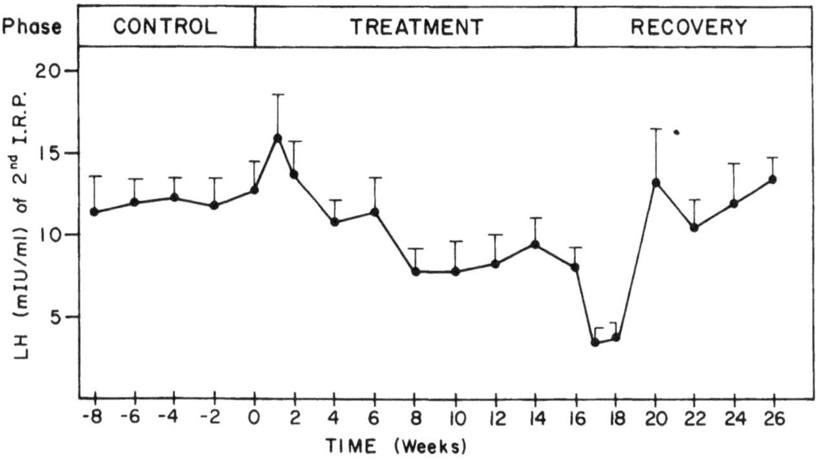

Fig. 2 Effect of combined treatment on basal LH concentrations. Data are mean ± S. E. M. n = 7. Reproduced with permission from Bhasin et al. [22].

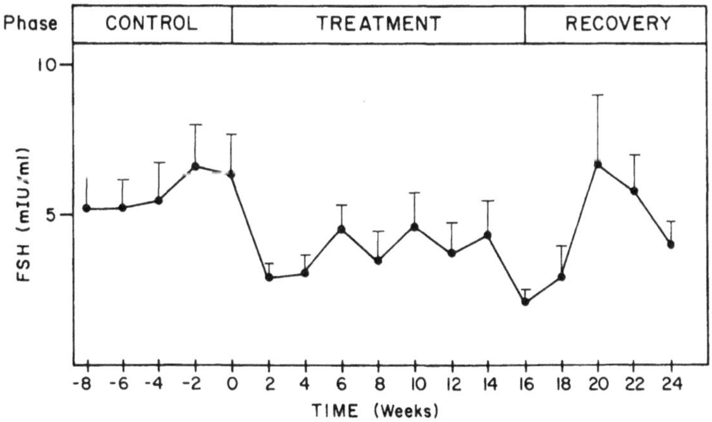

Fig. 3 Effect of combined treatment on basal FSH concentrations. Data are mean ± S. E. M. n = 7. Reproduced with permission from Bhasin et al. [22].

Effects of combined treatment on 24 h integrated LH and FSH responses on d1, 10, 28, 56 and 112 were assessed by calculating the areas under the curve on these days above d0 baseline. The stimulatory effcts of the agonist abate by d28 (fig. 4). Despite this loss of stimulatory response, only a very modest inhibition of integrated LH and FSH responses below baseline can be seen even as late as d112. Another method of assessing integrated LH secretion is to measure urinary LH, which has been shown to

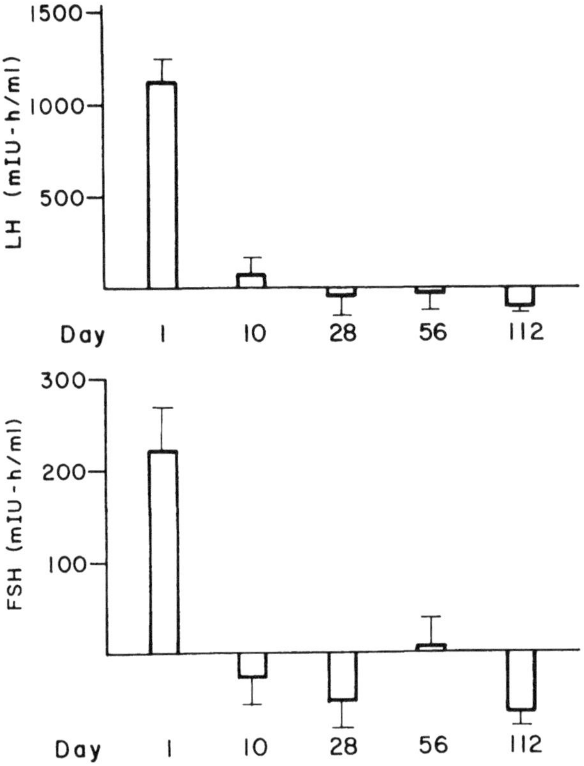

Fig. 4 Effect of combined treatment on 24h. integrated LH and FSH concentrations. 24h. integrated LH and FSH concentrations were assessed by calculating areas under the curve, above d0 (control) baseline. Data are mean ± S. E. M. n = 7. Reproduced with permission from Bhasin et al. [22].

accurately reflect 24 h LH secretion. 24 h urinary LH in subjects treated with the combined regimen, after an initial phase of stimulation, returns to baseline by d10–28 but does not show significant inhibition below d0 baseline at any time (fig. 5). Thus, integrated immunoreactive LH secretion, assessed by measuring the areas under the curve or by 24 h urinary LH, shows no significant inhibition during the 16-week treatment period. In light of these observations, it is intriguing that the sperm counts fell by approximately 90% in 6 out of 7 subjects. In separate studies in subjects treated with similar dosages of GnRH agonist alone for 28 days, serum testosterone concentrations were noted to decrease far more than could be explained by the modest decrease in serum gonadotropins, measured by standard radioimmunoassays. These data indicate that the antigonadal effects of the GnRH agonist in the human male cannot be fully explained on basis of down-regulation of pituitary gonadotropin secretion alone; additional mechanisms need to be invoked. Prelimi-

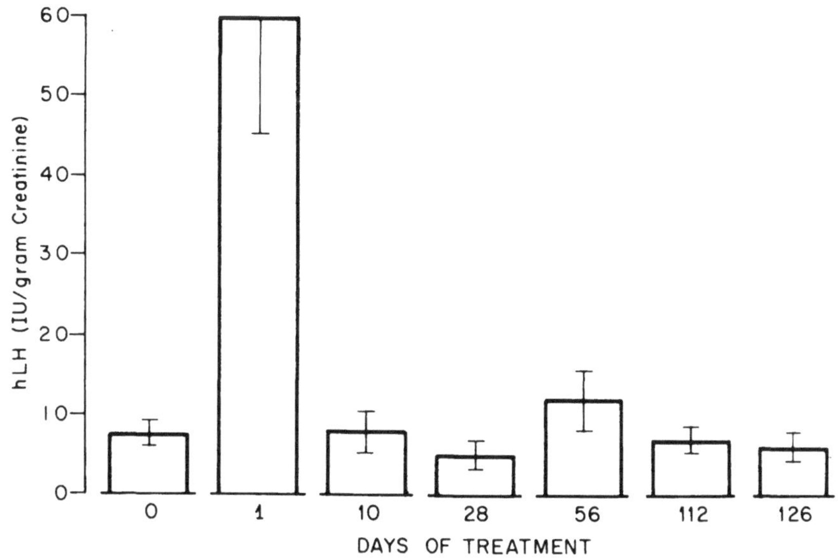

Fig. 5 Effect of combined treatment on 24h. urinary LH concentrations. Data are means ± S. E. M. n = 7. Reproduced with permission from Bhasin et al. [22].

nary data from our and other laboratories suggest that GnRH agonist treatment may result in secretion of qualitatively different LH species with diminished biologic activity [24, 25]. Other possibilities include loss of pulsatile pattern of gonadotropin secretion, direct inhibition at the gonadal level and secretion of a circulating inhibitor of LH action.

The failure of combined regimens employing intermittent injections of GnRH agonist appears related at least in part to imcomplete suppression of gonadotropins because complete hypophysectomy predictably leads to azoospermia. This may be due to several factors including the possibilities that: 1. human male may be biologically resistant to the inhibitory effects of the GnRH agonist; 2. the dose of the agonist could have been inadequate and 3. the regimens of intermittent daily injection may fail to provide constant and optimum blood levels.

Of these, the latter appears likely since the serum concentrations of the GnRH agonist, measured by radioimmunoassay, decline to undetectable levels by 12 h after the agonist injection. Furthermore, studies in rhesus monkey have shown that constant infusion of GnRH agonist results in far greater suppression of gonadotropins and spermatogenesis than regimens of intermittent injection [26]. This hypothesis, if borne out by our current investigations in the human male using constant subcutaneous injections, could be followed by studies evaluating biodegradable or removable long-term implants of GnRH agonist combined with testosterone.

References

[1] Heller, C. G., Y. Clermont: Recent Prog. Horm. Res. **20** (1964) 545–575.

[2] Bardin, C. W., C. A. Paulsen: In "Textbook of Endocrinology" (Ed. R. H. Williams), Chapter 6, pp. 293–354. W. B. Saunders Co., Philadelphia 1981.

[3] Swerdloff, R. S.: In "Campbell's Urology" (Ed. J. H. Harrision), 4th edition, pp. 125–133. W. B. Saunders Co., Philadelphia 1978.

[4] Cunningham, G. R., V. E. Silverman, I. Thornby et al.: J. Clin. Endocrinol. Metab. **49** (1979) 420.

[5] Leonard, J. M., C. A. Paulsen: In "Hormonal Control of Male Fertility" (Ed. D. J. Patanelli), p. 223. DHEW Publ. No. (NIH) 78–1097, 1978.

[6] Nieschlags, E., H. Hoogen, M. Bolk et al.: Contraception **18** (1978) 607.

[7] Paulsen, C. A., J. M. Leonard, E. C. Burgess et al.: In "Hormonal Control of Male Fertility" (Ed. D. J. Patanelli), p. 17. DHEW Publ. No. (NIH) 78–1097, 1970.

[8] Schearer, S. B.: In "Hormonal Control of Male Fertility" (Ed. D. J. Patanelli), p. 257. DHEW Publ. No. (NIH) 78–1097, 1978.

[9] Steinberger, E., K. D. Smith, L. J. Rodriguez-Rigau: Int. J. Androl. (Suppl.) **2** (1978) 748.

[10] Swerdloff, R. S., A. Palacios, R. D. McClure et al.: Int. J. Androl. (Suppl.) **2** (1978) 731.

[11] Swerdloff, R. S., L. A. Campfield, A. Palacios et al.: J. Steroid Biochem. **11** (1979) 663–670.

[12] Auclair, C., P. A. Kelly, D. H. Coy et al.: Endocrinology **101** (1977) 1890.

[13] Bergquist, C., S. J. Nillius, R. Beight et al.: Acta Endocrinol. **91** (1979) 601–608.

[14] Linde, R. B., G. C. Doelle, N. Alexander et al.: New Engl. J. Med. **305** (1981) 663–667.

[15] Rabin, D., R. Linde, G. Doelle et al.: In "LH-RH Peptide as Female and Male Concentraceptives" (Eds. G. Zatuchini, J. Shelton, J. Sciarra), pp. 296–306. Harper and Row, Philadelphia 1981.

[16] Heber, D., R. S. Swerdloff: Endocrinology **108** (1981) 2019–2021.

[17] Heber, D., R. S. Swerdloff: Science **209** (1980) 936.

[18] Hsueh, A. J. W., P. B. C. Jones: Endocrine Review **2** (1981) 437.

[19] Heber, D., S. Bhasin, B. Steiner et al.: J. Clin. Endo. Metab. (1974), in press.

[20] Bhasin, S., D. Heber, B. Steiner et al.: Clin. Endocrinol. (1984), in press.

[21] Bhasin, S., D. Heber, B. Steiner et al.: Fertil. Steril **40** (1983) 418.

[22] Bhasin, S., D. Heber, M. Peterson et al.: J. Clin. Endocrinol. Metab. (1984), submitted.

[23] Doelle, G. C., N. Alexander, R. M. Evans et al.: J. Androl. (1984).

[24] Kelly, S., F. Labrie, A. Dupont: The 65th Endocrine Society Meeting. San Antonio, Texas. June 8–10, 1983.

[25] Evans, R. M., G. C. Doelle, J. Lindener et al.: The Endocrine Society Meetings. San Antonio. Texas. June 8–10, 1983.

[26] Akhtar, F. B., G. R. Marshall, E. J. Wickings et al.: J. Clin. Endocrinol. Metab. **56** (1983) 534.

LH-RH analog therapy of precocious puberty

O. H. Pescovitz, F. Comite, C. Foster, D. Loriaux, G. B. Cutler, Jr.

Introduction

When the clinical features of puberty appear before the age of 8 in girls or 9 in boys, it is termed precocious puberty. There are three major mechanisms of precocious puberty: central precocious puberty (CPP), peripheral precocious puberty, and peripheral precocious puberty leading to secondary central precocious puberty. Central precocious puberty is initiated by hypothalamic-pituitary-gonadal activation, which is the mechanism that causes normal puberty. Most cases of central precocious puberty are idiopathic or caused by CNS lesions such as hamartomas, third ventricular cysts, astrocytomas or gliomas. The most common lesion is a benign hamartoma of the hypothalamus.

Peripheral precocious puberty does not involve activation of the hypothalamic-pituitary-gonadal axis. Secondary sexual characteristics result from an elevation in sex steroids that originates in either the adrenal gland or the gonad. Adrenal or gonadal lesions such as tumors, congenital adrenal hyperplasia (CAH), or McCune-Albright syndrome [1] usually account for peripheral precocious puberty. Familial male precocious puberty and hCG-secreting tumors are also causes of peripheral precocious puberty in boys.

Secondary central precocious puberty involves activation of the hypothalamic-pituitary-gonadal axis secondary to peripheral precocious puberty. The best described example in this category is central precocious puberty secondary to CAH [2].

Until recently, conventional therapy for precocious puberty was limited to the use of progestational agents which inhibited gonadotropin secretion by direct negative-feedback at the hypothalamic or pituitary level [3, 4]. Although these agents cause cessation of menses and some regression of secondary sexual characteristics, they usually have no effect on the rapid rate of bone age maturation and the accelerated growth rate that accompany precocious puberty [5–8]. In addition, significant side effects, including adrenal suppression [5, 6, 8, 9], Cushingoid features [6], and chromosomal abnormalities [10], have been observed.

Continuous infusions of LH-RH have been shown to inhibit the relase of LH and FSH [11, 12]. Recently, potent long-acting agonist analogs of luteinizing hormone releasing hormone (LH-RH_a) have been developed that initially stimulate but subsequently inhibit the relaese of pituitary gonadotropins [13, 17]. The mechanism by which this inhibition occurs appears to involve an uncoupling of the LH-RH receptor and the pituitary response. The ability of these LH-RH analogs to inhibit gonadotropin secretion has provided a new therapy for precocious puberty [18]. We describe here the results of therapy in a) central precocious puberty: 15 girls with idiopathic precocious puberty and 6 boys with hypothalamic hamartomas; b) peripheral precocious puberty: 5 girls with McCune-Albright syndrome, and c) secondary central precocious puberty: 4 children with congenital adrenal hyperplasia.

Methods

LH-RH_a

The LH-RH_a, D-Trp^6-Pro^9-Net-LH-RH, was provided by Drs. Jean Rivier and Wylie Vale of the Salk Institute, San Diego, CA. It was dissolved in normal saline and 10% mannitol to ensure long-term stability [19], and was stored at −20° C. Each batch was bioassayed prior to use and no loss of biologic activity was demonstrated after 12 months of storage or after repeated freeze-thaw cycles, refrigeration, or mild heating [20]. The patients were instructed to keep the preparation refrigerated until use. The LH-RH_a was administered by a single subcutaneous injection at a dose of 4 μg/kg/day.

Protocol

Patients were admitted to the Clinical Center of the National Institutes of Health. The protocol was approved by the Clinical Research Committee of the National Institute of Child Health and Human Development and by the Food and Drug Administration. We obtained informed consent from either parent and informed assent from older children. Pretreatment evaluation consisted of basal serum gonadotropin determinations every 20 minutes for four hours during the day (1000 to 1400) and night (2200 to 0200). Plasma testosterone (males) or estradiol (females) was measured four times (1000, 1400, 2200, and 0200). Serum hCG was measured to exclude ectopic hCG production, and plasma 17-hydroxyprogesterone and 11-deoxycortisol were measured to exclude congenital adrenal hyperplasia.

On day 2, 100 μg LH-RH was administered i.v. at time 0 and serum gonadotropins were measured at −30, −15, 0, 15, 30, 60, 90, 120, and 180 minutes. On day 3, we measured height 10 times using a stadiometer. An x-ray of the left hand and wrist was obtained for bone age, which was assessed by a radiologist who had no clinial information about the patients [21]. Computed tomography (CT) of the head and ultrasound of the adrenal glands were performed in each patient. The female patients had pelvic ultrasound and the males had testicular ultrasound studies. The patients were photographed to document the stage of pubertal development [22–24].

Hormone assays

Plasma luteinizing hormone (LH), follicle stimulating hormone (FSH), testosterone, estradiol, 17-hydroyprogesterone, and plasma renin activity were measured with modifications of previously described methods [25–29]. Delayed addition of trace after 3 days at 4° C reduced the limit of sensitivity for both LH and FSH to 0.5 mIU/ml (2nd International Reference Preparation of human menopausal gonadotropin).

Statistical analysis

All data are expressed as the mean ±S.E.M. unless otherwise stated. Statistical analysis was performed by Student's unpaired or paired t-test.

Results

Central precocious puberty

Idiopathic precocious puberty

Fifteen girls with idiopathic precocious puberty between the ages of 1–9 years were treated with LH-RH_a for a period of 6–18 months. They were Tanner II–V in pubertal development and nine had menses. All had accelerated growth rates, advanced bone ages, and elevated gonadotropin and estradiol levels. During LH-RH_a therapy, breast size decreased in 13/15 and pubic hair in 7/15 patients. Basal LH did not change significantly during therapy although basal FSH and both peak LH and peak FSH fell significantly ($p < 0.01$). Estradiol levels, growth rate, and the rate of bone age advancement also decreased significantly with LH-RH_a therapy (tab. 1) [30].

Table 1 Results of LH-RH$_a$ therapy in 15 girls with IPP

	Pre-therapy	On therapy	p*
Basal LH (mIU/ml)	9 ± 11	6 ± 2	NS
Basal FSH (mIU/ml)	11 ± 1	2 ± 1	<.01
Peak LH (mIU/ml)**	73 ± 15	5 ± 1	<.01
Peak FSH (mIU/ml)**	38 ± 8	4 ± 1	<.01
Estradiol (pg/ml)	41 ± 6	21 ± 3	<.01
Growth (cm/yr)	13 ± 1	7 ± 1	<.01
Δ Bone Age/Δ Chronologic Age	1.7 + 0.1	0.8 + 0.3	<.01

* Paired t-test of pretreatment and treatment results.
** Peak LH and FSH are the highest values observed during the LH-RH stimulation test.

Hypothalamic hamartoma

Six boys ages 1–6 years with true precocious puberty secondary to hypothalamic hamartomas have been treated with the LH-RH$_a$ [31]. The diagnosis of a hypothalamic hamartoma was made by computed tomography of the head which showed characteristic lesions ranging in size from 0.5 to 3 cm in diameter. The boys presented with Tanner II–IV pubertal development, pubertal growth rates, and advanced bone ages. They were treated with the LH-RH$_a$ for 6–12 months. Table 2 shows the response to LH-RH$_a$ therapy. Basal and peak LH and FSH, testosterone, testis volume, and growth rate decreased significantly during treatment. The rate of bone age advancement per year decreased from 3.2±0.9 to 0.8±0.2 ($p<0.01$). Pubic hair, facial hair, and erections decreased in all boys.

Table 2 Results of LH-RH$_a$ therapy in 6 boys with hypothalamic hamartomas

	Pre-Rx	6m.	12m.	p*
Basal LH (mIU/ml)	12 ± 2	4 ± 7	5 ± 8	<.005
Peak LH (mIU/ml)	78 ± 16	4 ± 0.5	5 ± 0.5	<.005
Basal FSH (mIU/ml)	9 ± 2	1 ± 0.1	1 ± 0.3	<.01
Peak FSH (mIU/ml)	19 ± 4	1 ± 0.2	1 ± 0.4	<.005
Testosterone (ng/dl)	509 ± 62	45 ± 30	68 ± 5	<.005
Testis volume (ml)	14 ± 3	9 ± 2	7 ± 1	<.005
Growth rate (cm/yr)	17 + 3	10 + 1	6 + 1	<.01

* Paired t-test of pretreatment and treatment (12 month) results.

Peripheral precocious puberty

McCune-Albright syndrome (MAS)

Five girls ages 1–5 years with MAS were treated with LH-RH_a, one for 3 months and four for 1 year. All presented with menses and characteristic bone lesions (polyostotic fibrous dysplasia). Three of the five had café au lait pigmentation. They had Tanner II–IV pubertal development. Accelerated growth rates and advanced bone ages were present in 4 of the 5 girls. LH-RH_a therapy failed to cause regression of secondary sexual characteristics or to stop menses. Basal and peak gonadotropins were below prepubertal normals before therapy [32] and did not change significantly with therapy (tab. 3). Estradiol levels fluctuated widely in 3 of the 5 patients. Values ranged from <12 pg/ml to >1000 pg/ml during the treatment course. Thus, these patients with MAS and peripheral precocious puberty did not appear to respond to treatment with the LH-RH_a [32].

Table 3 LH-RH_a therapy of 5 girls with MAS

	Pre-therapy	On therapy	p*
Basal LH (mIU/ml)	1.6 ± 0.3	3.0 ± 0.2	NS
Basal FSH (mIU/ml)	1.1 ± 0.5	1.0 ± 0.2	NS
Peak LH (mIU/ml)	3.6 ± 1.1	2.8 ± 0.1	NS
Peak FSH (mIU/ml)	5.3 ± 2.8	1.2 ± 0.3	NS

* Paired t-test of pretreatment and treatment results.

Secondary central precocious puberty

Central precocious puberty secondary to congenital adrenal hyperplasia (CAH)

Four children (3 boys and 1 girl) with CAH and central precocious puberty were treated with LH-RH_a [2]. They had the diagnosis of CAH made between the ages of three and six years. These patients were treated with standard doses of hydrocortisone and fludrocortisone. A diagnosis of central precocious puberty was made because of testicular enlargement in the boys, breast development in the girl, progressive pubic hair development, accelerated growth rates, and rapid bone maturation. Plasma sex steroid levels were elevated for age and gonadotropin levels were within the normal pubertal range both basally and in response to LH-RH stimulation. They were treated with LH-RH_a for 6–18 months in addition to the standard hydrocortisone and fludrocortisone therapy for CAH.

LH-RH_a significantly decreased basal plasma LH and FSH, peak LH and FSH responses to native LH-RH (fig. 1), and testosterone levels (fig. 2).

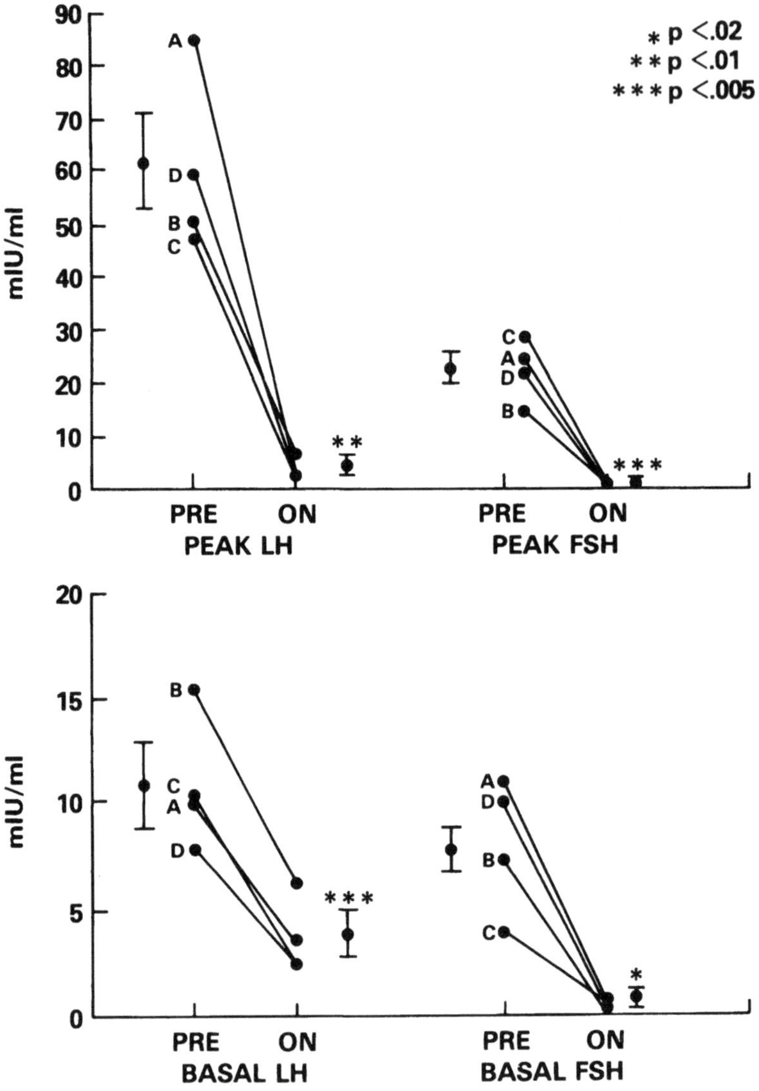

Fig. 1 Basal and peak (LHRH-stimulated) plasma LH and FSH levels in 4 children with congenital adrenal hyperplasia and central precocious puberty before ("Pre") and during ("On") 6–18 months of treatment with $LHRH_a$. The basal LH and FSH values for each patient (fig. 1, bottom) are the mean of 26 measurements obtained at 20 minute intervals from 1000 to 1400 and from 2200 to 0200. The peak values (fig. 1, top) are the highest LH and FSH levels achieved during an LHRH stimulation test.

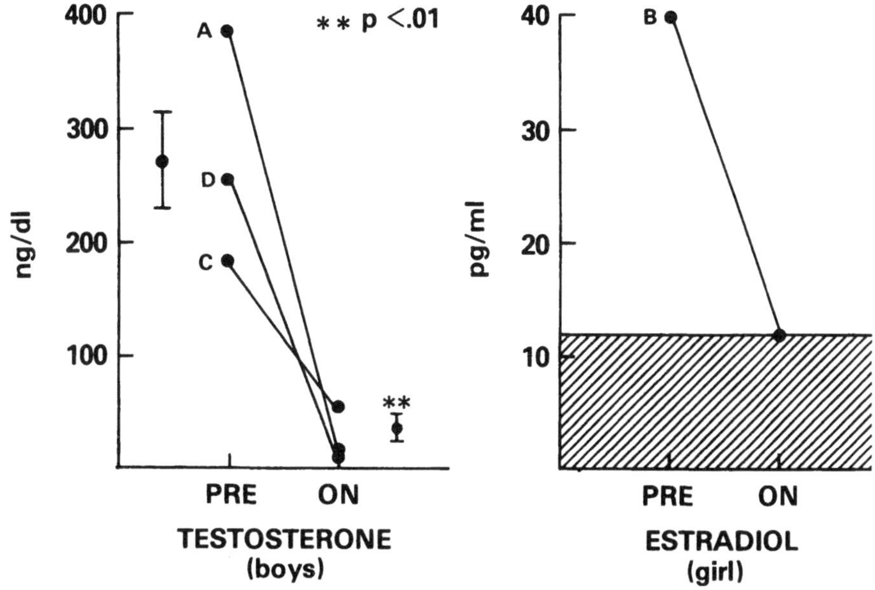

Fig. 2 Plasma sex steroid concentrations in 4 children with congenital adrenal hyperplasia and central prococious puberty before and during 6–18 months of treatment with $LHRH_a$. The testosterone levels for each of the three male patients (left panel) are the mean of four measurements at 1000, 1400, 2200, and 0200. The estradiol levels (right panel) are the mean of four measurements at the same times in the female patient. The hatched area represents the detection limit of the assay.

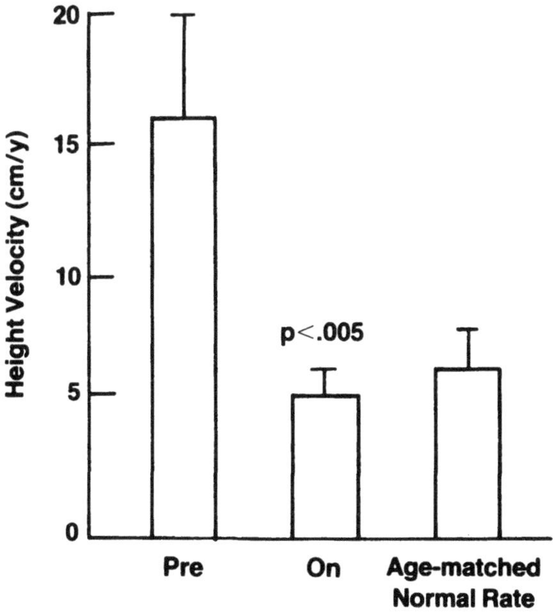

Fig. 3 Effect of $LHRH_a$ therapy on linear growth rate in 4 children with congenital adrenal hyperplasia and central precocious puberty.

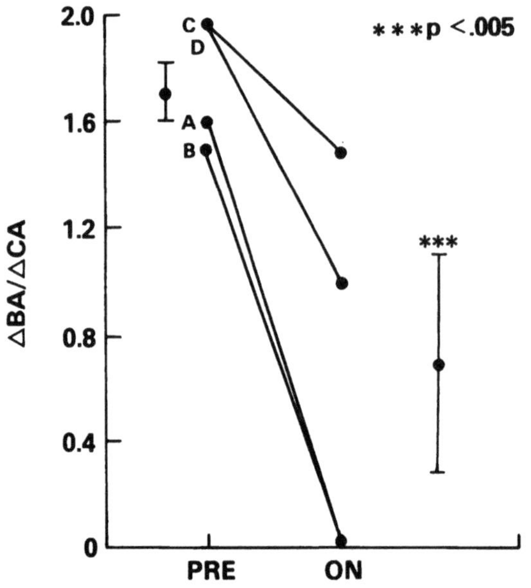

Fig. 4 Effect of $LHRH_a$ therapy on the rate of bone age advancement in 4 children with congenital adrenal hyperplasia and central precocious puberty. The rate of bone age advancement (ΔBA/ΔCA) prior to treatment represents the patient's pre-treatment bone age divided by his/her chronologic age. (Serial bone ages were not available during the pre-treatment period). The rate of bone age advancement during treatment represents each child's increase in bone age during treatment divided by the duration of treatment (6–18 months).

Testis size decreased in the males and breast development regressed in the female. $LH\text{-}RH_a$ therapy led to significant decreases in linear growth rate (fig. 3) and in the rate of bone age advancement (fig. 4).

Discussion

Long-acting analogs of LH-RH are a new and highly effective method for treating central precocious puberty. To date, all patients who have presented with hypothalamic-pituitary-gonadal activation, as indicated by elevated basal and LH-RH-stimulated gonadotropins, have responded to the $LH\text{-}RH_a$ with a suppression of both gonadotropins and sex steroids. Treatment has resulted in regression of secondary sexual characteristics, a return of growth to normal prepubertal rates, and significant decreases in the rate of bone age maturation. Patients who had central precocious puberty secondary to peripheral precocious puberty appear to have responded in a similar fashion. The children who had only peripheral precocious puberty without evidence of hypothalamic-pituitary activation (the 5 girls with McCune-Albright syndrome) do not appear to have responded to $LH\text{-}RH_a$ therapy. Sex steroid levels continued to be elevated and there was no regression of secondary sexual characteristics.

We conclude: 1. The etiology of precocious puberty should be determined whenever possible. 2. Patients who have central precocious puberty should be offered a trial of LH-RH_a. 3. No adverse side effects of LH-RH_a have been noted, although longer observation is necessary before the ultimate safety and effectiveness of this new therapy can be assessed.

References

[1] Foster, C. M., J. L. Ross, T. Shawker: J. Clin. Endocrinol. Metab. **58** (1984) 1161–1165.
[2] Pescovitz, O. H., F. Comite, F. Cassorla et al.: J. Clin. Endocrinol. Metab. **58** (1984) 857–861.
[3] Rifkind, A. B., H. E. Kulin, C. M. Cargille et al.: J. Clin. Endocrinol. Metab. **29** (1969) 506–513.
[4] Styne, D. M., M. M. Grumbach: In: Reproductive Endocrinology (S. S. C. Yen, R. Jaffee, eds.), pp. 189–240. W. B. Saunders, Philadelphia 1978.
[5] Kaplan, S. A., S. M. Ling, N. G. Irani: Am. J. Dis. Child. **116** (1968) 591–598.
[6] Richman, R. A., L. E. Underwood, F. S. French et al.: J. Pediatr. **79** (1971) 963–971.
[7] Lee, P. A.: Am. J. Dis. Child. **135** (1981) 443–445.
[8] Mathews, J. H., C. A. L. Abrams, A. Morishima: J. Clin. Endocrinol. Metab. **30** (1970) 653–658.
[9] Sadeghi-Nejad, A., S. L. Kaplan, M. M. Grumbach: J. Pediatr. **78** (1971) 616–624.
[10] Camacho, A. M., D. L. Williams, J. M. Montalvo: J. Clin. Endocrinol. Metab. **34** (1972) 279–286.
[11] Knobil, E.: Rec. Prog. Horm. Res. **36** (1980) 53–88.
[12] Belchetz, P. E., T. M. Plant, U. Nakai et al.: Science **202** (1978) 631–633.
[13] Happ, J., P. Scholz, T. Weber et al.: Fertil. Steril 30 (1978) 674–678.
[14] Crowley, W. F., W. Vale, I. Z. Beitins et al.: Sixty-first Annual Meeting of the Endocrine Society, Los Angeles 1979, Abstract no. 16, p. 76.
[15] Bengquist, C., S. J. Nillius, L. Wide: J. Clin. Endocrinol. Metab. **49** (1979) 472–474.
[16] Bengquist. C., S. J. Nillius, L. Wide: Lancet **2** (1979) 215–217.
[17] Linde, R., G. C. Doelle, N. Alexander: N. Engl. J. Med, **305** (1981) 663–667.
[18] Comite, F., G. B. Cutler, Jr., J. Rivier et al.: New Engl. J. Med. **305** (1981) 1546–1550.
[19] Dermody, W. C., J. R. Reed: N. Engl. J. Med. **295** (1976) 173.
[20] Winterer, J., D. Chatterji, F. Comite et al.: Contraception **27** (1983) 95–200.
[21] Greulich, W. W., S. I. Pyle: Radiographic Atlas of Skeletal Development of the Hand and Wrist. Stanford University Press, Stanford 1959.
[22] Marshall, W. A., J. M. Tanner: Arch. Dis. Childh.**44** (1969), 291–303.
[23] Marshall, W. A., J. M. Tanner: Arch. Dis. Childh. **45** (1970) 13–23.
[24] Tanner, J. M.: Growth at Adolescence. Blackwell, Oxford 1978.
[25] Odell, W. D., G. T. Ross, P. L. Rayford: J. Clin. Invest. **46** (1967) 248–255.
[26] Nieschlag, E., D. L. Loriaux: Z. Klin. Chem. Biochem. **10** (1972) 164–168.
[27] Cargille, C. M., P. L. Rayford: J. Lab. Clin. Med. **75** (1970) 1030–1040.
[28] Odell, W. D., P. L. Rayford, G. T. Ross: J. Lab. Clin. Med. **70** (1967) 973–980.
[29] Zachmann, M., A. Prader, H. P. Kind: Helv. Pediatr. Acta. **29** (1974) 61–72.
[30] Comite, F., F. Cassorla, O. Pescovitz et al.: Pediatr. Res. **17** (1983) 161 A.
[31] Comite, F., O. H. Pescovitz, K. Reith et al.: J. Clin. Endocrinol. Metab. (in press).
[32] Foster, C. M., F. Comite, O. H. Pescovitz, J. Clin. Endocrinol. Metab. (in press).

Treatment of prostatic cancer with LH-RH analogues and control of therapy by cytology and DNA cytophotometry

R. Nagel, V. Borgmann, H. Al-Abadi, M. Schmidt-Gollwitzer †

Introduction

The studies of Huggins and Hodges [1] in 1941 established as a fact that the suppression or withdrawal of androgen slows down the growth of prostatic cancer for some time. Since then, bilateral orchiectomy for withdrawal of testicular androgen (with or without additional estrogen therapy) has been applied widely as a palliative primary treatment for locally advanced, inoperable carcinomas of the prostate. Androgen withdrawal by castration, however, is not accepted by all patients, and it was found that indirect suppressions of androgen production by substances imitating the effect of estrogens may produce cardiovascular side effects [2].

When, in 1971, Schally and coworkers [3] succeeded in isolating, characterizing and synthesizing the endogenous decapeptide LH-RH, it was expected to open a new approach to the treatment of fertility disturbances [4–9]. However, neither the natural LH-RH nor the newly developed synthetic LH-RH analogue, which is more potent and produces a more persistent effect than the former, have fulfilled these expectations due to a possible dose and time-dependent paradoxical antifertility effect [10–14].

The research took a new direction when animal studies with rats showed a substantial reduction of the amount of serum testosterone as well as the weight of the ventral prostate seminal vesicles and testes to result on continuous injection of high doses of the potent LH-RH analogue Buserelin (D-Ser-[TBU]^{6}-EA^{10}-LH-RH, HOE 766*) [12, 13]. In men, too, prolonged administration of the LH-RH analogue induced inhibition of testosterone synthesis, though incomplete, which appeared to offer new possibilities in the treatment of androgen-dependent conditions in the field of urology.

In 1981, Rredding and Schally [11] succeeded in inhibiting prostatic cancer growth by prolonged administration of the potent LH-RH analogue in small-scale experi-

* Fa. Hoechst AG, West Germany.

ments with rats. This effect suggested employment of the drug in the primary treatment of locally advanced or metastasing cancer in men as well. Especially in view of the side effects and complications of estrogen therapy, which had emphasized the need of a more tolerable carcinostatic drug, the LH-RH analogue Buserelin virtually offered itself as a means of inhibiting androgen-dependent cancer growth in the prostate. In the same year, the first clinical trial with Buserelin was undertaken by Labrie and Faure [6], and on June 1, 1981, the authors started the first dose-finding study which was completed in November, 1981 [15].

Patients and methods

In the Department of Urology at the Free University of Berlin, Charlottenburg, Medical Center, 51 patients with locally advanced prostatic cancer were treated with the LH-RH analogue Buserelin from June 1981 to September 1983. 47 patients had a locally advanced state C carcinoma (T3, NO/+, MO), while only 4 patients had a stage D carcinoma (T3, NO/+, M1) with bone metastases.

As to the grades of malignancy, 10 of the 51 patients had grade I, 32 of them had grade II, and 9 had grade III carcinomas. 4 of the grade II patients had metastases (M1).

36 of the 51 patients were treated for more than 6 months, 22 of the former for periods of one year to more than 2 years.

The response of the locally advanced carcinoma without bone metastases (stage C) or other clinical symptoms to any therapy can be established solely by the regressive changes in the tumor itself, which is possible only through histology, cytology and DNA cytophotometry. With orchiectomy, DES or antiandrogen therapy, tumor response can be evaluated definitely and accurately after 6 months. If no regressive changes are manifest in the tumor itself at this point and therapy is continued, local tumor progression or metastasing is likely to occur in the near future.

For the sake of a true evaluation of the therapy, only the 36 patients who were treated for more than 6 months shall be reported on. They all had stage C carcinomas.

Since this institution was the first in West Germany to employ Buserelin in the treatment of prostatic cancer, various dosaged and medication intervals were first investigated with 9 patients, from June 1 through October 1981, in order to find the appropriate dose regimen for rapid and sustained reduction of serum testosterone to the level seen in castrated men.

As shown in table 1, Buserelin was given subcutaneously in 2 or 3 daily doses for periods varying from 3 to 14 days. Thereafter, therapy was usually continued with 3 intranasal doses daily of 200 mcg each. After 3 weeks, all dose regimens except one

Table 1 Buserelin, initial dose regimen

6/1/1981 – 30/10/1981	n = 9
n	**Dosage**
3	2 • 1000 mcg/s.c./day 1– 3 → 3 • 200 mcg/day/i.n.
2	3 • 1000 mcg/s.c./day 1– 6 → 3 • 200 mcg/day/i.n.
4	2 • 100 mcg/s.c./day 1–14 ↗ **2 • 200 mcg/day/i.n.** ↘ 3 • 200 mcg/day/i.n.
	Current dose regimen
	3 • 500 mcg/s.c./day 1– 7 → 3 • 400 mcg/day/i.n.

produced a decrease in serum testosterone to such levels as found in castrated men, and maintained this "castrate" level for months, independent of the duration and dosage of the initial subcutaneous injection. It was only the intranasal application of 200 mcg Buserelin twice daily that proved insufficient for keeping the serum testosterone level within this range, despite a preceding 2 weeks' sequence of subcutaneous injections of 200 mcg daily.

Based on these dose-finding studies and an agreement among several medical centers, the following standard dose regimen was adopted in mid-1982 and so far has been used with 32 patients: Subcutaneous injection of 3 times 500 mcg daily for 7 days, followed by long-term intranasal application of 3 daily doses of 400 mcg each.

Based on the results of all our dose-finding studies, we started, in July 1983, with the *primary intranasal treatment* of 8 patients who had *not* received initial subuctaneous injections [16] (tab. 2).

Table 2 Buserelin, primary intranasal treatment

July 1983	n = 8
Dosage	
3·400 mcg/ i.n. /day 1–28 → 3·300 mcg/day/ i.n.	

The idea was to investigate whether it was possible to reduce serum testosterone within 3 or 4 weeks to the "castrate" level reached with combined subcutaneous and intranasal administration. If this were true, patients could be spared hospitalization.

The dose regimen for exclusively intranasal application is this: 3 daily doses of 400 mcg each for 28 days, and after that 3 daily doses of 300 mcg.

Hormone analyses

During the first 2 weeks of therapy, blood samples were taken twice daily at 8 a.m. and 4 p.m., and thereafter once weekly at 8 a.m., in order to determine serum levels of testosterone, LH, prolactin and FSH by radioimmuno assays. In addition to the usual blood tests, serum thyroxin, T3, and cortisol were measured every 4 weeks.

The normal serum testosterone levels as established by radioimmuno assays range from 2.5 to 10 ng/ml in sexually mature men. Testosterone levels in a control group of 40 surgically castrated men with prostatic cancer, aged 60 to 80 years, ranged from 0.1 to 0.8 ng/ml (mean value 0.28 ng/ml).

Clinical follow-up examinations

All patients underwent the examinations listed in table 3 at intervals of 4 weeks, 3 months and 6 months. As the 36 patients had non-metastasing, locally advanced prostatic carcinomas without clinical symptoms (stage C; T3, NO/+, MO), the response to Buserelin therapy, i.e. the cytological regression grade, could be established reliably only by cytology and DNA cytophotometry in the tumor itself.

Table 3 Follow-up examinations during Buserelin therapy

every 4 weeks	every 3 months	every 6 months
Blood Chemistry	Bone Scan	IVP
Rectal Palpation	Rectal Ultrasound	Cat Scan
Weight	Chest Film	
Physical Status	**Aspiration Biopsy** **DNA Cytophotometry**	Punch Biopsy

Results

Hormone studies

Prior to long-term treatment, the serum levels of testosterone and of the gonadotropic substances LH and FSH of all patients were found to be within standard range.

Therapy-induced changes were observed only with LH and testosterone. All other values remained standard and were evidently not affected by Buserelin therapy.

LH levels as measured over a period of 12 months show (fig. 1) that, after the usual increase during the first 2 weeks of therapy, a definite drop to subnormal values sets in after the third week.

After 3 weeks of Buserelin therapy with a sequence of subcutaneous injections of 2 daily doses of 1,000 mcg, 3 daily doses of 1,000 mcg, or 2 daily doses of 100 mcg each, followed by intranasal application of 3 daily doses of 200 mcg, serum LH levels fell to lower than normal (below 5 mIU/ml), and serum testosterone decreased

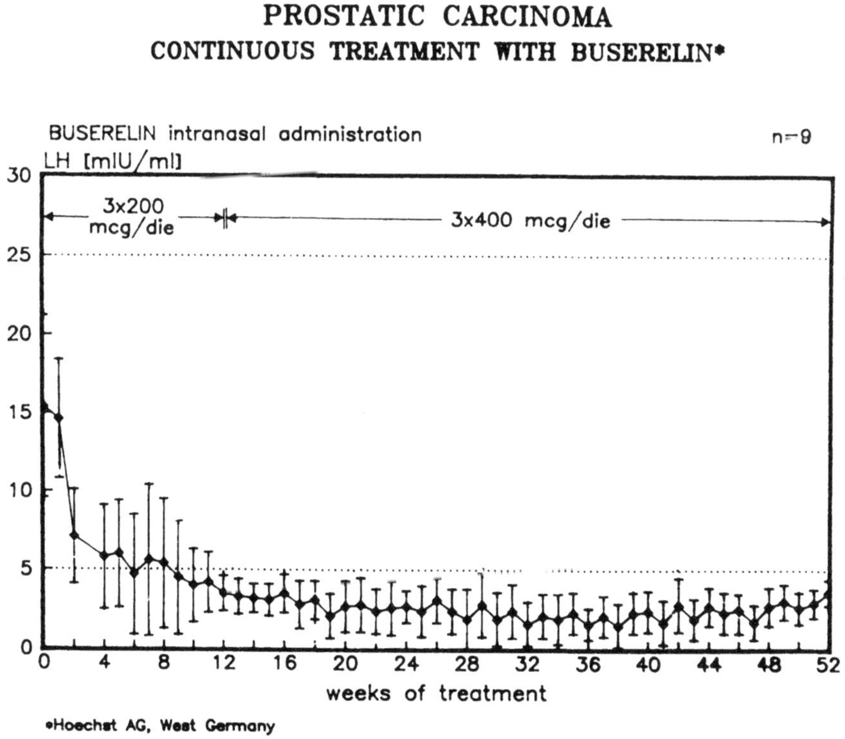

Fig. 1 LH levels of 9 patients during Buserelin therapy.

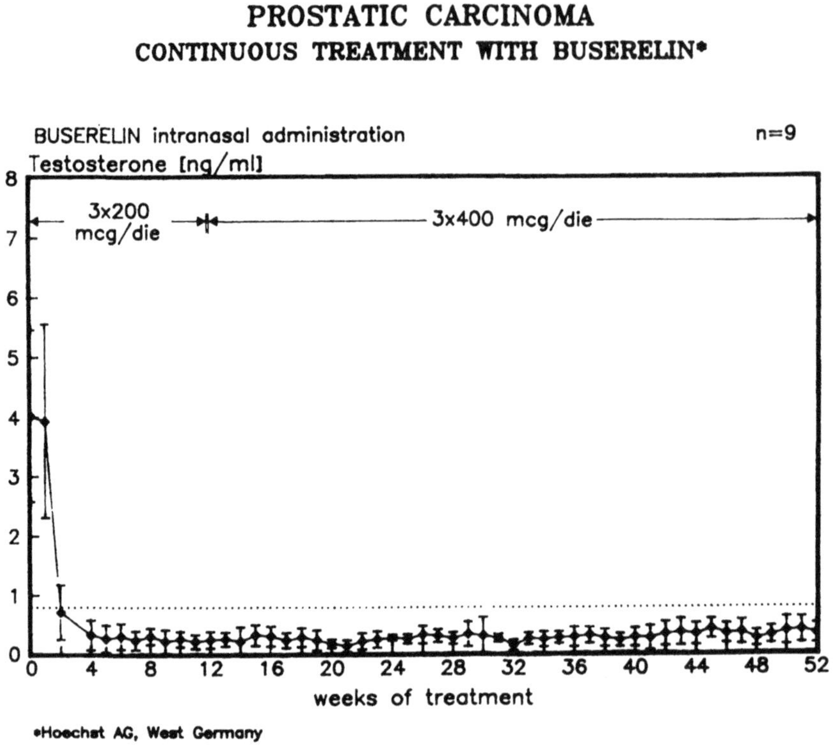

Fig. 2 Serum testosterone levels of 9 patients during Buserelin therapy.

to less than 0.8 ng/ml. These levels were reliably maintained, without exception, in all patients over observation periods of up to 2 years and longer.

Figure 2 shows the serum testosterone levels of 9 patients after at least 12 months of Buserelin therapy. All patients showed significant "castrate" values within standard variation. None of them had signs of clinical or cytological progression. 3 of them were treated for 24 months.

2 patients received intravenous infusions of 1500 mcg Buserelin daily for 3 days, as it had been suggested that continuous infusion of high doses might bring about an accelerated fall of serum testosterone levels. Initial infusion and continuation of therapy with intranasal application of 3 daily doses of 400 mcg Buserelin proved to have no such advantage over other dose regimens. It rather turned out to be merely inconvenient for the patients, for even after continuous infusion it takes 3 weeks until serum testosterone finally falls to "castrate" level. Therefore, this kind of administration is of no clinical importance.

The study of 8 patents receiving primary intranasal treatment with 3 daily doses of 400 mcg for 28 days and, thereafter, 3 times daily 300 mcg has shown so far (fig. 3)

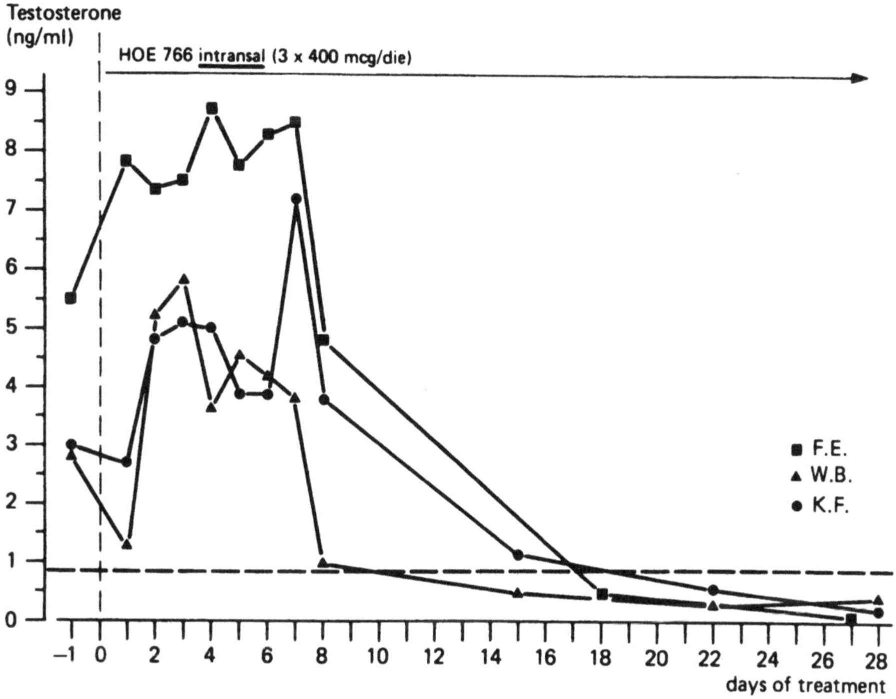

Fig. 3 Serum testosterone levels of 8 patients under primary intranasal therapy with Buserelin.

that the decrease of serum testosterone to "castrate" level sets in within 4 weeks of exclusively intranasal application.

Obviously serum testosterone reduction by intranasal application is the same as with combined subcutaneous and intranasal administration. These results confirm our assumption that subcutaneous injection – and hence hospitalization – is not necessary.

Cytology

The rating of tumor response to Buserelin was based on the cytological regression grade found on fine-needle aspiration biopsy, and on the changes of DNA content in the tumorous nuclei measured by single-cell cytophotometry. As the patients were in stage C and had neither bone metastases nor clinical symptoms, these were the only parameters with which to objectify the effect of Buserelin on the primary tumor, particularly since the serum testosterone level cannot be taken as an indicator of therapy effect because clinical progression does not cause a renewed increase.

Occasional punch biopsies showed exactly the same results as aspiration biopsy with regard to regression grades. Years ago, the accordance between the results of aspiration and punch biopsies was shown by the authors to be 97%, with punch biopsy being taken as 100% which, of course, is a purely theoretical assumption.

The cytological regression grading defines the regression of the primary tumor induced by any form of therapy and does not identify therapy-specific regression.

The most important signs of regression are found in the *nucleus* (pyknosis, decrease in size, rarefaction, disaggregation of chromatin) and in the *nucleoles* (decrease in size, disappearance).

The cytological criteria for regression correspond with those stated by Alken, Dhom et al. [17] in 1975 for regression grading by histological examination. The cytological regression grading as adopted by the Uro-Pathological Group in West Germany distinguishes 6 grades:

Regression grades II to VI indicate good to sufficient therapy response of the tumor, established by the typical cytological changes. These regression grades do not require any change of therapy.

Regression grades VIII and X signal that therapy response is poor, or that there are no regressive changes in the tumor at all.

Based on our experiment with 300 patients and more than 1,000 control aspiration biopsies under 6 different types of therapy, we can state that regression grades VIII and X signal that tumor progression (metastates) is likely to occur within just a few months if therapy is not changed. The difference between good (grade II to VI) and poor regression (grade VIII or X) ist statistically significant.

Intrapersonal reproducibility amounts to approx. 90%, interpersonal reproducibility has been shown to be 80 to 85%.

Figures 4a, b show, as an example, the cytological findings in a case of good response after 12 months of Buserelin therapy which was confirmed by the DNA cytophotogram (fig. 6).

K. P., 75 years old: Typical grade II carcinoma before Buserelin therapy. The nuclei were irregularly displaced and hyperchromatic, the nucleoles were prominent, some were no longer round; some nuclei even had 2 nucleoles (fig. 4a).
After 12 months of Buserelin therapy, the nuclei ere distinctly smaller, the entire cell cluster was rarefied; nucleoles were hardly visible and had partly disappeared (fig. 4b). Because of the good therapy response, Buserelin therapy was continued. The patient has been in stable condition without any signs of progression for 24 months.

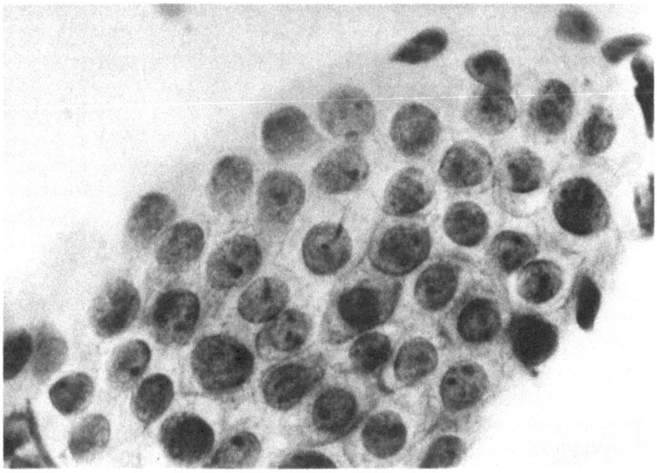

Fig. 4a Moderately differentiated prostatic carcinoma prior to Buserelin acetate-therapy. Cytoplasmatic contors partly still alveolate, but blurred at the border. Irregularly displaced and partly polymorphous nuclei. Marked nuclear hyperchromasy, clearly prominent nucleoles, often more than 1 nucleole in one nucleus. x 630.

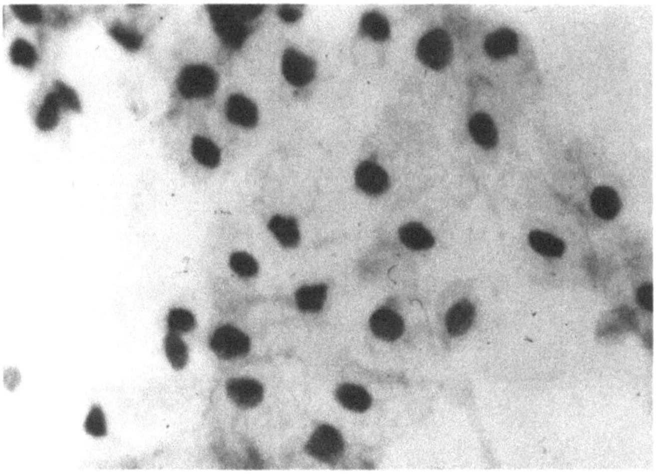

Fig. 4b Same case, after 6 months of therapy. Marked regression of tumorous cells. The nuclei are clearly smaller, nucleoles hardly visible. Nuclear pyknoses and rarefaction against the background of partly disaggregated cytoplasm. Regression grade IV. x 630.

In contrast to this, figures 5a, b shows the results in a case of almost non-existent therapy response.

E. H., 71 years old: Grade II carcinoma without metastases. Prior to Buserelin therapy, the nuclei were highly polymorphous and irregularly displaced, the nucleoles were prominent and mostly no longer round, and some nuclei had several nucleoles (fig. 5a).

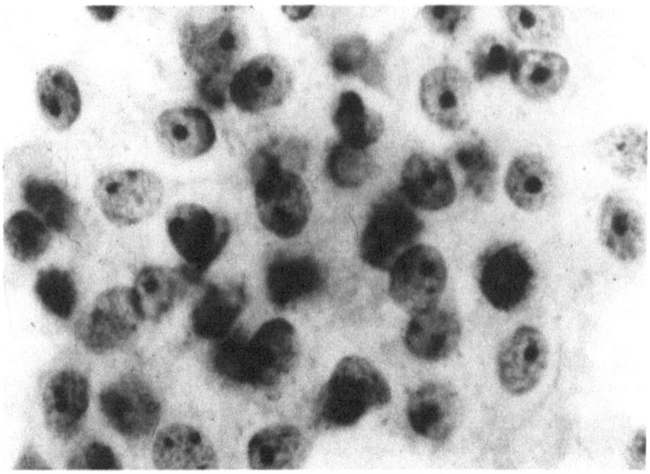

Fig. 5a E. H., 75 years, stage C (T 3), grade II carcinoma. Hyperchromatic and polymorphous nuclei.
The nucleoles are prominent and no longer round, partly 2 nucleoles in a nucleus. Papanicolaou. x 630.

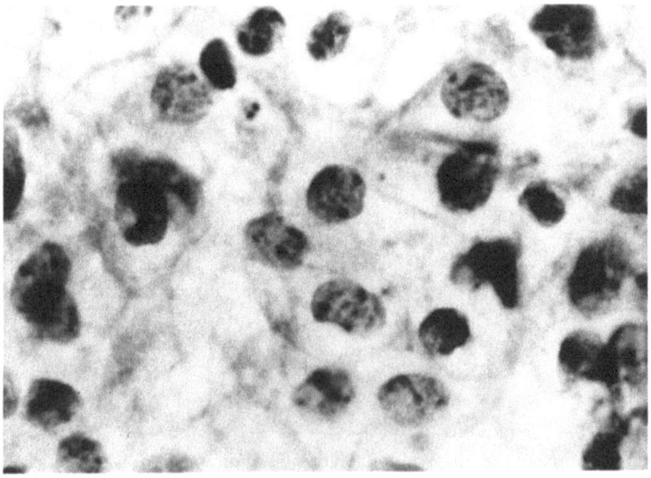

Fig. 5b Same patient, after 6 months of Buserelin therapy. Still highly polymorphous and hyperchromatic nuclei, several prominent nucleoles. No regressive changes as compared with primary cytology, no therapy effect. Regression grade X. Papanicolaou. x 630.

After 12 months of Buserelin therapy, there was a prevalent nuclear polymorphy, still numerous prominent nucleoles which were no longer round, often more than 2 nucleoles in one nucleus. There were no regressive changes at all compared with primary cytology; regression grade X (fig. 5b). Therefore it was necessary to cross over to secondary EMCYT (estramustine

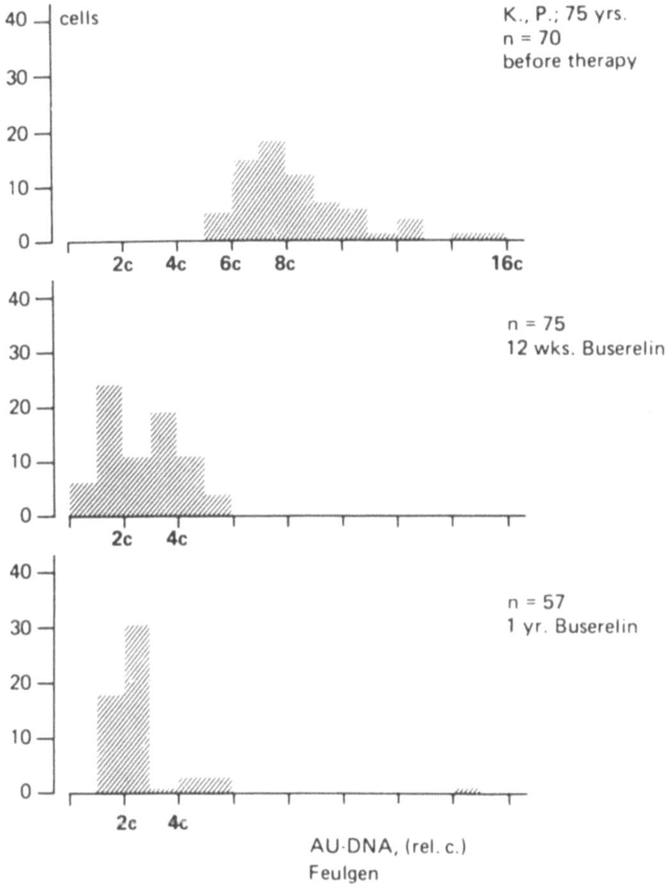

Fig. 6 DNA cytophotogram for moderately differentiated prostatic carcinoma, grade II, during Buserelin therapy: Already after 3 months, a clear shift of the DNA frequency peak to the left, into the 2c and 4c range, is seen with this therapy. After 1 year of therapy, the frequency peak is clearly in the diploid range, with some values spreading to 6c.

phosphate) therapy after 7 months. After 6 months of EMCYT therapy, the cytological finding was equally poor, and confirmed by the DNA cytophotogram (fig. 7). At the same time, local tumor progression occurred accompanied by tumor break-through into the urinary bladder so that therapy had to be changed to a third drug, cyclophosphamide. The patient was treated with cyclophosphamide until, 26 months after starting Buserelin therapy, he died of the primary disease. The poor response to primary and secondary therapy is especially striking in the DNY cytophotograms (fig. 7).

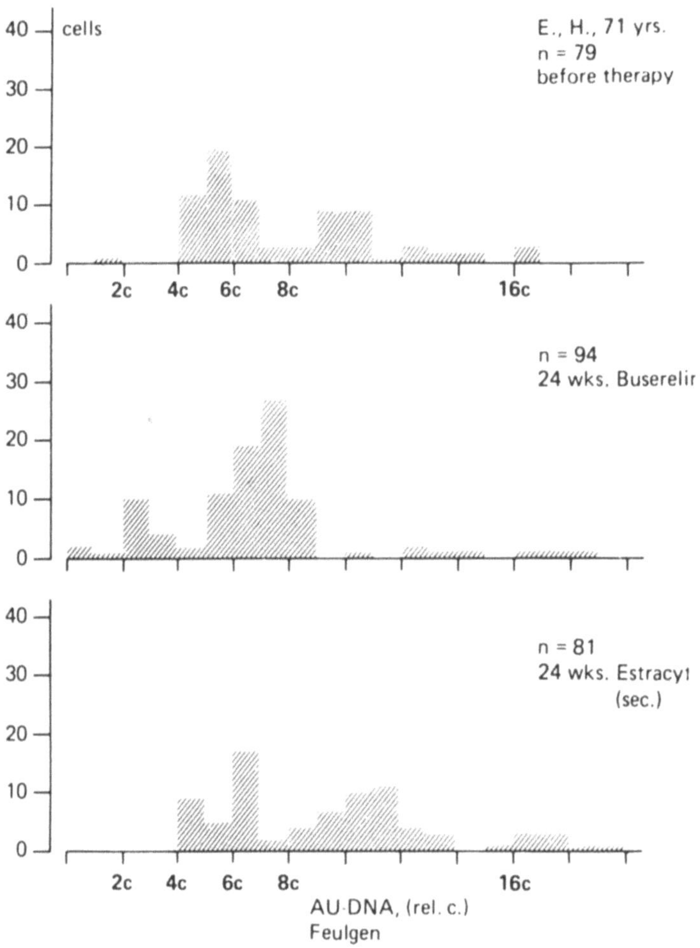

Fig. 7 DNA cytophotogram for moderately differentiated prostatic carcinoma, grade II, under secondary EMCYT therapy after resistance to LH-RH analogue. Before primary therapy, the DNA frequency peak was near 5c, a second peak was near 9c, with some values spreading up to 16c. After 6 months of Buserelin therapy, the DNA frequency peak was near 7c, with a second peak near 2c. After cross-over to EMCYT therapy, the tumor appears clearly aneuploid.

DNA single cell-scanning cytophotometry

While cytology gives a morphological – and that is a qualitative – rating of therapy response, the analysis of the nucleus through single-cell cytophotometry affords a quantitative rating of regression in the primary tumor. Both methods, particularly DNA cytophotometry, can contribute greatly towards a better understanding of biological tumor activity.

It has been known for years that tumor cell populations, corresponding to a change in the number of chromosomes towards aneuploidy, show a higher DNA content than normal tissues. This finding has been confirmed over and again by examinations of carcinomas of different organs, especially the mammas, lungs, and urinary bladder.

These results can easily be applied to the carcinoma of the prostate whose DNA content of the tumorous nuclei differs significantly from that of the adenoma, as shown for the first time by Sprenger and coworker [18] in 1975, later by Zetterberg [19], and also by the authors' experience.

As far as we know we were the first to undertake not only *sequential analyses* of the response of the DNA content of tumorous nuclei in prostatic carcinomas but also to investigate this under various therapeutic measures.

A statistically significant drop of the grade of ploidy from aneuploid towards diploid occurs in prostatic carcinomas when therapy is successful. If an aneuploidy remains unchanged during therapy, a negative clinical course of the disease may be predicted. Morever, therapy-resistant carcinomas of the prostate differ in their nuclear DNA content significantly from carcinomas with positive therapy response.

It is obvious from the studies made so far that nuclear DNA cytophotometry, though it is time-consuming as 60 to 80 individual tumorous nuclei have to be measured per patient, is a further reliable and especially good parameter for establishing therapy response in the prostatic carcinoma, and thus for realizing a prognostically oriented therapy.

Method

The cytophotograms demonstrate the deviation of malignant nuclei from the diploid (2c) set of chromosomes of normal cells. This means that for each patient, the DNA content of normal leukocytes (standard = 2c) has to be measured first and then compared with that of the tumorous nuclei. The values obtained by this comparison are given on the abscissa, in so-called Arbitrary Units (AU), and the exact number (n) of nuclei measured each time appears on the ordinate. Accordingly, 2c means diploid, 4c tetraploid, and 8c octaploid.

Results of DNA cytophotometry

The prognostic value of DNA cytophotograms for Buserelin therapy is the same as for any other therapy; it is statistically significant and can be reproduced in the sample at any time. Figures 6, 7, and 8 show the cytophotograms of 3 patients with different therapy responses.

K. P., 75 years old, grade II carcinoma (fig. 6):

Prior to therapy, there was a broad DNA peak in the 8c range, with values spreading up to 16c. After 12 weeks of therapy, a clear shift to the left, into the 4c and 2c range, is seen indicating that a response of the tumor may be expected although a definite evaluation is, in principle, only possible after 24 weeks of therapy. This finding was confirmed by the cytophotogram taken after 1 year of Buserelin therapy, showing a slim peak in the 2c range and only very few values between 4c and 6c. The cytophotograms correspond with the cytological findings on aspiration biopsy and the clinically stable condition of the patient after 15 months of therapy.

E. H., 71 years, grade II carcinoma (fig. 7):

Prior to therapy, the DNA frequency peak was near 5c, with further peaks near 9c, and some values reaching beyond 16c. After 24 weeks of Buserelin therapy, there still was a distinct

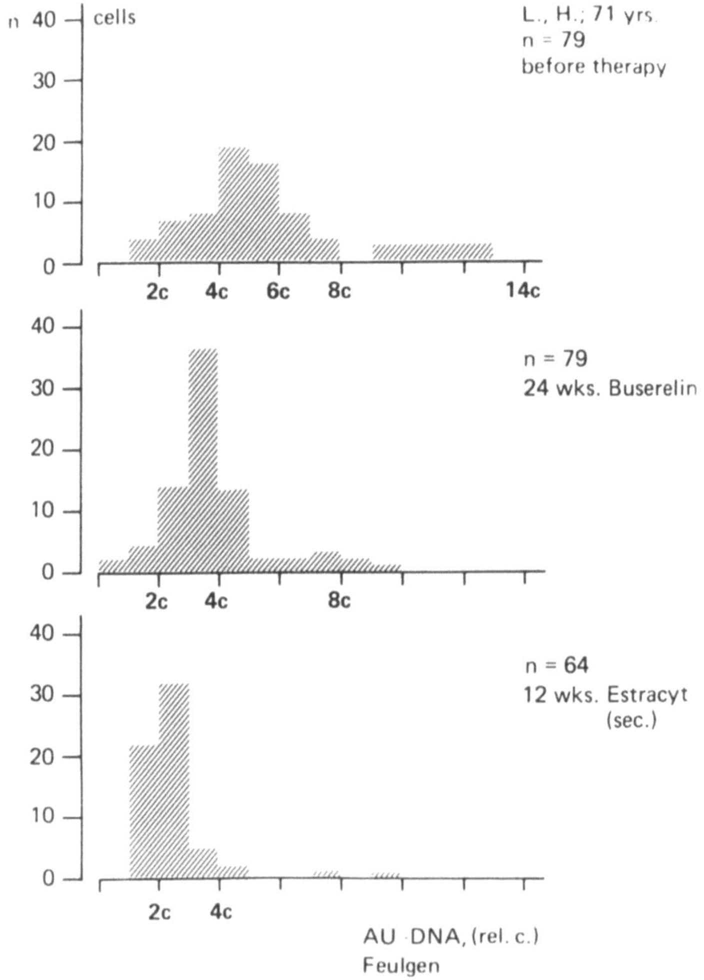

Fig. 8 DNA cytophotogram for moderately differentiated prostatic carcinoma, grade II (T3), prior to therapy, after 24 weeks of Buserelin therapy and, because of poor cytological regression grade, after 12 weeks of secondary EMCYT therapy. After 12 weeks of EMCYT therapy, there is a slim DNA frequency peak near 2c whereas before this therapy, the tumor showed a frequency peak near 4c, with values spreading up to 8c and even 13c.

DNA frequency peak near 8c, with values spreading up to 16c which, after this period of treatment, is an ominous sign. It also corresponded with the cytological finding. Therapy was changed to EMCYT some months later. After 24 weeks of secondary EMCYT therapy, there was still a marked aneuploidy of the tumor, with widely scattered values between 4c and 16c, i.e., resistance to this drug as well. This finding was clinically confirmed by local tumor progression with break-through into the urinary bladder. At that time, however, there was no evidence of distant metastases. Nevertheless, therapy was modifed by cross-over to cyclophosphamide, the third drug. Despite this change of therapy, the patient died, after 8 months of cyclophosphamide treatment, of wide-spread metastases and uncontrollable bleeding from the bladder.

L. H., 71 years, grade II carcinoma (Fig. 8):
Prior to Buserelin therapy, the DNA frequency peak was between 4c and 6c with some values spreading to 14c. After 24 weeks of Buserelin therapy, the cytophotogram showed a statistically non-significant shift to the left, into the 4c range, with numerous values spreading to 8c and beyond. Therapy response was rated poor, hence therapy was changed to EMCYT. After 12 weeks of secondary therapy with EMCYT, there was a significant frequency peak in the diploid (2c) range, i.e., response to secondary therapy was good, and accordingly, the patient has remained clinically stable for 20 months. EMCYT is the only therapy with which tumor response can be established already after 3 months.

Cytological and clinical results

These results of the 36 patients reated for 6 to 28 months are based mainly on cytological regression grading and DNY cytophotometry; the clinical course of the disease is, of course, taken into consideration as well.

The experience with this study has proven again that approx. 20% of locally advanced carcinomas are not hormone-dependent and do not respond to androgen withdrawal, as demonstrated by the lack of regressive changes.

31 of the 36 patients who were treated for 6 to 28 months showed the good to sufficient regression grades II to VI and responded positively to therapy, i.e., no clinical progression did occur. 5 patients were considered therapeutic failures as they showed poor or no regression at all, i.e., grade VIII or X. 4 of them were changed to secondary EMCYT therapy after 7, 7, 12 and 13 months. 1 patient was treated with Buserelin for 12 months, with EMCYT for 6 months, and crossed over to cyclophosphamide after 18 months until, after another 8 months, he died of the primary disease.

In 3 of these cases, response to secondary therapy was good. At the time of crossover, the serum testosterone levels of all 4 patients were clearly within castrate range. This is the reason why the testosterone level cannot be taken as a parameter for therapy effect.

4 patients had primary bone metastases. 2 of them have so far been treated only for a few months, so therapy response cannot be judged yet. One of them was free from pain shortly after starting therapy. Another patient, who has been treated for 13 months and was also pain-free shortly after starting therapy, has been in clinically stable condition despite unchanged metastatic state. The fourth patient died from myocardial infarction after 9 months; he had wide-spread metastases. Apart from him, 3 more patients died: 1 after 26 months, of the primary disease, after secondary EMCYT and tertiary cytostatic therapy had failed (tumor break-through into the urinary bladder). 2 died after 9 and 21 months; they had had no metastases and died from heart failure.

Side effects

The major side effects produced by Buserelin are hot flushes, which may be initial or permanent, sweats, and itching in the nose. In no case did the side effects require the discontinuation of therapy. All patients did, however, suffer the expected loss of libido and potency.

Out of the 51 patients treated, 2 complained of itching in the nose, 7 had sweats. 20 patients suffered from hot flushes, which were only initial in 10 cases but permanent in the other 10 cases.

Discussion

The therapy of the locally advanced prostatic carcinoma with or without metastases in the non-symptomatic stage still is a controversial matter, particularly with regard to the question of when to start therapy. Especially in the United States it is advocated not to start therapy before symptoms (bone pains, obstruction) do occur. In many European countres, on the other hand, immediate orchiectomy and/or estrogen therapy for stage C (T3) carcinomas still is common practice.

As *the potent LH-RH analogue Buserelin leads to a reduction of serum testosterone to the level found in castrated men and,* with sufficient dosage, *can also be maintained within this range over prolonged periods of time,* Buserelin offers itself for the treatment of locally advanced prostatic cancer and enables us to avoid orchiectomy and estrogen therapy with its side effects.

So far our studies have shown that at least the stage C (T3) carcinoma requires *close bioptic control* in order that tumors not responding to androgen withdrawal be discovered *before* metastates occur.

5 of 36 patients did not respond to androgen withdrawal, and 3 of them showed good response only after secondary EMCYT therapy. For each patient, control as-

piration biopsies were made at intervals of 3 to 6 months, and DNA cytophotometry every 6 months. The therapy study with 36 patients in stage C who had neither metastases nor clinical symptoms was judged justified since aspiration biopsy, together with the cytological methods, affords a unique means of examining the tumor itself, and, moreover, we have had extensive experience with these methods (more than 300 patients/1,000 bioptic controls).

Only 36 out of 51 patients were taken into his study. According to the authors' experience with Buserelin therapy, the control criteria valid for orchiectomy and estrogen therapy also apply to Buserelin therapy, as in principle, Buserelin belongs to the same type insofar as it causes androgen reduction to values similar to those of castrated men. *With this therapeutic approach, the regression grade – and hence therapy response – can definitely be established by cytology after 6 months,* whereas EMCYT therapy permits regression grading as early as 3 months after initiating therapy.

We have also proven that *rectal palpation results in false positive diagnoses in at least 50% of the cases,* especially when therapy response is positive, i.e., findings on palpation suggest that the tumor does not respond to therapy. A correspondence between the results of rectal palpation and cytology was found only in cases of poor or no regression. This explains why the often highly valued rectal palpation cannot be used as a parameter for therapy effect in clinical studies of new drugs for the non-metastatic carcinoma of the prostate.

1 patient with primary grade II carcinoma – though his serum testosterone level remained constant within "castrate" range – entered into local progression accompanied by a break-through of the tumor into the urinary bladder even after secondary EMCYT therpay so that he had to be treated with cyclophosphamide. He died of the primary disease after 26 months.

None of the 5 patients with resistance to Buserelin therapy showed any renewed increase in serum testosterone levels despite clinical progression or failure of the primary therapy. Therefore, *the serum testosterone level can by no means be taken as a parameter of therapy effects.*

This study has proven again that, since neither palpation nor testosterone levels are reliable, *cytology and DNY cytophotometry are the only true parameters for therapy control.*

Conclusion

This investigation of 36 patients, who were treated for more than 6 months, has proven the LH-RH analgue Buserelin to be potent enough to reduce serum testosterone to levels similar to those seen in castrated men within 3 weeks, and maintain this level for 2 years and longer under continuous therapy with intranasal application of the drug. Intranasal application is uncomplicated even for elderly patients; compliance has so far been very good as shown by short-term serum testosterone controls while side effects are rare and tolerable. It is a decisive advantage of Buserelin in the treatment of locally advanced prostatic cancer that – in the case of good therapy response – it offers an alternative to both orchiectomy with its psychical stress, and estrogen therapy with its possible cardiovascular side effects.

At this point it is not possible to draw any final conclusions as to the duration of this drug-induced castration effect – although it does not seem to differ substantially from that of orchiectomy or estrogen therapy.

In the present stage of investigation, patients in clinical stage C (T3) should be controlled as to the effect of Buserelin on the primary tumor by aspiration or punch biopsy at least every 6 months, since 5 of 36 patients in our study had a hormone resistance or clinical progression despite the fact that their serum testosterone levels remained within the range found in castrated men, i.e., up to 20% of all advanced prostatic carcinomas must generally be expected not to be androgen-dependent.

Judging from the results so far achieved it is to be expected that Buserelin will prove equivalent to the therapies commonly used in the primary treatment of prostatic carcinomas. Apart from this, Buserelin is an excellent means of testing whether a carcinoma will primarily respond to hormone therapy.

It remains to be shown by further well-designed clinical and biochemical studies whether a combination of Buserelin with other drugs is superior to Buserelin alone in the primary treatment of advanced prostatic carcinomas.

References

[1] Huggins, C., R. E. Stevens, C. V. Hodges: Arch. Surg. **43** (1941) 209.
[2] Veterans Administration Cooperative Urological Research Group: Treatment and survival of patients with cancer of the prostate. Surg. Gynaecol. Obstet. **124** (1967) 1011.
[3] Schally, A. V., Y. Arimura, R. M. G. Baba et al.: Biochem. Biophys. Res. Commun. **43** (1971) 393.
[4] Bergquist, C., S. J. Nillius, T. Bergh et al.: Acta Endocrinol. **91** (1979) 601.
[5] Cusan, L., C. Auclair, A. Belanger et al.: Endocrinology **104** (1979) 1369.
[6] Faure, N., A. Lemay, A. Belanger et al.: In "LHRH Peptides as Female and Male Contraceptives" (Eds. G. I. Zatuchni, J. D. Shelton, J. J. Sciarra), p. 307. Harper and Row, Philadelphia 1981.
[7] Hardt, W., M. Schmidt-Gollwitzer, M. von der Ohe et al.: Geburtsh. Frauenheilk. **41** (1981) 791.
[8] Schmidt-Gollwitzer, W. Hardt, K. Schmidt-Gollwitzer et al.: Contraception **23** (1981) 187.
[9] Wiegelmann, W., H. G. Solbach, H. K. Kley et al.: Horm. Metab. Res. **9** (1977) 521.
[10] Auclair, C., P. A. Kelly, D. H. Coy et al.: Endocrinology **101** (1977) 1890.
[11] Redding, T. W., A. V. Schally: Proc. Natl. Acad. Sci. USA **78** (1981) 6509.
[12] Rivier, C., J. Rivier, W. Vale: Endocrinology **105** (1979) 1191.

[13] Sandow, J., W. von Rechenberg, G. Jerzabek et al.: Acta Endocrinol. **94** (1980) 489.
[14] Sandow, J., R. M. Clayton, H. Kuhl: In "Endocrinology of Human Infertility: New Aspects", p. 221. Serono Symposium, Oxford 1980. Academic Press, New York 1981.
[15] Brogmann, V., W. Hardt, M. Schmidt-Gollwitzer et al.: Lancet (1982) 1097.
[16] Borgmann, V., R. Nagel, H. Al-Abadi et al.: Prostate **4** (1983) 553.
[17] Alken, C. E., G. Dhom, W. Straube et al.: Urologe A **14** (1975) 112.
[18] Sprenger, E., L. Volk, W. W. Michaelis: Beitr. Path. **153** (1974) 370.
[19] Zetterberg, A., P. L. Esposti: Acta Cytol. **20** (1979) 46.
[20] Leistenschneider, W., R. Nagel: Eur. Urol. **6** (1980) 111.
[21] Leistenschneider, W., R. Nagel: Scand. J. Urol. Nephrol. Suppl. **55** (1980) 197.

Clinical experience (up to 40 months) with the LH-RH agonist Buserelin in the therapeutic approach to prostatic cancer

N. Faure, A. Lemay, B. Laroche, G. Robert, R. Plante, M. Thabet, R. Roy, C. Jean, A. T. A. Fazekas

Introduction

Cancer of the prostate is the second or third most common cause of cancer deaths in males in North America [1]. Orchiectomy or the administration of estrogens are the traditional modes of palliative therapy for patients with metastatic disease [2, 3]. However, the current modes of androgen suppression can have relative contraindications, psychologically or on the cardiovascular systems respectively [4].

The potential achievement of "chemical castration" has been investigated through the development of potent LH-RH agonists [5]. The suppression of testicular androgens has been achieved in several animal species and in man using these synthetic compounds [6–9].

We have previously reported early results of a phase II study the purpose of which was to define the effective dosage of the LH-RH agonist D-Ser $(TBU)^6$, des-Gly-NH_2^{10} LH-RH ethylamide, (HOE 766 or Buserelin), which would suppress and maintain testicular androgen inhibition [9, 10]. We report here on long-term safety data (up to 40 months) and on clinical efficacy of Buserelin administered for a period of 3 to 21 months to a group of 29 patients with a stage D prostatic carcinoma.

Material and Methods

Protocol

Twenty-nine patients with a metastatic prostate carcinoma (stage D1: 6; stage D2: 23) received 500 µg subcutaneously (SC) of Buserelin every eight hours for seven days followed by 400 µg intranasally (IN) every eight hours, or a dose varying between 50 and 200 µg SC daily (3 patients). Twenty-three patients had never received any other therapy except for surgical prostatectomy. In six other patients, previous therapy with estrogen and/or irradiation had been stopped at least three and eight months, respectively, before starting Buserelin.

Before the initiation of Buserelin administration, complete history, physical examination, and informed consent were obtained. Details of the urinary symptomatology, occurence of pain, description of general status, level of activity were carefully recorded then as well as at the monthly visits. The subjective evaluation of all the patients was done by the same investigator. Objective parameters were also measured before therapy and at regular intervals thereafter: rectal exam and transrectal ultrasonography (after one, three, six months, etc.), bone scan (every three months), chest X-ray (every three months), and any other radiography (metastatic series, intravenous pyelography) when necessary.

Endocrine parameters were also measured weekly for the first month and monthly thereafter (LH, FSG, testosterone) or every three months (17-OH-progesterone, DHT, 17 β-estradiol).

A group of 10 patients at various stages of cancer have been entered in the early dose-range finding studies. They have now been treated with Buserelin for periods of 22 to 40 months. The complete 3 monthly laboratory evaluation is being used to gather long-term safety data. Four other patients, now off therapy, had been treated for periods of 16 to 26 months.

Laboratory safety tests

Hematological (CBC, platelets), biochemical (serum glucose, BUN, uric acid, creatinine, cholesterol, total protein, SGOT, SGPT, alkaline and total acid phosphatase, prostatic acid phosphatase (by RIA), sodium, potassium, chloride, inorganic phosphorus), and hormonal (cortisol, prolactin, thyroxine) studies as well as urinary analysis were performed before therapy and at regular intervals during the treatment. These data gathered regularly have been used to demonstrate the safety and absence of significant side effects associated with long-term LH-RH agonist therapy.

Histological studies of the testis

Histologic examination of the testis of ten patients castrated for various reasons after 0.5 to 12 months of therapy with Buserelin was performed. The microscopic findings were compared with 18 age-matched controls (six patients with prostatic cancer in whom orchiectomy was performed and who had not received any other treatment and 12 patients who died from another cause).

Results

Pituitary-testicular axis inhibition

Following the dose-range finding studies, a sequential combined regimen was chosen using the SC and IN routes. In order to attain rapid pituitary desensitization, 500 μg of Buserelin was administered three times a day SC for one week. The practical intranasal route of administration could then be instituted at the dose of 400 μg intranasally.

After the first week of therapy, the serum testosterone was similar to baseline (fig. 1), and in 13 out of 28 patients, testosterone was higher than the baseline value by a mean of 1.59 ng/ml (see insert). However, at the second week of therapy, the mean serum testosterone was inhibited to 35.4% of control ($P < .01$). The mean levels were inferior to 1.0 ng/ml within 3 weeks. The sensitivity of our testosterone assay is 0.4 ng/ml. No escape could be demonstrated once the serum levels were lowered.

Serum LH showed a 61.8% decrease after three months of therapy and remained at the lower limit of sensitivity of the assay thereafter ($p < 0.01$). FSH serum levels were

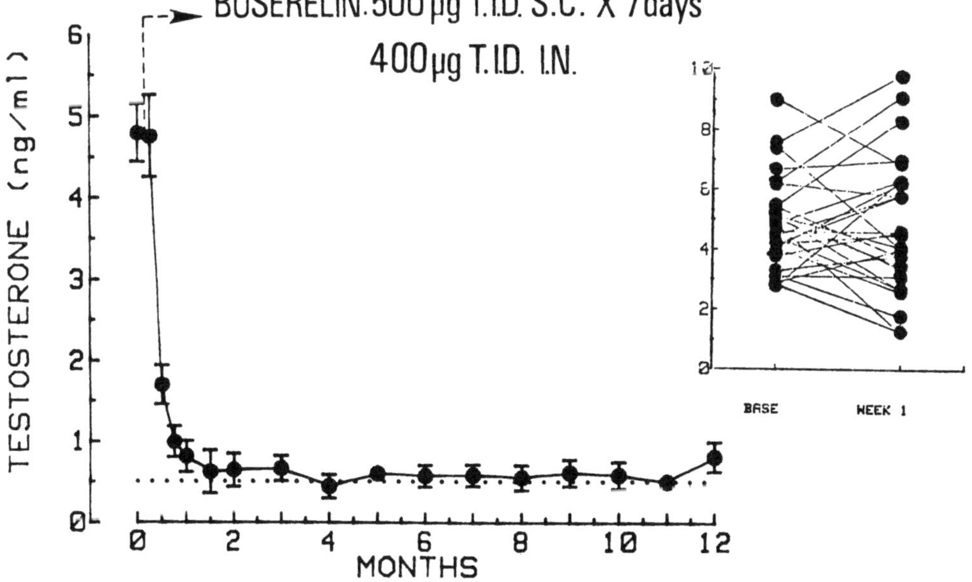

Fig. 1 Mean ± SEM basal and testosterone in 28 patients with stage D prostatic carcinoma who were treated daily with Buserelin (500 μg SC every eight hours for seven days followed by 400 μg intranasally every eight hours). Insert: Individual serum testosterone levels before and after the first 7 days of buserelin (SC).

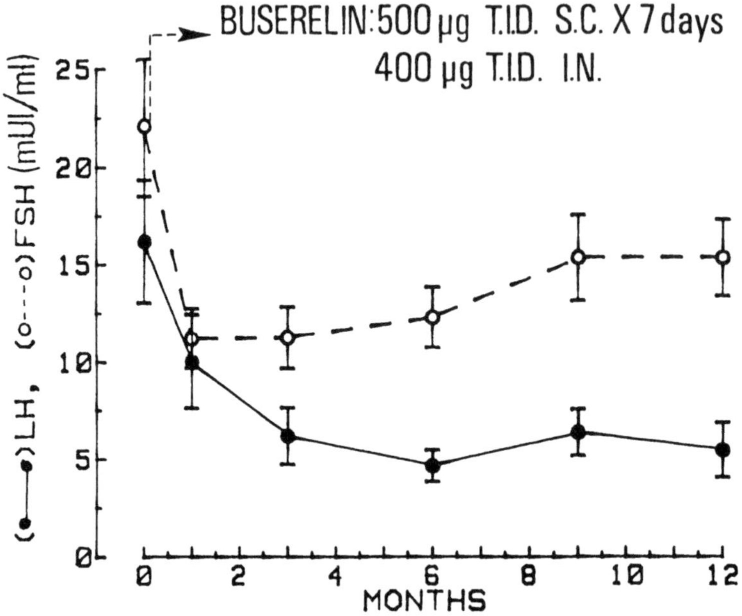

Fig. 2 Mean ± SEM basal serum LH and FSH in 28 patients with prostatic cancer treated with Buserelin (500 µg SC every eight hours for seven days followed by 400 µg intranasally every eight hours).

inhibited at the same interval ($p < 0.01$) but the levels showed a tendancy to rise after 9 months (p: NS) (69.5% of baseline vs 50.9% at 9 and 3 months respectively) (fig. 2).

Figure 3 shows the increase in LH serum levels 3 hours after the first, second and fourth injections of Buserelin as well as during the chronic IN therapy. The data show clearly that pituitary response is already 82% inhibited after the second dose of Buserelin. The pituitary remains refractory as long as the therapy is continued.

Clinical efficacy of LH-RH agonist treatment

Table 1 lists the subjective and objective parameters used to evaluate the clinical efficacy of Buserelin therapy. Each of these parameters could be of different value for evaluation of the treatment. The results are expressed as percentage of the number of patients presenting with an anomaly of these parameters at the start of therapy and who were evaluated every 3 months.

The efficacy of Buserelin treatment is best evaluated by the overall clinical assessment, which is a global impression taking into account all the parameters both subjective and objective. After 3 to 6 months of Buserelin treatment, 76 and 77% of

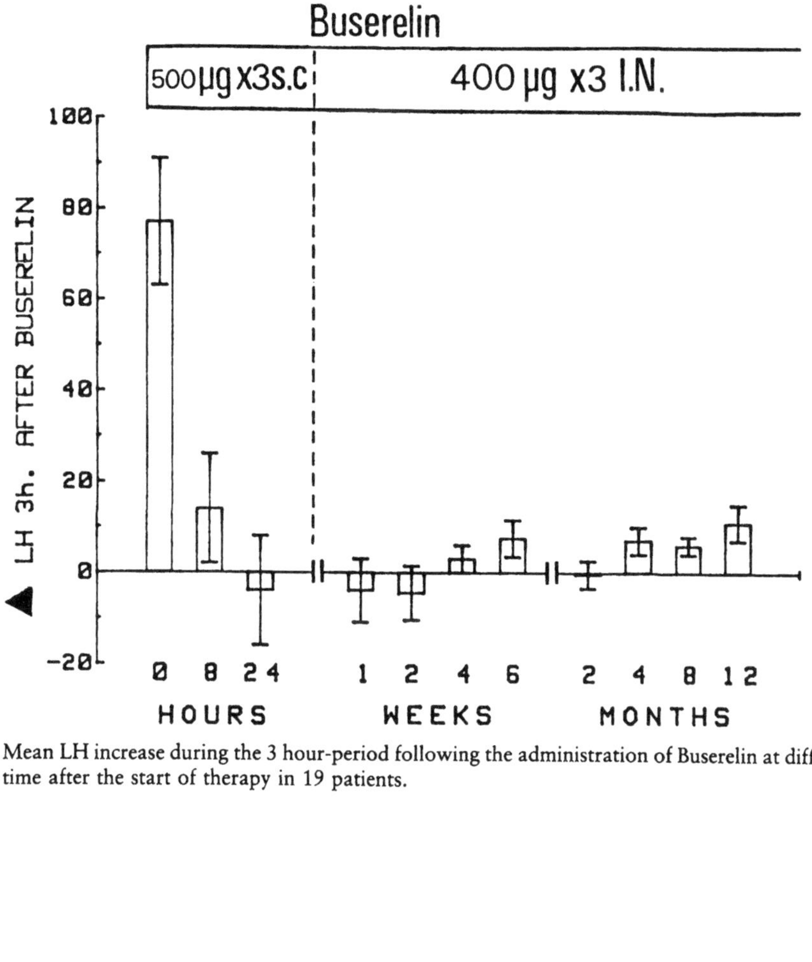

Fig. 3 Mean LH increase during the 3 hour-period following the administration of Buserelin at different time after the start of therapy in 19 patients.

Table 1 Clinical efficacy

	Month 3				Month 6				Month 9				Month 12			
	n[1]	I	S	D	n	I	S	D	n	I	S	D	n	I	S	D
Subjective Parameters																
Bone Pain	13	61%	8%	31%	10	60%	10%	30%	8	38%	12%	50%	3	66.6%	33.3%	–
Prostatism	27	33%	59%	8%	21	38%	52%	10%	14	22%	64%	14%	7	29%	57%	14%
Objective Parameters																
Bone scan	21	14%	57%	29%	17	35%	30%	35%	10	40%	30%	30%	8	25%	37,5%	37,5%
Prostate size	24	42%	58%	–	19	53%	47%	–	15	47%	53%	–	7	57%	43%	–
Prost. Acid Phosph.	18	61%	33%	6%	14	72%	14%	14%	9	78%	11%	11%	4	100%	–	–
Alkaline Phosphatase	10	20%	50%	30%	8	25%	37.5%	37.5%	5	20%	40%	40%	1	–	100%	–
Overall Assessment	29	31%	45%	24%	22	32%	45%	23%	15	33.3%	33.3%	33.3%	10	40%	40%	20%
Deaths (from cancer)			2 pat.				1 pat.				1 pat.					
Change of therapy			1 pat.								2 pat.					

[1] n = number of patients presenting an abnormality of the parameters at the start of therapy and evaluated at each time interval
I = Improvement; S = Stabilization; D = Deterioration of the disease process

the 29 patients showed a regression or stabilization of their disease while 24 to 23% respectively did not respond to the androgen suppressive therapy. Three patients died from the disease during the first 6 months, another died from a cardiovascular condition and the therapy was stopped in one patient because of no response.

During the following 3 month-periods (9 and 12 months) 15 and 10 patients could be evaluated: 66 and 80% showed a positive response or a stabilization of their condition respectively and the remaining third and fifth deteriorated. At the 9th month of therapy, one patient, who had previously responded, escaped from the hormonal treatment. One patient died and the treatment was stopped in 2 other patients.

Side effects and safety of long-term use of LH-RH agonists

Hematological and biochemical parameters (cf Material and Methods) evaluated regularly up to 40 months did not show any significant change that could be attributed to the agonistic analogue. All the values remained within normal limits or did not change significantly from the levels measured prior to the start of treatment. The occurrence of a decrease in hemoglobin levels occasionally found correlated with the progression of the disease (data not shown).

Buserelin administration had no significant effect on serum levels of cortisol and thyroxine measured every 3 months for up to 40 months. Serum prolactin was measured every three months for periods up to nine months and was not affected by LH-RH agonist.

No side effect associated with Buserelin administration was noticed except those related to decreased androgen formation such as hot flushes and gradual decrease in potency in the patients who were sexually active at the beginning of treatment.

Histologic studies of the testis

The histologic sections of the testis from LH-RH agonist-treated patients as well as castrated controls were reviewed single blind by the pathologist. Three general histologic patterns could be defined: Class 1: spermatogenesis arrest at the spermatid level, occasional spermatozoa in the seminiferous tubules, decrease in the number of Leydig cells that are isolated or in small clusters; Class 2: spermatogenesis arrest at the spermatocyte II level, occasional spermatids and very rarely a spermatozoa in the lumen of the tubules, marked decrease in the number of Leydig cells showing occasional signs of degeneration; Class 3: complete absence of spermatogenesis, only Sertoli cells in the seminiferous tubules, very rare and degenerated Leydig cells. No sign of toxicity could be found, there was no microinfarct and no evidence of calcifications (fig. 4).

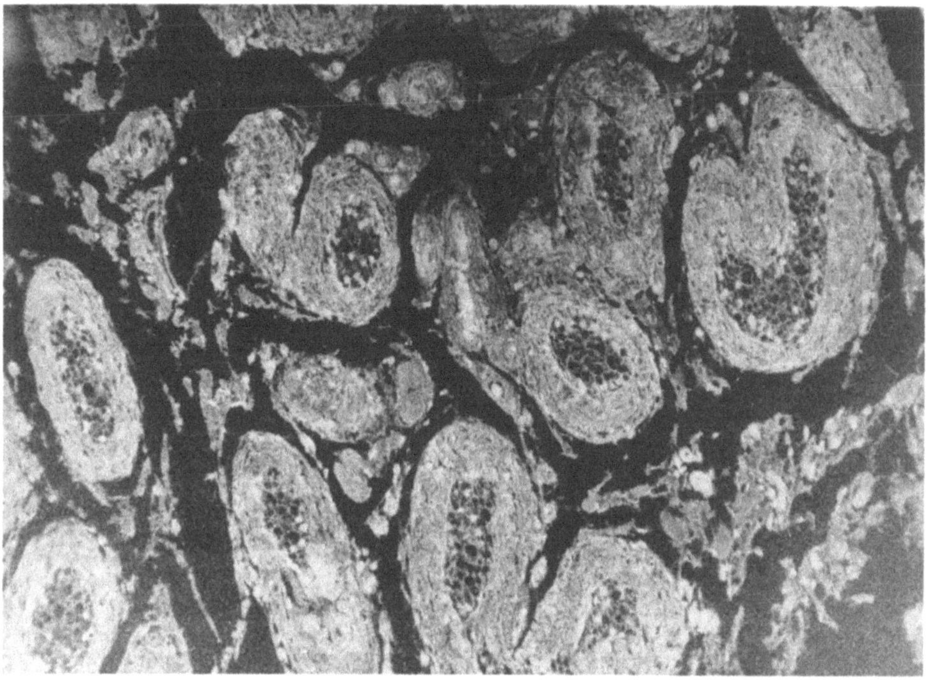

Fig. 4 Testicular histology showing complete absence of spermatogenesis (Sertoli cells only) and disappearance of Leydig cells in a patient castrated after 12 months of Buserelin administration (50 μg daily SC).

The six prostate cancer controls (no previous therapy) were all Class 1 and in the autopsy controls (no cancer) there were eight Class 1, three Class 2, and one Class 3 histologic aspects of the testis. In the patients treated with Buserelin, there seemed to be a correlation between the duration of therapy and the decrease in spermatogenesis: all six patients treated for 0.5 to 6 months were Class 1, one patient treated for 6 months was Class 2, and all patients treated for 7 to 18 months were Class 3.

Discussion

Practical regimen for inducing hypogonadotropic hypogonadism

Intranasal administration of Buserelin following 7 days of subcutaneous injections induces a rapid and significant decrease of circulating levels of testosterone (within 2 weeks) followed within 6 weeks by a more profound inhibition to levels similar to those found after orchiectomy (fig. 1). When achieved, the suppression is maintained as long as therapy is continued. In only one patient out of 29 studied for periods of time up to 18 months, testosterone levels showed a temporary slight increase (1.3–1.7 ng/ml) during months 3 to 6.

The suppression of serum testosterone can be explained by inhibition of gonadotropin secretion. An important stimulation of LH and FSH is seen after the first administration of the LH-RH agonist (fig. 2). The repetitive administration of pharmacological doses of Buserelin causes an immediate and marked decrease of LH levels and pituitary response, and lowers progressively basal levels of LH and FSH (figs. 2, 3). The serum LH levels measured are at the lower limit of sensitivity of the radioimmunoassay.

The down-regulation of the pituitary response is reversible since there is a prompt return to normal stimulation after cessation of therapy [9]. Thus, in man, the main mechanism responsible for testicular inhibition could be the achievement of a temporary and reversible state of hypogonadotropic hypogonadism. This is further supported by the demonstration that the testosterone response to exogenous HCG is preserved during chronic LH-RH agonist treatment in transexuals [11]. The question of a possible direct effect of LH-RH agonists on the testis is not resolved in the human.

Clinical efficacy of LH-RH agonist treatment

The clinical evaluation of the 23 not previously treated patients and of the 6 previously treated patients shows no difference in the response to therapy between these 2 groups. Three of the previously treated patients responded to therapy and 3 did not and showed a progression of the disease.

The overall clinical assessment as well as the response to the different criteria studied, both objective and subjective, show that the response of patients with metastatic carcinoma to chronic LH-RH agonist administration appears quite similar to the responses reported after conventional therapy (tab. 1). Although these numbers are small and the period of observation is short, beneficial effects of LH-RH agonist treatment would compare with surgical castration and estrogen treatment, as most authors have reported a positive response in 65 to 80% of patients [12–14].

In our study, 2 patients presented an increase in bone pain during the first week of treatment. Testosterone values at 1 week were already decreasing below starting levels in these 2 patients. At week 1 of treatment with 500 μg of Buserelin SC every eight hours, an increase of testosterone (mean 1.59 ng/ml: range 0.3–3.5 ng/ml) was found in 46% of patients (fig. 1). This small increase in serum testosterone was not accompanied by a clinical flare-up. At week 2, serum testosterone was significantly decreased in all patients. An increase in serum levels of testosterone during the first few days of therapy accompanied by subjective signs of a possible "tumor flare" during that period has been described to occur in about 10% of patients [15]. It is possible that a short-lived rise in testosterone in the first few days of therapy would lead to a temporary increase in bone pain in some patients. One way to avoid these problems would be to start the therapy with the addition of an antiandrogen that could neutralize peripherally the effects of the initial surge of testicular androgens.

Side effects and long-term safety data

The only side effects related to the therapy are those that could be attributed to the decrease of testicular androgens. In our experience, all patients sexually active at the start of Buserelin treatment showed a gradual decline in their potency toward the cessation of sexual intercourse. The occurrence of hot flushes was variable and temporary in spite of continuation of therapy and persistence of androgen inhibition.

The LH-RH agonist Buserelin is devoid of any effect on other pituitary hormone as assessed by the serum levels of prolactin, thyroxine, and cortisol measured regularly for more than three years (except for prolactin, which has been evaluated for a maximum of twelve months) (data not shown).

A complete evaluation of hematological and biochemical parameters has been monitored every one to three months in all the patients receiving Buserelin therapy. No effect could be attributed to Buserelin treatment, all change in these parameters being explained by the progression of the metastatic disease or by another preexisting health condition.

Histologic studies

From our short series, it seems that overall, the most marked changes on spermatogenesis are correlated to prolonged and profound suppression of testicular steroidogenesis. Compared with age-matched control, LH-RH agonist decreases spermatogenesis and has no deleterious effect [16]. Failure to demonstrate any apparent toxic effect of chronic administration of LH-RH agonist on human testis supports the possible use of these compounds as a reversible approach in male contraception. However, it should be mentioned that in these two studies, chronic LH-RH treatment was administered to men aged 60 or more and some effects could be possibly overlooked because of the histologic changes in the testis associated with age.

From our experience and from that of others, it seems that one of the major advantages of LH-RH agonist treatment in prostate cancer is its specificity of action, absence of adverse side effects and of clinical chemistry changes for periods up to 40 months. The sequential administration of Buserelin by subcutaneous and intranasal routes used in our studies was found to be practical and the compliance of the patients was excellent.

LH-RH agonist treatment appears as a valuable medical alternative to conventional homronal therapy in prostatic cancer. Profound and sustained inhibition of serum androgen levels obtained within 3 to 4 weeks is followed by a beneficial effect on the disease as compared to other regimens for the first year of treatment. Comparative multicenter trials will be needed to delineate the place of this therapeutic approach.

References

[1] Klein, L. A.: N. Engl. J. Med. **300** (1970) 824–833.
[2] Huggins, C., R. E. Steven, C. V. Hodges: Arch. Surg. **43** (1941) 209–223.
[3] Bailar III, J. C., D. P. Byar: Cancer **26** (1970) 257–261.
[4] Hedlund, P. O., H. Gustafsson, S. Sjogren: Scand. J. Urol. Nephrol. Supp. **55** (1980) 103–105.
[5] Corbin, A., B. J. Bex: Acta Eur. Fertil. **11** (1980) 113–130.
[6] Sandow, J., W. Rechenberg, G. Jerzabek et al.: Acta Endocrinol. 294 (1980) 489–497.
[7] Bélanger, A., C. Auclair, L. Ferland et al.: J. Steroid. Biochem. **13** (1980) 191–196.
[8] Borgman, V., W. Hardt, M. Schmidt-Gollwitzer et al.: Lancet **I** (1982) 1097–1099.
[9] Faure, N., F. Labrie, A. Lemay et al.: Fertil. Steril. **37** (1982) 416–424.
[10] Faure, N., A. Lemay, B. Laroche et al.: The Prostate **4** (1983) 227–251.
[11] Tolis, G., A. Mehta, A. M. Comaru-Schally: J. Clin. Invest. **68** (1981) 819–822.
[12] Resnick, M. I., J. T. Grayhack: Urol. Clin. North Am. **2** (1975) 141–161.
[13] Menon, M., P. C. Walsh: Prostate Cancer (Edited by S. Murphy), pp. 175–200. PSG Publishing Co., Littleton 1970.
[14] Murphy, G. P., N. H. Slack: Urol. Clin. North Am. **3** (2980) 631–638.
[15] Santen, R. J., B. Warner, J. Smith: LH-RH and its analogs (Edited by B. H. Vickery, J. J. Nestor, E. S. E. Hafez) MTP Press, Lancaster. In press.
[16] Rajfer, J., R. S. Swerdloff, D. Heber: Fertil. Steril. **39** (1983) 440–441.

Antigonadal properties of LH-RH agonists: therapeutical applications in human

M. Schmidt-Gollwitzer †, W. Hardt, V. Borgmann

Introduction

The hypothalamic pituitary system is responsible for proper gonadal function. Secretion of the gonadotropins is on the one hand maintained by the release at regular intervals of gonadotropin releasing hormone (pulsatile secretion of LH-RH), and on the other hand positively or negatively modulated by the sexual steroids [77].

Unphysiologically high concentrations of LH-RH are followed, after an initial stimulation phase due to a reduction in pituitary receptors, by both a decrease in gonadotropin secretion and dissociation of the LH/FSH ratio. This pathological mechanism can be accentuated by the biologically more effective LH-RH agonists [9]. Repeated application leads to a secondary reduction of gonad function [10]. This paradoxical antigonadal effect of LH-RH agonist offers new prospects for fertility control and ablative endocrine therapy.

In this article, the results of our clinical experimental studies with the potent LH-RH agonist Buserelin are summarized.

Antigonadal effect

Single dose application of the LH-RH agonist Buserelin* leads to a more prolonged and marked secretion of gonadotropins, compared with the effects of natural LH-RH [3]. The pituitary reaction in sexually mature women is most vigourous at midcycle, maximal release occurring after an interval of 2 to 8 hours. Release of LH is substantially higher than that of FSH (fig. 1). Application over several days produces a marked decline in pituitary reaction, accompanied by almost complete suppression of FSH secretion.

* The LH-RH agonist Buserelin was kindly supplied by Dr. M. von der Ohe, Hoechst AG, Frankfurt a. M., Germany.

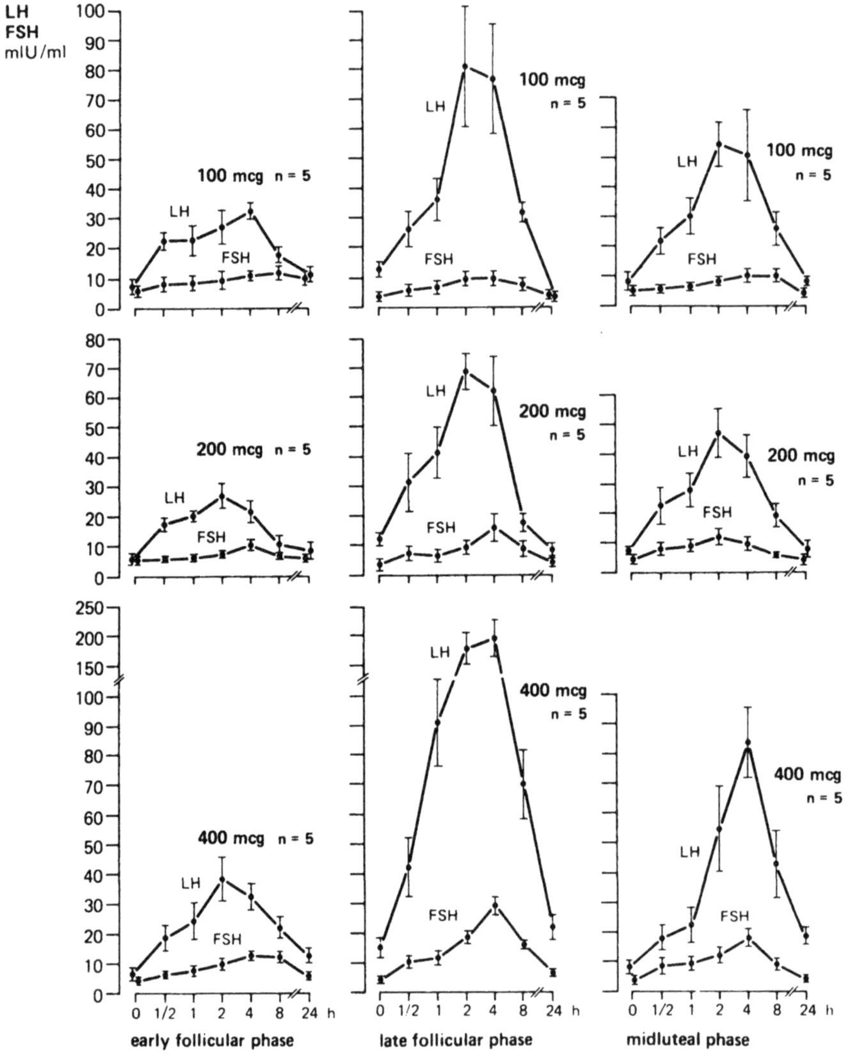

Fig. 1 Stimulation profiles of gonadotropins during different phase of the normal menstrual cycle after intranasal application of different doses of Buserelin (0, 1/2, 1, 2, 4, 8, 24 hours after stimulation).

Concommitant with the release of gonadotropins, single dose application of the LH-RH agonist leads to stimulation and several days' application to reduction of sexual steroid production (fig. 2). It is thus possible to exert a regulatory influence on the cyclic ovarian function. Intranasal (i.n.) application of the LH-RH agonist provides a clinically acceptable method, in contrast to intravenous or subcutaneous application.

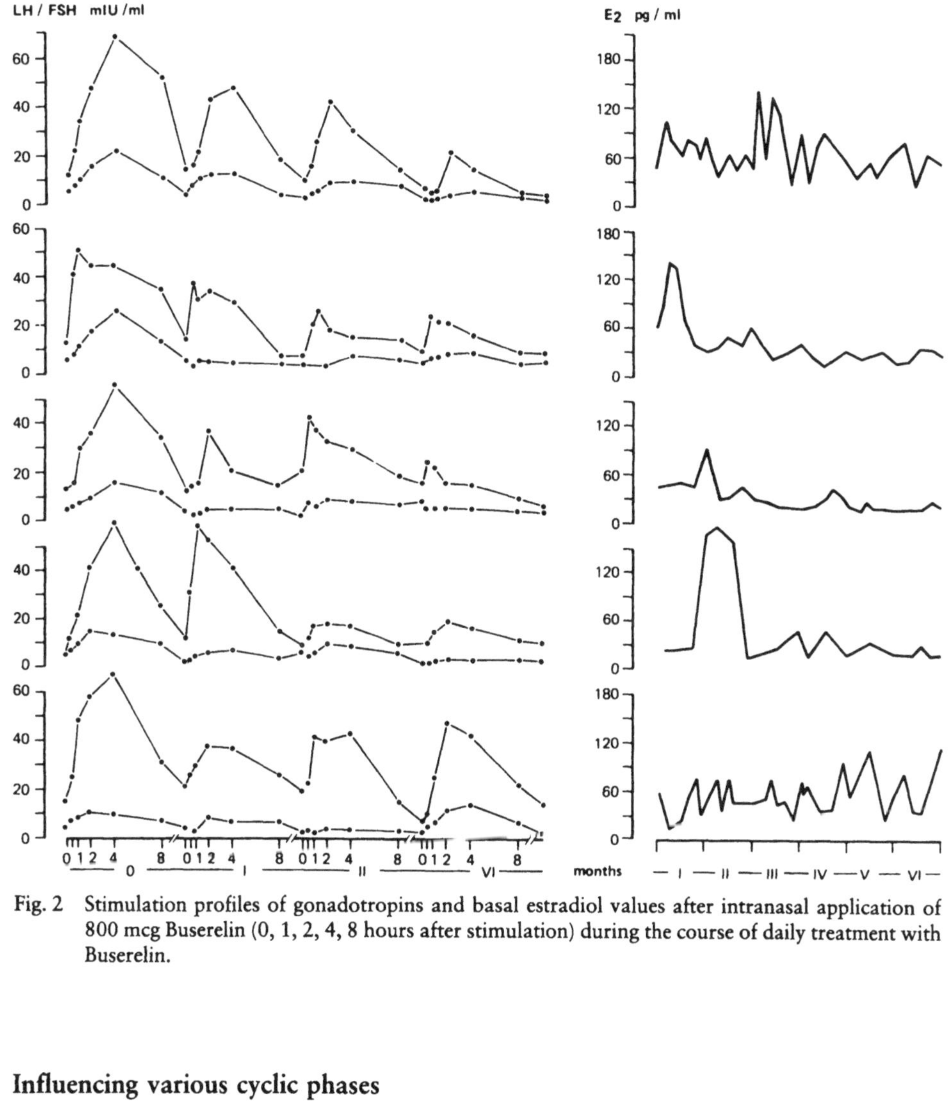

Fig. 2 Stimulation profiles of gonadotropins and basal estradiol values after intranasal application of 800 mcg Buserelin (0, 1, 2, 4, 8 hours after stimulation) during the course of daily treatment with Buserelin.

Influencing various cyclic phases

Whereas luteolysis, leading to abortion, can be induced by the LH-RH agonists in animal experiments (rats, guinea-pigs, primates), the results obtained with fertile women are by no means so straightforward and promising. Although the initial enhancement of progesterone synthesis is succeeded by a poststimulatory decline, the progesterone levels remain in some women within the range typical for normal corpus luteum function (fig. 3).

Even highly dosed subcutaneous application (100% compared to 1–2.5% resorption after intranasal application) at various stages of the luteal phase, failed to produce concrete evidence of a sure luteolytic effect of the LH-RH agonist in humans, either

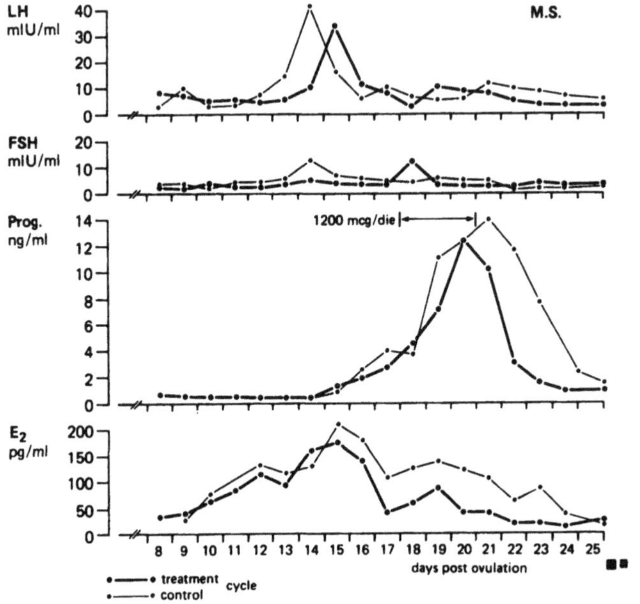

Fig. 3 Hormone profiles during the control cycle and the course of midluteal treatment with 1200 mcg Buserelin intranasally. Normal corpus luteum function during and after treatment with Buserelin.

in terms of the measured progesterone values or in terms of significant shortening of the luteal phase (fig. 4).

Furthermore, the reduction of progesterone synthesis induced by the agonist can be reversed by human chorionic gonadotropin, and the luteal phase prolonged beyond the normal duration (fig. 5). Even in cases where a pregnancy has occurred immediate reactivation of the corpus luteum can be expected. Thus, the idea of postovulatory contraception using LH-RH agonists, put forward by Caspar et Yen and Lemay et al. is not a practicable approach [2, 8].

Compared to the stable corpus luteum function, the more complex process of follicle ripening appears to be more susceptible to the influence of LH-RH agonists. Follicle ripening can be disturbed by the drug as a function of both time and dose. Low doses (up to 200 mcg/day i.n.), starting at menstruation, produce a fall in the estradiol level following an initial stimulation. The treatment thus leads to delay of ovulation, which in the low dose range depends on the duration of the application. The succeeding corpus luteum function ist not impaired (fig. 6). Higher doses (400 mcg/day i.n.), on the other hand, applied over the same period, more frequently lead to impairment of the corpus luteum function, and after 20-day application, to inhibition of ovulation, which, however, is dependant on beginning treatment early. To

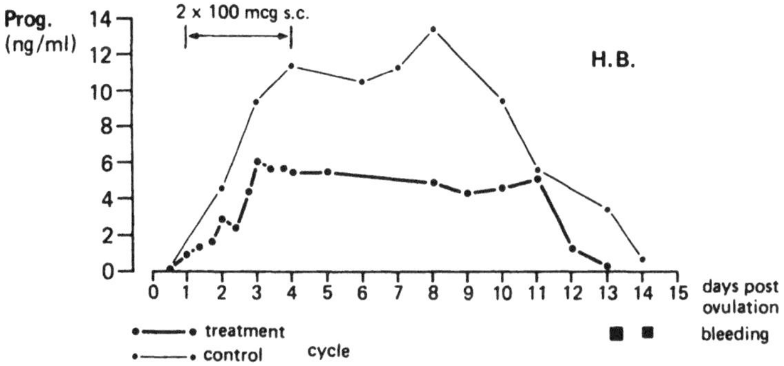

Fig. 4 Progesterone values during the control cycle and the course of early luteal treatment with 200 mcg buserelin s. c.

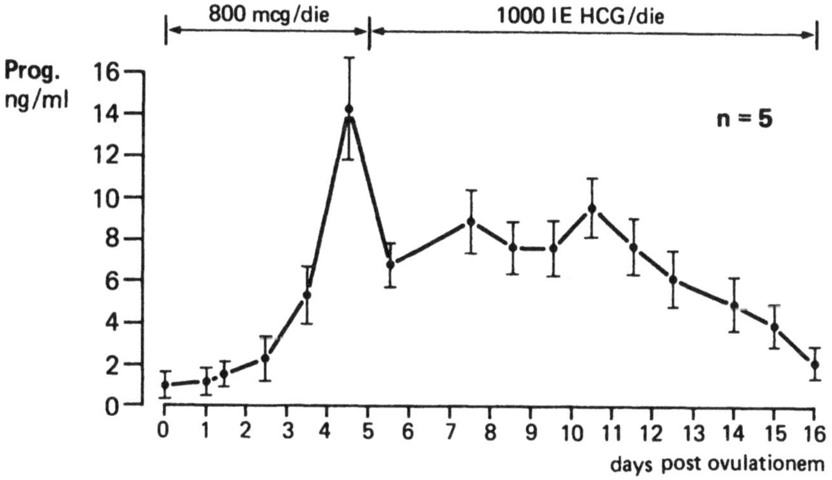

Fig. 5 Prolongation of corpus luteum function with human chorionic gonadotropin after treatment with Buserelin.

obtain reproducible inhibition of ovulation, medication must be commenced before the 5th day of cycle, otherwise the process of selection of the dominant follicle can no longer be interrupted with certainty (fig. 7). The inhibiting effect, particularly after the 7th day, then becomes an ovulation inducing effect.

Delay or inhibition of ovulation results in menstrual bleeding at unpredictable times, showing that control of the cycle is no longer possible. The short-term effect on follicle ripening as a means of long-term fertility control is thus shown to be scarcely practicable. The extent to which the proven inhibition of ovulation can be maintained over longer periods, remains to be clarified.

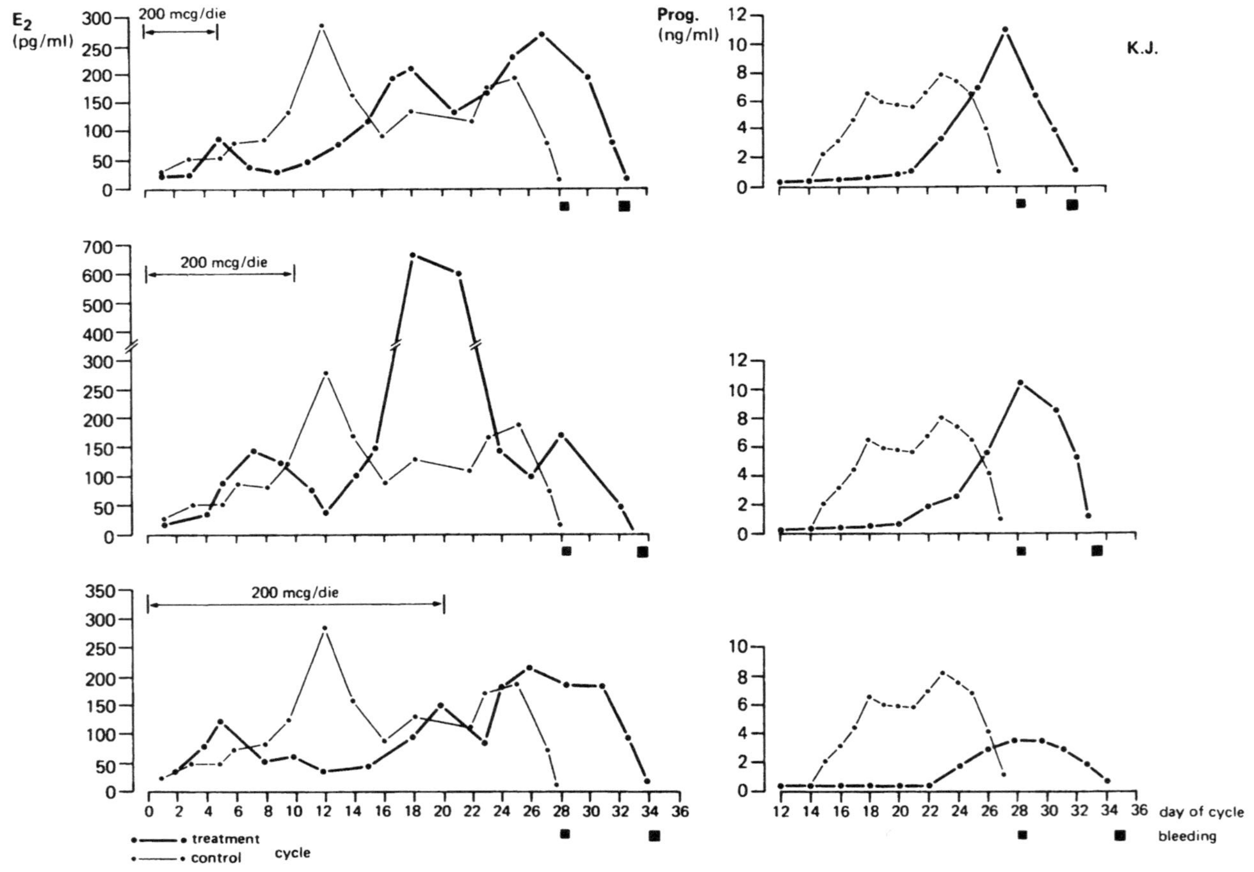

Fig. 6 Hormone profiles of sexual steroids during and after treatment with Buserelin during follicular phase (200 mcg/d intranasally).

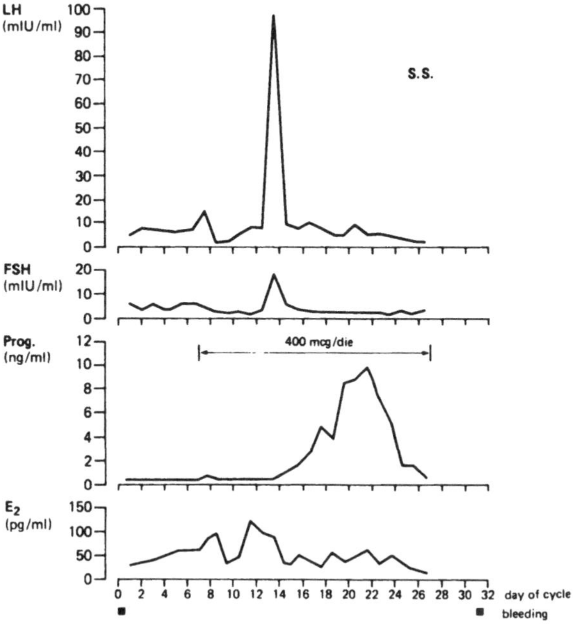

Fig. 7 Hormone profiles during the course of treatment with 400 mcg Buserelin. Starting of therapy: 7th day of cycle. Normal corpus luteum function.

Continuous Medication

Continuous treatment, as a function of dose, can be used to inhibit ovulation over a period of months or years. With doses up to 200 mcg, progesterone values in as many as 85% of the therapy months were found indicative of either certain anovulation, luteinization of non-ruptured follicles or severe corpus luteum insufficiency. Increased dosage to 400 mcg daily produces this condition in 97% of therapy months (tab. 1) [11]. For doses above 400 mcg, anovulation can be shown in practically 100% of the medication months.

Table 1 Distribution of serum progesterone levels of 79 volunteers during the course of treatment with different doses of Buserelin

Dose (mcg/die)	Progesterone			Months	
	< 1	1–3	3–6	> 6	
100	34 (46%)	17 (23%)	14 (19%)	9 (12%)	74
200	121 (67%)	33 (18%)	22 (12%)	5 (3%)	181
400	136 (87%)	16 (10%)	4 (3%)	0 (0%)	156
800/1200	38 (95%)	2 (5%)	0 (0%)	0 (0%)	40

In contrast to the inhibition of ovulation, which is clearly dose-dependant, the effect on estrogen production, even at contraceptive levels of the LH-RH agonist, is very variable. Whereas in a number of cases an abrupt restriction of estrogen secretion with consequent amenorrhea at an early stage was found, the majority showed, albeit with decreasing tendency, considerable variations in the estradiol level up to levels of the preovulatory phase (fig. 8).

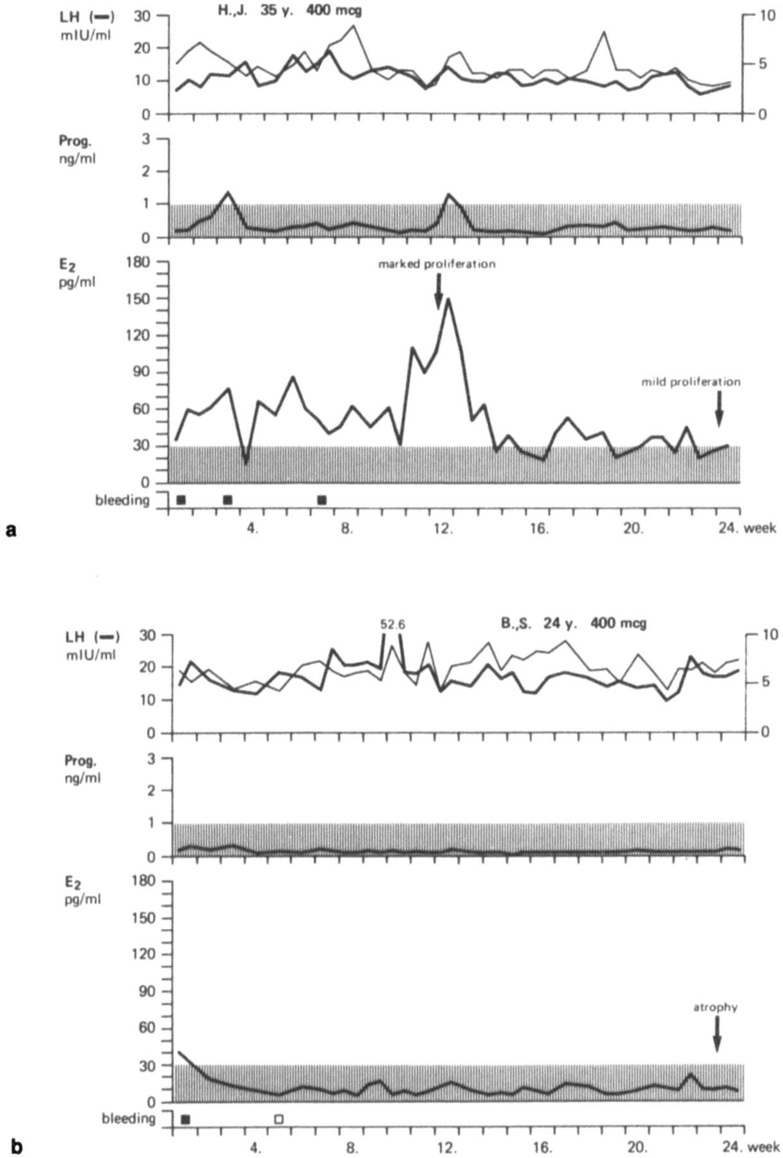

Fig. 8 Typical hormone profiles during the continous treatment with 400 mcg Buserelin intranasally. a) marked fluctuation of estradiol values, b) sustained suppression of estradiol values.

This indicates that the effect on the follicle ripening mechanism at contraceptive doses is individually very variable, with two thirds of the women showing mainly irregular bleeding patterns, resulting from desynchronized endometrium formation. Endometrium biopsies repeated during different therapy months indicate both phases of prolonged and enhanced endometrium stimulation as well as phases of insufficient or non existent stimulation (inactivity or atrophy) (tab. 2). Atypical endometrium hyperplasia was found in no cases. Declining estrogen secretion further resulted in a corresponding reversal of the initially present hyperplastic changes in the endometrium [4].

Table 2 Distribution of bleeding pattern of 79 volunteers during the course of treatment with different doses of Buserelin (Regular bleeding: intervals of 3 to 6 weeks, irregular bleeding: more than 6 weeks)

Dose	Bleeding Pattern			N
(mcg)	no	irregular	regular	
100	1	4	9	14
200	11	3	14	28
400	7	14	7	28
800/1200	3	6	0	9

Clinical application

The possibility of long-term fertility control and ablative endocrine therapy with LH-RH agonists has been confirmed by our studies. Acceptance of the intranasal method of application was found to be very high. In addition, experimental findings confirm that this agonist has no measurable effect on essential metabolic functions – in contrast to the sexual steroids conventionally used for contraception.

Contraception

Continuous medication is, however, accompanied by loss of control of menstrual bleeding (tab. 2). Since a decrease in estrogens down to pre- or postmenopausal levels is generally to be expected in the course of treatment, phases of uninhibited estrogen effects on the endometrium, except in occassional cases, are unlikely; more probable are the results of longterm estrogen deficiency. It thus became desirable to develop a new treatment schedule which guarantees the contraceptive as well as estrogenic effect on the one hand, and permits better cycle control on the other.

Our approach was to determine to what extent cycle control could be achieved by discontinuous medication (3 weeks treatment, 1 week's break). In view of the persistent disturbance of follicle ripening by the above mentioned 20-day treatment, it was assumed that intercurrent ovulation would hardly be likely during one week's

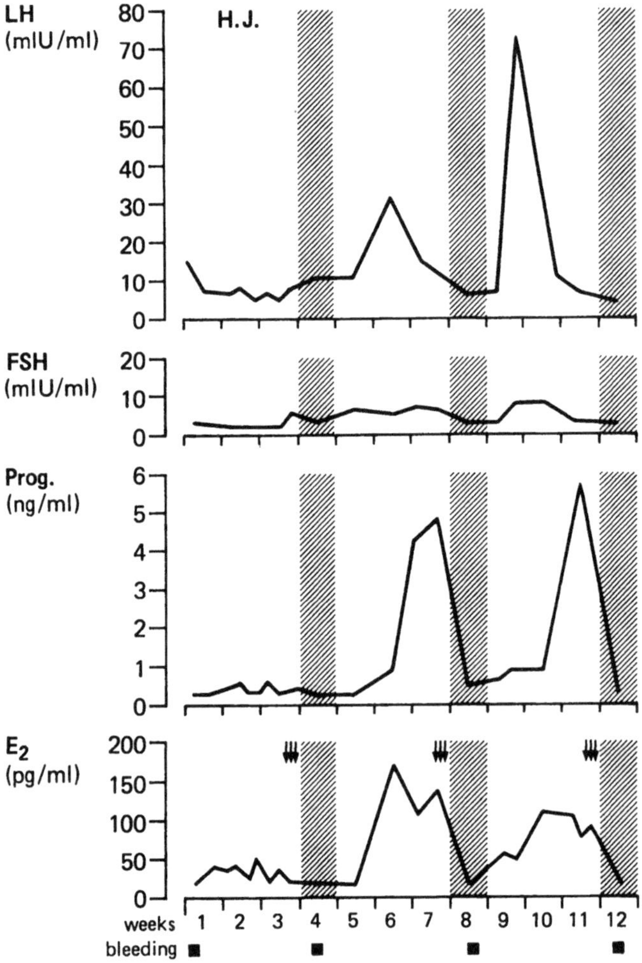

Fig. 9 Discontinuous treatment with 400 mcg Buserelin with gestagen-induced bleeding (arrow = 10 mg norethisterone enanthate). Normal withdrawal bleedings.

break. To ensure regular menstruation during the treatment breaks, the discontinuous LH-RH medication was combined with a short-term gestagen therapy (20th–22nd day). The results of the clinical tests with 21 volunteers over 101 months of treatment show this approach to be feasible [5].

At doses of 400 mcg, the contraceptive effect was maintained in spite of the week's break. In contrast to the continuous treatment (33% regular bleeding) the discontinuous medication, with additional gestagen therapy, produced a regular bleeding pattern in the majority of women (80% of the volunteers, fig. 9). In 20% of the group, however, early ovarian suppression occurred in spite of discontinuous treat-

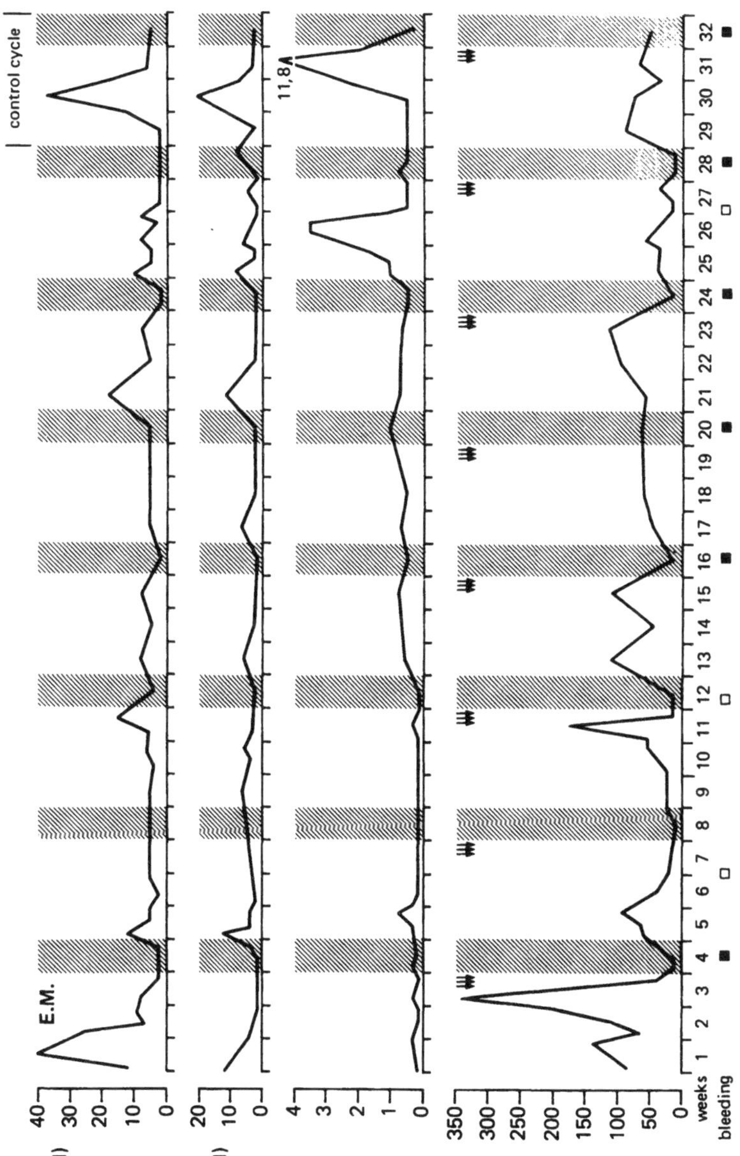

Fig. 10 Discontinuous treatment with 400 mcg Buserelin with gestagen-induced bleeding (arrow = 10 mg norethisterone enanthate). Occurrence of irregular bleeding.

ment, resulting in intermittent bleeding, with or without menstruation in the break, or amenorrhea (fig. 10). Biopsies revealed that the degree of endometrium proliferation was insufficient to allow induction of menstruation by gestagen treatment. In the majority of women, however, hormone levels and biopsies before, during and after menstruation showed cyclic estrogen secretion as well as proliferation, transformation and desquamation of the endometrium in accordance with the findings expected during a normal cycle (tab. 3).

Table 3 Morphological findings of the endometrium during the discontinuous treatment with Buserelin with gestagen-induced bleeding

Time of endometrial biopsy	Morphological finding	N
before gestagen treatment	moderate proliferation	5
	early secretory transformation	1
after gestagen treatment (during pause)	secretory transformation with desquamation	13
after withdrawal bleeding	early proliferation	8

Thus the risk of uninhibited estrogen influence on the endometrium appears to be avoidable by combination of the LH-RH treatment with gestagen therapy which produces menstruation.

Discontinuous medication thus appears to represent a practicable fertility control procedure. This is currently being tested for its clinical usefulness in a multi-center study.

Ablative Endocrine Therapy

Ablative endocrine therapy in the cause of benign or malignant hormone-dependent disorders, can lead to an improvement in the condition by interruption of the gonad function. The conventional procedures, such as operative or radiogenic castration are definitive and should only be carried out when the hormone sensitivity of malignant disorders has been established with certainty. In order to determine this dependance, as well as for the treatment of benign conditions, such as endometriosis or precocious puberty, reversible procedures for gonad suppression are desirable. High doses of sexual steroids are only of limited acceptability in view of their not inconsiderable side effects.

With high doses of the LH-RH agonist Buserelin (800–1200 mcg/day), intranasally administered, steroidogenesis in both men and women can be suppressed for prolonged periods [1, 6]. The measured testosterone or estradiol values correspond to these found after surgical gonadectomy (fig. 11).

The time required for complete pharmacological castration in women is longer than that in men, or at least unpredictable within certain limits (2–12 weeks). After termination of treatment, the gonad function reverts to normal within a short time (2–8 weeks) (fig. 11).

Our experience so far with the LH-RH agonist Buserelin is that the suppression of testosterone secretion in men with metastasizing prostate carcinomas can be maintained as long as required. The degree of remission achieved by this pharmacological castration corresponds to that obtained by definitive surgical castration [1]. Above all, the possibility of testing the hormone dependence of the tumor before performing irreversible surgical castration, as well as the therapeutic possibilities of this psycho-

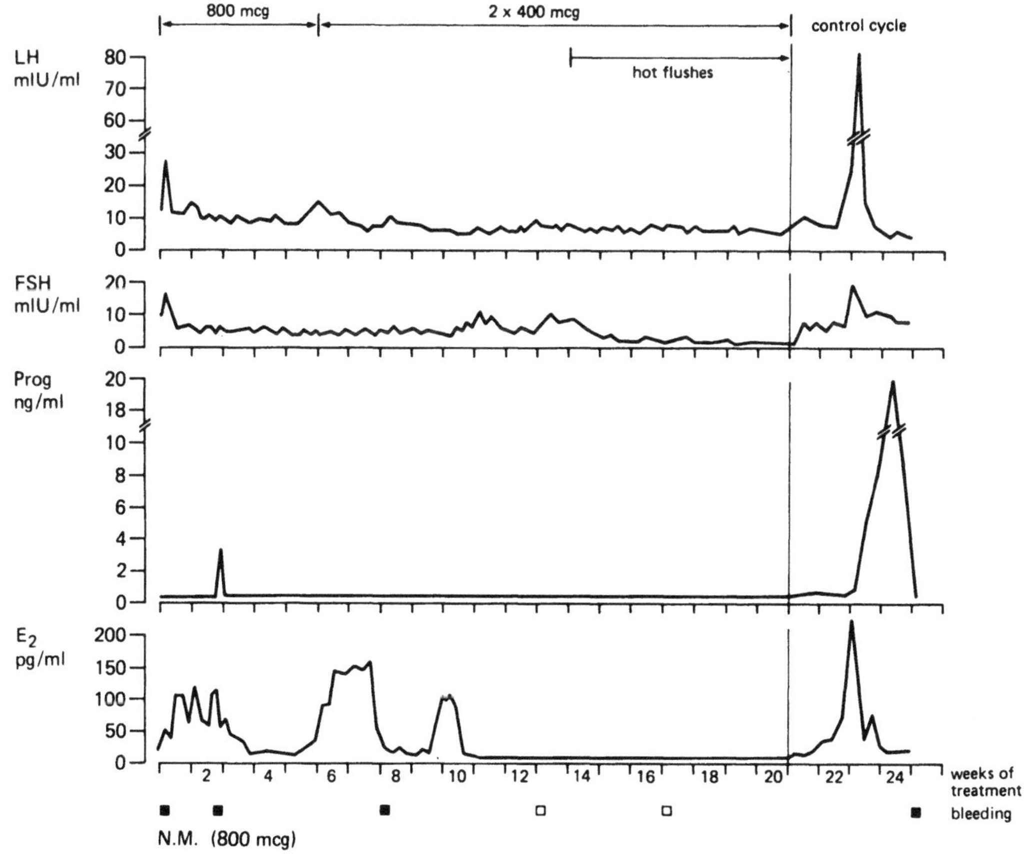

Fig. 11 Reversible pharmacological castration with 800 mcg Buserelin. Normal reproductive function after cessation of therapy.

logically less distressing procedure, have substantially extended the scope of treatment for this disorder.

Decisive advantages have been gained in the treatment of endometriosis. It is now possible to suppress completely ovarian steroidogenesis without any of the side effects normally associated with use of the related sexual steroids. Even though operative treatment provides the only final cure for endometriosis, a primary conservative attempt at treatment with drugs is both desirable and reasonable, particularly for younger women who wish to have children. This reversible pharmacological castration, which we have been able to demonstrate for the first time, is clearly superior to other drug treatments so far available in view of the high efficiency, reversibility and the absence of side effects, and is expected to become the method of choice within the foreseeable future [6].

In conclusion, the development of the LH-RH agonists have given rise to partly unexpected therapeutical possibilities for influencing the gonad function. They can be used for fertility control and for ablative endocrine therapy of hormone dependent disorders. In view of their specific pituitary point of attack, the rapid reversibility of its effects and non-interference with metabolic processes, these drugs are likely to take an important place in the future as an interdisciplinary therapeutic tool.

References

[1] Borgmann, V., W. Hardt, M. Schmidt-Gollwitzer et al.: Lancet **1083** (1982) 1097–1099.
[2] Casper, R. F., S. C. C. Yen: Science **205** (1979) 408–410.
[3] Dericks-Tan, J. S. E., E. Hammer, H.-D. Taubert: J. Clin. Endocrinol. Metab. **45** (1977) 597–599.
[4] Hardt, W., M. Schmidt-Gollwitzer, M. von der Ohe et al.: Geburtsh. Frauenheilkunde **421** (1981) 791–796.
[5] Hardt, W., K. Schmidt-Gollwitzer, J. Nevinny-Stickel et al.: Geburtsh. Frauenheilk. **42** (1982) 874–877.
[6] Hardt, W., M. Schmidt-Gollwitzer: Clin. Endocrinol. **19** (1983) 613–617.
[7] Knobil, E.: Recent Progr. Horm. Res. **36** (1980) 53–88.
[8] Lemay, A., F. Labrie, A. Belanger et al.: Fertil. Steril. **32** (1979) 646–651.
[9] Sandow, J., W. von Rechenberg, G. Jerzabek et al.: Fertil. Steril **30** (1978) 205–212.
[10] Schmidt-Gollwitzer, K., W. Hardt, G. Rebholz et al.: Acta Endocrinol. Suppl. **225** (1979) 357.
[11] Schmidt-Gollwitzer, M., W. Hardt, K. Schmidt-Gollwitzer et al.: Contraception **23** (1981) 187–196.

Contraceptive use of LH-RH agonists

S. J. Nillius

Introduction

Anti-fertility properties of the luteinizing hormone-releasing hormone (LH-RH) agonist D-Ser(TBU)^6-EA^{10}-LH-RH (Hoe 766, Hoechst AG) were found during clinical trials with this analogue for induction of ovulation. In acute studies in women with amenorrhea the LH-RH agonist proved to be highly potent and long-acting [1]. However, during chronic administration of the superagonist the stimulatory effect on the gonadotropin secretion and gonadal function decreased [2]. It was not possible to induce full follicular maturation and ovulation in amenorrheic women by daily subcutaneous (s.c.) administration of the LH-RH agonist [3]. These observations initiated contraceptive studies with the superagonist in regularly menstruating women.

A review of our clinical trials with D-Ser(TBU)^6-EA^{10}-LH-RH (LRH-Ag) for inhibition of ovulation, induction of inadequate luteal function, luteolysis and early abortion in women is given in this paper.

Inhibition of ovulation

Daily s.c. administration of 5 µg of the LRH-Ag was shown to inhibit ovulation in regularly menstruating women [4]. This is illustrated by figure 1, which shows results of 84 days of s.c. LRH-Ag treatment resulting in complete inhibition of ovulation. Three anovulatory bleedings occurred during this time, indicating that follicular growth with estrogen secretion took place. During the following days of daily intranasal treatment with 174 µg of LRH-Ag the menstrual-like bleedings were preceeded by slightly elevated serum progesterone levels. Luteinization of follicles or inadequate luteal phases occurred with the intranasal treatment during the first three cycles followed by two presumptively ovulatory cycles [5].

The intranasal route of administration proved to be practical for further exploration of this new approach to birth control. Daily doses of between 87–600 µg administered by a nasal spray were given to 39 healthy women to study the effect on ovulation. The results suggested that a daily intranasal dose of at least 400 µg had to be administered for reliable inhibition of ovulation [6]. The first contraceptive study with intranasal superagonist in 27 regularly menstruating women showed that daily

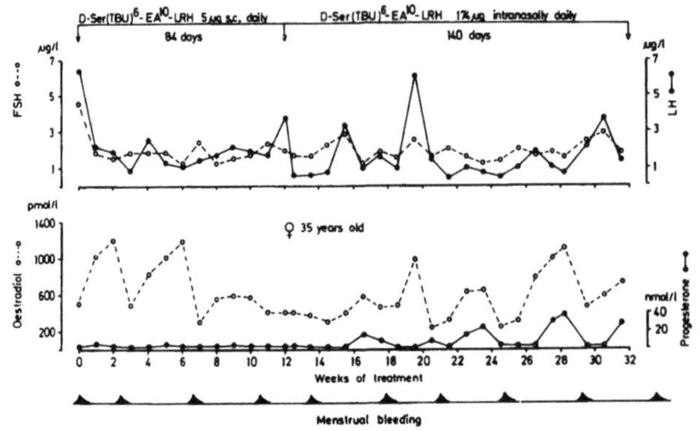

Fig. 1 Serum levels of follicle-stimulating hormone (FSH), lutenizing hormone (LH), estradiol and progesterone during daily s. c. LRH-Ag therapy followed by daily intranasal treatment of a 35-year-old healthy woman. Ovulation was inhibited by the s. c. dose of 5 µg of LRH-Ag, while the daily intranasal dose of 174 µg proved insufficient for complete suppression of ovulation, as shown by the reappearance of cyclical progesterone secretion during treatment. (Reproduced from Nillius et al. [5], with permission.)

Intranasal dose (µg)	Subjects (no)	Treatment months (no)	Anovulatory treatment months (no)
200	10	149	149
400	37	290	288
600	24	125	124
Total	71	564	561

Fig. 2 A summary of results from 71 female volunteers treated with single intranasal daily doses of 200–600 µg of the LRH-Ag for 3–21 months. (Data from Nillius and Bergquist [8].)

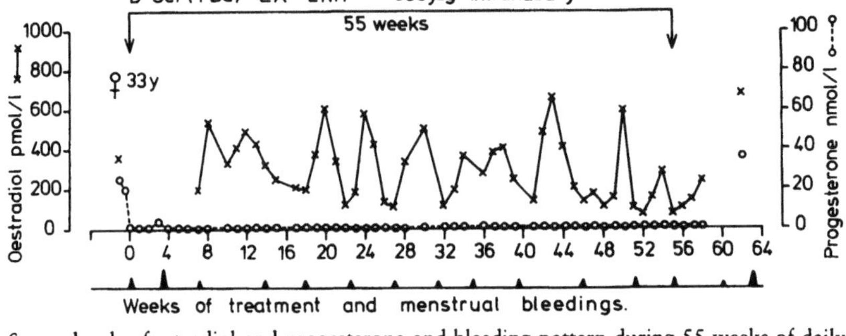

Fig. 3 Serum levels of estradiol and progesterone and bleeding pattern during 55 weeks of daily treatment with 600 µg LRH-Ag intranasally in a 33-year-old volunteer. Estradiol x——x; progesterone O- - - -O. (Reproduced from Bergquist et al. [10], with permission).

doses of 400 or 600 μg given over 3–6 months provided safe and effective birth control by inhibiting normal ovulation in all but 2 of 89 treatment months [7].

The contraceptive effectiveness of daily intranasal LRH-Ag treatment was confirmed during 564 treatment months in 71 female volunteers (fig. 2). Only 3 normal ovulatory menstrual cycles occurred at the initiation of the treatment with the first nasal spray, which was technically deficient. Twenty-seven women received 400 μg and 24 women 600 μg LRH-Ag daily by this nasal spray [9]. An improved, more efficient nasal spray was later developed by Hoechst (Frankfurt/Main). Ten women received 200 μg and another then 400 μg LRH-Ag daily, administered by the new nasal spray. Normal ovulatory cycles were not observed in any of these women. No pregnancies occurred.

The bleeding pattern during treatment of the first group of 51 volunteers varied. Fairly regular cyclical uterine bleedings occurred in 18 women, 23 women had oligomenorrhea and the remaining 10 women developed amenorrhea during the treatment. The total bleeding index, i.e. the number of bleeding episodes per month, was 0.44 [9]. No serious bleeding disturbances occurred during the prolonged LRH-Ag therapy. Three volunteers reported spottings of 10–20 days duration during the first three months of treatment. Dysfunctional uterine bleeding, i.e. prolonged and heavy bleeding, did not occur [9].

Estradiol and progesterone patterns during 55 weeks of daily intranasal LRH-Ag therapy of a woman with regular cyclical uterine bleedings during the treatment are shown in figure 3. Ovulation was consistently inhibited, as shown by the low serum progesterone levels throughout the treatment. Follicular growth and maturation occurred, as evidenced by the cyclical estrogen secretion reaching low normal preovulatory serum estradiol levels. Twelve menstrual-like bleedings occurred during the more than year-long treatment.

Amenorrhea developed in about 20% of the volunteers. A 55-week treatment course resulting in amenorrhea is illustrated in figure 4. Follicular maturation and ovulation were suppressed throughout the prolonged treatment. The serum estradiol level fluctuated within the normal early follicular phase range. A menstrual bleeding preceded by normal ovulation occurred 35 days after the long-term treatment.

Return of ovulation after cessation of prolonged treatment was remarkably rapid (figs. 3 and 4). Ovulatory menstrual bleedings in the first group of 51 volunteers occurred after 33 days, on average (median). The 10 women with amenorrhea during treatment had their first ovulatory bleeding somewhat later (46.8 days) than the 41 women with uterine bleedings during treatment (32,8 days, $p < 0.01$). Five women who subsequently wanted to become pregnant had no difficulties in conceiveing [9].

The rapid resumption of ovulation after discontinuation of a more than two-year-long LRH-Ag therapy of a woman with amenorrhea throughout the prolonged treat-

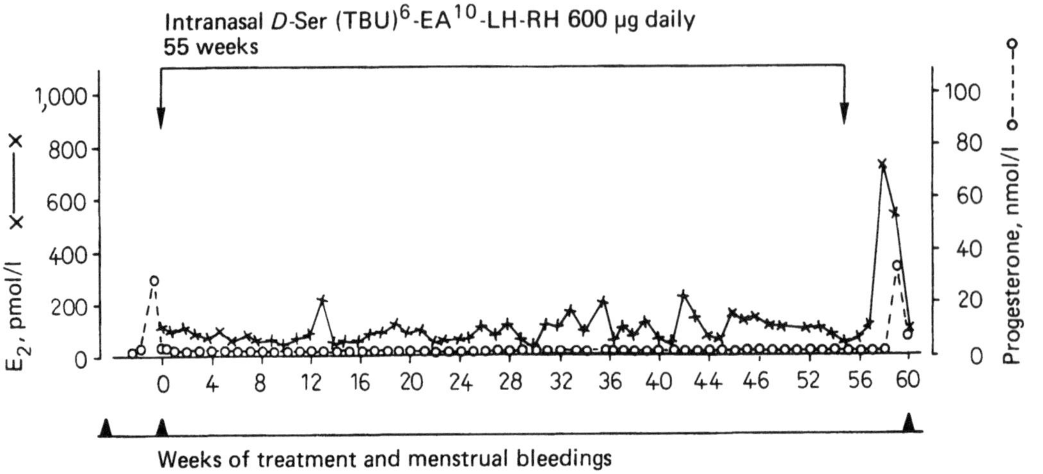

Fig. 4 Serum levels of estradiol (E_2) and progesterone during 55 weeks of daily LRH treatment with 600 µg LRH-Ag intranasally in a 23-year-old volunteer with amenorrhea during treatment. (From Bergquist, C. et al.: Long-term intranasal luteinizing hormone-releasing hormone agonist treatment for contraception in women. Fertil. Steril. 38:190, 1982 [9]. Reproduced by permission of the publisher, The American Fertility Society, Birmingham, Alabama.)

ment is illustrated in figure 5. Follicular maturation and ovulation was completely inhibited by the daily intranasal treatment. The serum estradiol level remained in the normal early follicular phase range. No clinical symptoms or signs of estrogen deficiency occurred.

No side effects except the bleeding disturbances caused by the induced anovulation (see above) were observed. The bleeding irregularities and amenorrhea were well accepted by all volunteers. However, they may be a drawback to this contraceptive method in developing countries. No signs of hyperplastic changes were noted in 50 endometrial biopsy specimens [12 and unpublished results]. The predominant histologic picture was one of inactive or weak proliferative glands with slightly atrophic stroma.

A major advantage of using chronic LH-RH agonist therapy instead of steroid treatment for inhibition of ovulation is the fact that the LH-RH analogues have specific actions on the hypothalamic-pituitary-gonadal system and lack systemic effects. They are therefore not likely to cause metabolic derangements and other generalized adverse effects.

It has been suggested by Schmidt-Gollwitzer et al. [13] and others [14, 15] that intranasal LRH-AG treatment should be combined with oral progestogen therapy to ensure better cycle control and prevent possible untoward effects on the endometrium by the unopposed estrogen secretion. The results from these studies are too preliminary to draw any definitive conclusion. The cycle may be more regular but the

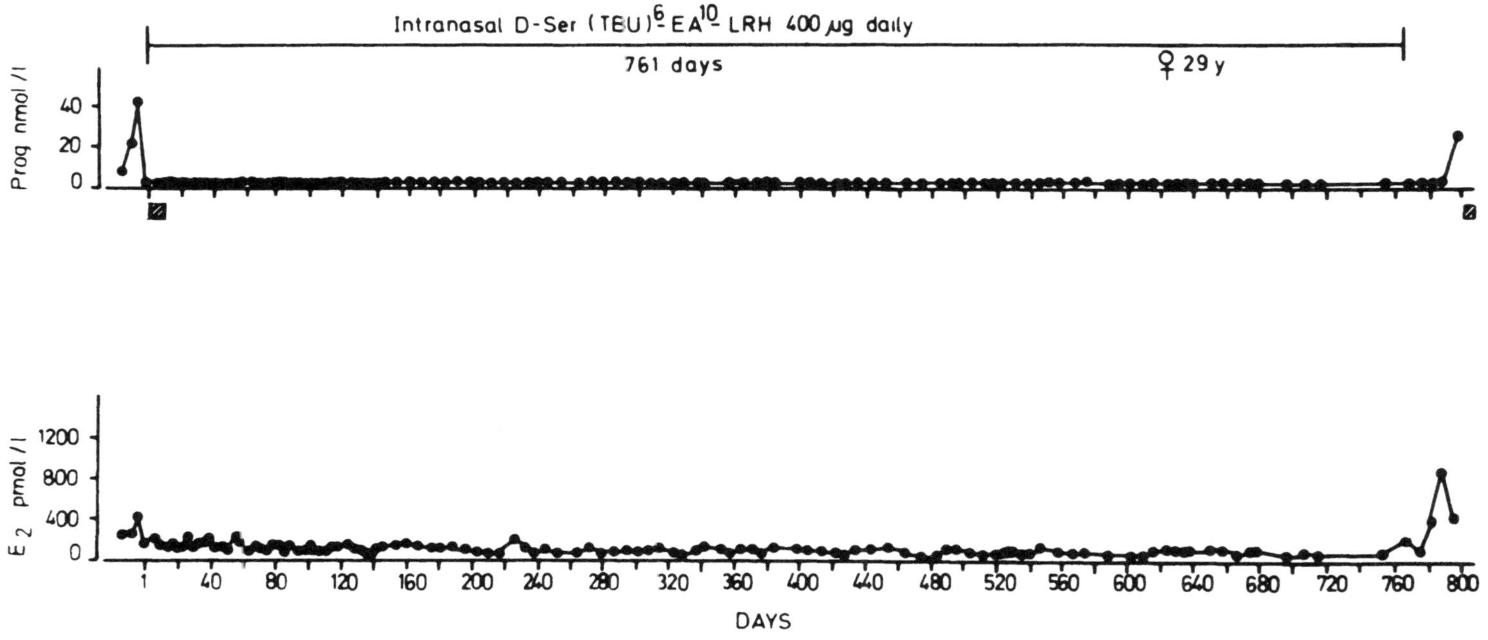

Fig. 5 Serum levels of progesterone (top) and estradiol (below) during 761 days of daily therapy with 400 µg of LRH-Ag intranasally in a 29-year-old volunteer with amenorrhea throughout treatment. ■ Menstrual bleeding. (Reproduced from Bergquist et al. [11], with permission.)

addition of progestogen causes new side effects, which made two of ten volunteers in our pilot study discontinue the combined treatment (Bergquist et al., unpublished observations). The average estrogen secretion seems to be more marked during interrupted combined LRH-Ag-progestogen regimens. The progestogen doses added are often lower than the doses recommended in textbooks for complete secretory transformation of the endometrium. It is in this connection important to remember that the sequential oral contraceptives afford less protection against adenocarcinoma of the endometrium than the combined oral contraceptives [16].

During continuous LRH-Ag treatment there is a significant reduction in the mean estradiol levels during the course of long-term therapy [9, 17]. The estradiol levels and the bleeding pattern agree with the histologic picture of inactive or weak proliferative endometrium. We did not observe marked hyperproliferative activity. Early signs of hyperplastic changes were noted by another group of investigators [17]. However, the finding decreased as treatment progressed. Recently, anti-steroidal effects of an LH-RH agonist have been described in the rat [18]. Another superagonist has been found to diminish the estradiol binding sites both in intact and ovariectomized-hypophysectomized rats [19]. Such actions might explain the inactive or weak proliferative activity of the endometrium in spite of low-normal serum estrogen levels in woman on chronic LH-RH agonist therapy for inhibition of ovulation.

It seem too early to abandon the continous intranasal treatment with only LRH-Ag for inhibition of ovulation and contraception in women. Further studies with careful monitoring of effects on the bleeding and endometrial patterns are clearly warranted. At present the clinical data are insufficient to decide if therapy with LRH-Ag alone or LRH-Ag and progestogen is the treatment of choice.

To sum up, daily intranasal LRH-Ag administration is a practical and acceptable new method of birth control which has proved to provide safe, effective and rapidly reversible contraception in women. If adequate doses are given, normal ovulatory cycles do not occur during the treatment due to LRH-Ag induced desentiziation of the pituitary processes responsible for gonadotropin release [8]. Ovulation and fertility are rapidly regained after cessation of prolonged treatment.

Induction of inadequate luteal function

Normal follicular growth and maturation are prerequisites for adequate corpus luteum function. In an attempt to disrupt the normal gonadotropin secretory pattern and disturb early follicular growth, we administered 5–25 μg of the LRH-Ag for 1–5 consecutive days in the very early follicular phase of the menstrual cycle. During the treatment cycles of the 12 volunteers, the luteal phase did not differ in length or progesterone concentrations from those of the control cycles However, the highest doses resulted in a marked desensitization of the pituitary gonadotropin secretion (fig. 6) followed by a prolongation of the follicular phase [20]. These results are in contrast to those of another group of investigators [21] who administered 50 μg of the superagonist D-Trp^{6}-EA^{10}-LRH s.c. daily during the first three days of the menstrual cycle. The results were a prolongation of the follicular phase, a sustained decrease in serum FSH, a reduced preovulatory rise of estradiol and a smaller midcycle surge of LH than normal. Five of their volunteers also developed short or inadequate luteal phases. Thus, this potential approach to peptide contraception has to be further studied to resolve the discrepancy between the results of the two trials.

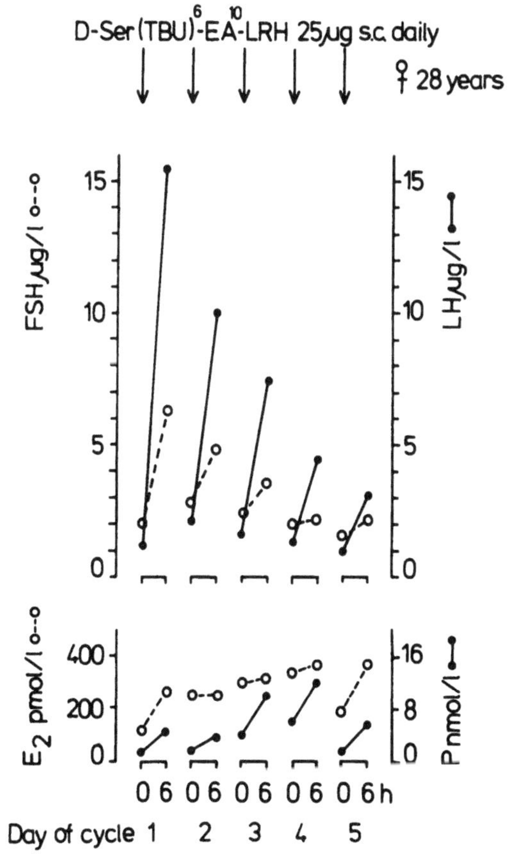

Fig. 6 Pituitary desensitization in a 28-year-old normal woman, illustrated by decreasing gonadotropin responses to the LRH-Ag during 5 days of s. c. treatment with 25 μg LRH-Ag daily during the early follicular phase of the menstrual cycle. (Reproduced from Skarin et al. [20]; with permission.)

Induction of luteolysis

Administration of LRH agonists on each of two consecutive days during the mid-luteal phase of the menstrual cycle can induce luteolysis in women with early decline of the serum progesterone level and premature onset of menstruation (fig. 7) [22, 23, 24]. None of the volunteers in the luteolytic studies were exposed to the risk of pregnancy. The critical time or "window" for luteolysis to occur is narrow [25, 26]. Successful luteolysis was induced in 26 of 27 cycles (96%) when the superagonist D-Trp^6-EA^{10}-LRH (50 µg s.c. once or twice) was administered on or after day 5 after the LH peak. However, when treatment began within 5 days of the LH peak, the agonist failed to induce luteolysis in 10 of 13 cycles [25]. Thus, a serious drawback to the luteolytic approach to peptide contraception is the fact that the timing of the LRH agonist administration is so critical for its effectiveness.

Furthermore, exogenous human chorionic gonadotropin (HCG) prevents the luteolytic effect of the superagonists [24, 27] (fig. 7). Concomitant administration of superagonists and HCG not only prevents luteolysis but stimulates the progesterone secretion and prolongs the luteal phase of the treatment cycle. It is doubtful that LH-RH agonists can be useful as post-ovulatory luteolytic agents in women.

Induction of early abortion

The possible abortifacient effects of potent LH-RH agonists were studied in early human pregnancy [28]. Repeated doses of the LRH-Ag were administered intravenously (i.v.) for 4 days to volunteers requesting legal abortion. The LRH-Ag treatment did not induce any changes in the estradiol or progesterone levels in comparison with the serum levels observed during normal early human pregnancy. The HCG levels in serum continued to rise during and following the treatment and the pregnancies were terminated by suction curettage. The histopathological investigation of the uterine contents revealed normal pregnancy tissue. Failure to interrupt early human pregnancy is illustrated in figure 8, which shows hormone results from a volunteer in early pregnancy (46 days after the last menstrual period) given the huge i.v. dose of 1500 µg or LRH-Ag. Two other clinical trials have been performed in women in early pregnancy in attempts to induce abortion [27, 29]. None of these studies, performed with different superactive long-acting LRH agonists, has been successful. Thus, the luteolytic effect caused by superagonists in the non-pregnant luteal phase of the human menstrual cycle is clearly prevented by endogenous HCG secreted during early pregnancy.

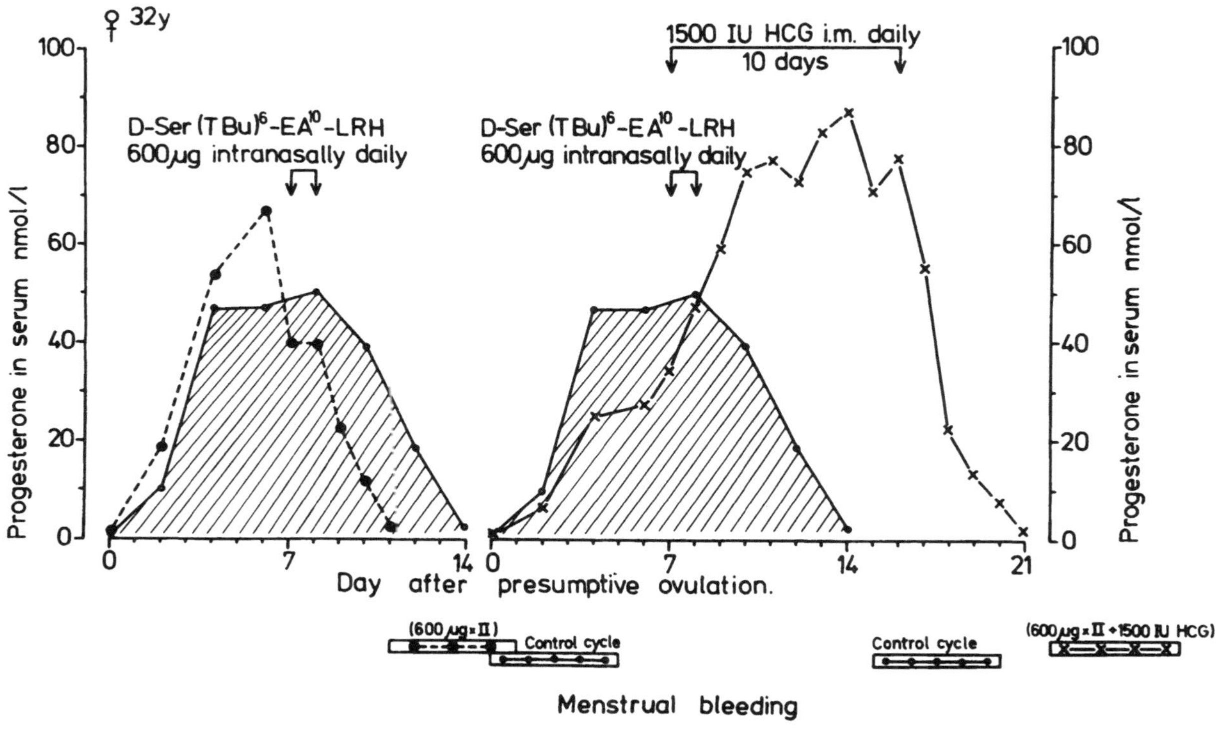

Fig. 7 Serum progesterone levels and length of the luteal phases during one control cycle (shaded area) and two treatment cycles with the LRH-Ag only (left) and the LRH-Ag plus HCG (right). (Data from Bergquist et al. [24].).

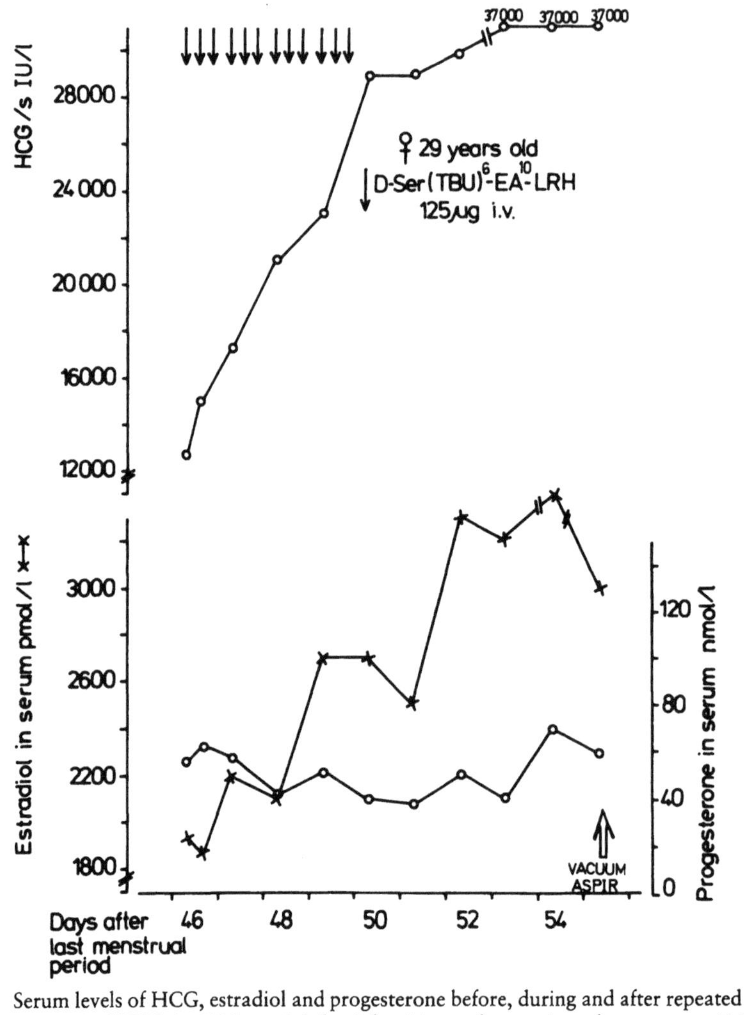

Fig. 8 Serum levels of HCG, estradiol and progesterone before, during and after repeated i. v. injections (arrows) of LRH-Ag (125 µg t.i.d. for 4 days) in a volunteer in early pregnancy (46 days after the last menstural period). (Reproduced from Skarin et al. [28], with permission.)

Summary

New approaches to female contraception based on the hypothalamic gonadotropin-releasing hormone have been proposed during recent years. They are paradoxically based on stimulatory rather than inhibitory analogues of LH-RH. Chronic administration of superactive LH-RH agonists leads to desensitization of the pituitary processes responsible for gonadotropin secretion. Luteolytic approaches to peptide contraception have been studied. However, the results are not very promising. The contraceptive effectiveness of such approaches has not been demonstrated. The luteolytic effect of present superagonists is prevented by exogenous and endogenous HCG. Whether LH-RH agonists can cause irreversible infertility by inducing corpus luteum insufficiency remains to be proven. Human ovulation can effectively be reversibly inhibited for long periods of time by continous intranasal LH-RH agonist therapy. This method of birth control has already been shown to provide safe, effective and acceptable contraception in women. Further clinical trials of this new lead to contraception are clarly warranted.

Acknowledgements

The author wishes to express his sincere gratitude to Hoechst AG, Frankfurt/Main, FRG, for generous supply of the LH-RH agonist and to Mrs. Karin Mattson for skilful technical assistance. The studies were supported by the international Committee for Contraception Research of the Population Council and the Swedish Medical Research Council (Grant No 13X-3145). The financial support provided to the former organization by the International Development Research Centre of Canada, The Ford Foundation, The Rockefeller Foundation and the Geo. J. Hecht Fund is gratefully acknowledged.

References

[1] Nillius, S. J., L. Wide: Ups. J. Med. Sci. **82** (1977) 21–26.
[2] Nillius, S. J., L. Wide: Acta Endocrinol. (Kbh.) Suppl. **212** (1977) 138.
[3] Skarin, G., S. J. Nillius, L. Wide: Ups. J. Med. Sci. **85** (1980) 103–112.
[4] Nillius, S. J., C. Bergquist, L. Wide: Contraception **17** (1978) 538–545.
[5] Nillius, S. J., C. Bergquist, L. Wide: Int. J. Fertil. **25** (1980) 239–246.
[6] Bergquist, C., S. J. Nillius, L. Wide: Contraception **19** (1979) 497–506.
[7] Bergquist, C., S. J. Nillius, L. Wide: Lancet **II** (1979) 215–217.
[8] Nillius, S. J., C. Bergquist: In "LH-RH and Its Analogs: Contraception and Therapeutic Applications" (Eds. B. H. Vickery, J. J. Nestor Jr., E. S. E. Hafez). MTP Press Limited, Lancaster 1983, in press.
[9] Bergquist, C., S. J. Nillius, L. Wide: Fertil. Steril. **38** (1982) 190–193.
[10] Bergquist, C., S. J. Nillius, L. Wide: Clin. Endocrinol. **16** (1972) 147–151.
[11] Bergquist, C., S. J. Nillius, L. Wide: Ups. J. Med. Sci. (1984), in press.
[12] Bergquist, C., S. J. Nillius, L. Wide et al.: Fertil. Steril. **36** (1981) 339–342.
[13] Schmidt-Gollwitzer, M. et al.: This book (1984).
[14] Lemay, A., N. Faure, F. Labrie et al.: Acta Endocrinol. (Kbh) Suppl. **250** (1983) 85.
[15] Kuhl, H., C. Jung, H.-D. Taubert: Acta Endocrinol. (Kbh) Suppl. **250** (1983) 76.
[16] Don Gambrell, R., C. Bagnell, R. Greenblatt: Review. Am. J. Obstet. Gynecol. **146** (1983) 696–707.
[17] Schmidt-Gollwitzer, M., W. Hardt, K. Schmidt-Gollwitzer et al.: Contraception **23** (1981) 187–195.

[18] Sundaram, K., Y.-Q. Cao, N.-G. Wang et al.: Life Sciences **28** (1981) 83–88.
[19] Pedroza, E., J. A. Vilchez-Martinez, D. H. Coy et al.: Biochem. Biophys. Res. Commun. **95** (1980) 1056–1062.
[20] Skarin, G., S. J. Nillius, L. Wide: Contraception **25** (1982) 31–39.
[21] Sheehan, K. L., R. F. Casper, S. S. C. Yen: Science **215** (1982) 170–172.
[22] Lemay, A., F. Labrie, A. Belanger et al.: Fertil. Steril. **32** (1979) 646–651.
[23] Casper, R. F., S. S. C. Yen: Science **205** (1979) 408–410.
[24] Bergquist, C., S. J. Nillius, L. Wide: Contraception **22** (1980) 341–347.
[25] Sheehan, K. L., R. F. Casper, S. S. C. Yen: Fertil. Steril. **37** (1982) 209–212.
[26] Lemay, A., N. Fare, F. Labrie et al.: Fertil. Steril. **39** (1983) 661.
[27] Casper, R. F., K. L. Sheehan, S. S. C. Yen: Contraception **21** (1980) 471–478.
[28] Skarin, G., S. J. Nillius, L. Wide: Contraception **26** (1982) 457–463.
[29] Tolis, G., A. M. Comaru-Schally, A. E. Mehta et al.: Fertil. Steril. **36** (1981) 241–242.

LH-RH analogs and luteal function of the rhesus monkey

J. P. Balmaceda, R. H. Asch

Introduction

The corpus luteum plays an important role in the reproductive function of primates, including the human. Inadequate luteal function is cited as the cause in a significant proportion of infertility cases and early pregnancy loss [1, 2]. Controlled modification of the luteal phase may also have important contraceptive applications.

It is well established that abnormal gonadotropin secretion patterns during the follicular phase can produce an insufficiency of the corpus luteum expressed in decreased progesterone (P) levels and a shortened life span. Specifically, decreased levels of follicle stimulating hormone (FSH) and of the FSH:LH (luteinizing hormone) ratio during the follicular phase are associated with lower P secretion in monkeys [3] and women [4]. In addition, studies in rhesus monkeys have demonstrated that suppression of FSH secretion in the early follicular phase can induce an abnormal luteal phase [5].

However, the factors that determine luteal function after ovulation are still the subject of controversy. Opinions differ on the relative importance of ovulatory gonadotropin levels versus local mechanisms involving estrogen and prostaglandin (PG) production by the corpus luteum.

The corpus luteum responds to exogenously administered human chorionic gonadotropin (hCG) or LH by increasing P secretion [6], and the use of antigonadotropic antiserum injected during the luteal phase has been reported to lower peripheral serum P levels and to shorten the corpus luteum life span [7]. On the other hand, recent studies have shown normal luteal phases in monkeys hypophysectomized after ovulation [8]. In addition, estrogen administered to rhesus monkeys can induce luteolysis without changing LH serum concentrations [9], and functional luteolysis is associated with local changes that include increasing concentrations of estradiol and PGF:PGE ratios in the aging corpus luteum. Moreover, hCG stimulation of P production is correlated with a reversal of the changes of PG production ratios [10].

In this chapter we present work done in our laboratories utilizing LH-RH analogs to study the variables that control luteal function in the rhesus monkey in search for possible clinical applications.

The primate model

The studies presented in this paper were performed using rhesus monkeys *(Macaca mulatta)*. In the past, we have accumulated experience in handling these animals and have become familiarized with their reproductive cycle. The rhesus monkey's menstrual cycle is of approximately the same length as that of the human female. The follicular and luteal phases are also of approximately the same duration as in humans. Finally, the temporal relation of gonadotropin and steroid peaks with ovulation, as well as the endocrine relationship between hypothalamus, hypophysis and ovaries, presents no significant differences from those described in women.

With the combined use of peripheral estrogen measurements and serial laparoscopy, we can determine the time of ovulation with an accuracy of ±12 h without interfering with the cycle. Surgical procedures performed on the genital tract of these animals were done using microsurgical techniques to minimize tissue damage, avoiding interference with the cycle and the formation of significant adhesions.

LH-RH agonists and the luteal function of the rhesus monkey

Administration of [D-Trp^6]-LH-RH during the luteal phase

The first experiment of the series was designed to evaluate the effect of a single dose of a potent LH-RH agonist, [D-Trp^6]-LH-RH, (10 μg) administered on different days of the luteal phase [11]. Animals received the agonist on post-ovulatory day 3, 5 or 7. Initiation of menses was determined by daily vaginal smears. Daily blood samples were obtained to determine levels of estradiol, P and LH. A significant shortening of the length of the luteal phase, as compared with the average for our colony, occurred in all animals injected on day 3 and in 4 of the 5 animals injected on day 5. No changes were detected on animals injected on day 7 (tab. 1).

In the second experiment, we studied the effect of hCG administration in two groups of animals injected with [D-Trp^6]-LH-RH during the luteal phase. Three animals received a single dose of 10 μg of the agonist on day 5 after ovulation, followed by daily injections of hCG from day 6 to 10 in increasing dosages (day 6 = 30 IU, day 7 = 60 IU, day 8 = 90 IU, day 9 = 180 IU, day 10 = 360 IU). A second group of 4 animals received daily injections of 10 mg of the agonist from day 6 to day 10 after ovulation and hCG following the same schedule as the first group. Human chorionic gonadotropin administered as above produced circulation levels of the hormone very similar to those of monkey chorionic gonadotropin (mCG) observed in early pregnancy in this species [10].

The results of both experiments are summarized in table 1. The administration of hCG completely abolished the luteolytic effect of the agonist and the length of luteal

Table 1: Effects of [D-Trp^6]-LH-RH (10 μg) administration on the luteal phase length of the thesus monkey

[D-Trp^6]-LH-RH	hCG	n	Individual Animals	X ± SEM
3		4	7-7-11-8	8.2 ± 0.9*
5		5	12-8-11-7-7	9.0 ± 1.0*
7		4	14-15-12-14	13.7 ± 0.6
5	6–10	3	14-14-15	14.3 ± 0.3
6–10	6–10	4	16-15-19-15	16.0 ± 1.0
	6–10	25		15.2 ± 0.8
Untreated colony		50		15.1 ± 0.6

phase observed was comparable to that observed in our untreated colony or in animals receiving only hCG.

In vitro studies on the effect of [D-Trp^6]-LH-RH on luteal cell function

The experiments described above proved that LH-RH super agonists could induce premature luteolysis. However, the site of action remained unclear, so the following experiment was undertaken to study the possibility of a direct effect of [D-Trp^6]-LH-RH on the luteal cell.

Corpora lutea were obtained at laparotomy performed in monkeys 6 to 8 days after ovulation, and were transported to the laboratory in Ham's F10-Hepes medium. The cells were dispersed and incubated in separate tubes as described by Stouffer and collaborators [12]. Each tube contained a different concentration of [D-Trp^6]-LH-RH ranging from 1 to 100 ng/ml. Progesterone production was measured in each tube before and after hCG (50 μg/ml) was added. No difference in P concentrations was observed among the tubes containing different concentrations of the agonist or when compared to controls. Moreover, the response to hCG stimulation was also similar in all the tubes [13].

Although these results were obtained *in vitro,* they strongly suggest a lack of direct effect of the LH-RH agonist upon the luteal cells.

The effect of [D-Trp^6]-LH-RH administration on hypophysectomized rhesus monkeys

A third model utilized to study the site of action for the luteolytic effect of LH-RH agonist was hypophysectomized animals in which ovulation was induced with administration of exogenous gonadotropins. If not through a direct effect on the corpus lutem, as suggested by the results of the *in vitro* studies, the luteolytic effect of [D-Trp^6]-LH-RH could be due to the alteration of gonadotropin secretion induced by these agonists. The absence of a functioning pituitary should then nullify this effect.

The study was performed in 3 animals hypophysectomized at least 9 months before the experiment that were receiving a weekly maintenance dose of methylprednisolone acetate (8 mg/kg) intravenously. The completeness of hypophysectomy was confirmed histologically in one animal that died of acute pancreatitis and that did not have any pituitary remnants in the sella turcica. All animals were amenorrheic. Lack of circulating LH levels was proven by using the mouse interstitial cell testosterone assay for LH-hCG determinations before and after the administration of 150 μg of LH-RH.

Ovulation was induced with human menopausal gonadotropins (Pergonal, Serono Laboratories, Inc., Randolph, MA) in two separate cycles in each animal. The animals received 37.5 IU of FSH and LH daily by intramuscular injections until peripheral serum estrogens reached 350 pg/ml or more. At this time, hCG (1000 IU) was administered. Ovulation occurred 36 to 48 h after the hCG injection. During the course of the first cycle, each animal received 10 μg of [D-Trp^6]-LH-RH on days 3 and 5 of the luteal phase. As shown in figure 1, no significant drop in serum P levels was observed and the length of the luteal phase remained within the limits observed for our colony, although this same regimen had been proved to be luteolytic in intact animals. Circulating P levels reached a peak between days 6 and 7, post-ovulation, and ranged from 4.6 to 6.3 ng/ml. Administration of 10 μg [D-Trp^6]-LH-RH on days 3 and 5, post-ovulation, did not suppress the normal increase of serum progesterone concentrations that occur during the first week post-ovulatory. The length of the luteal phases in the 3 treated animals was 13, 13 and 14 days, respectively. These results were not different from luteal phase duration in untreated animals in our colony, but were significantly longer than that observed in intact animals treated with [D-Trp^6]-LH-RH on days 3 and 5, post-ovulation [13].

On the second induced ovulatory cycle, 1 mg of [D-Trp^6]-LH-RH was infused directly into the utero-ovarian artery. This vessel is responsible for more than 90% of the ovarian circulation in the nonpregnant rhesus monkey [14]. The infusion was performed using a Harvard pump connected with Silasticm tubing to a 30 gauge needle inserted into the artery. The rate of the infusion was 0.17 ml/min, and it was maintained for 1 h. Blood samples were obtained from the ovarian vein (2 ml/sample) at −30, 0, 10, 20, 30, 40, 50, 60 and 90 min relative to initiation of the infusion. Systemic blood was drawn daily from the saphenous or femoral vein. Serum was utilized to measure P by radioimmunoassay.

The results of the ovarian infusion are presented in figure 2. No changes in progesterone concentrations on the serum obtained from the ovarian vein were encountered. Also, the luteal phase length and peripheral serum concentrations of progesterone were not different from what we described above for untreated cycles.

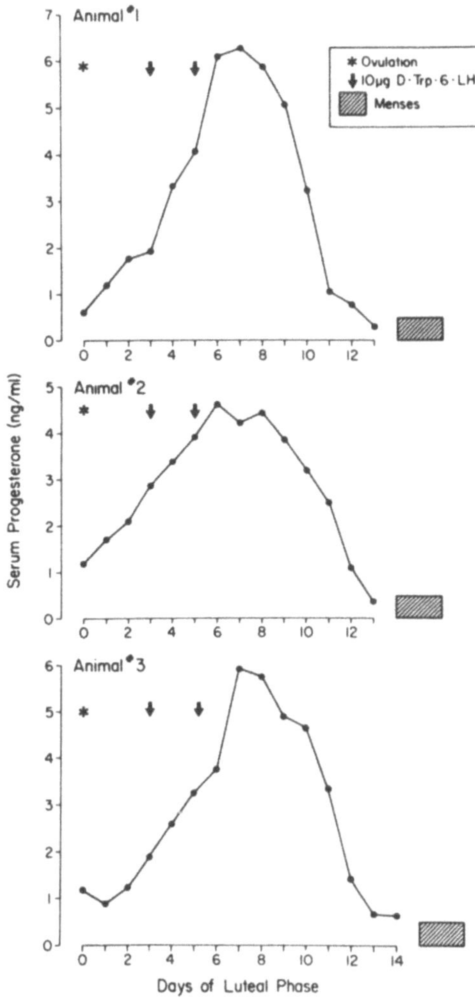

Fig. 1 Serum progesterone (P) concentrations and luteal phase lengths of induced ovulatory cycles in hypophysectomized rhesus monkeys treated with 10 µg [D-Trp[6]]-LH-RH on days 3 and 5 post-ovulation (R. H. Asch, et al.: Lack of luteolytic effect of D-Trp-LH-RH in hypophysectomized rhesus monkeys (*Macaca mulatta*) [13].).

The results of the experiments performed in hypophysectomized rhesus monkeys reinforced the information obtained by the *in vitro* experiments, strongly suggesting that luteolysis induced by the LH-RH agonist is not due to a direct effect at the gonads. The presence of a functioning pituitary appears to be essential for luteolysis to occur after the administration of [D-Trp[6]]-LH-RH.

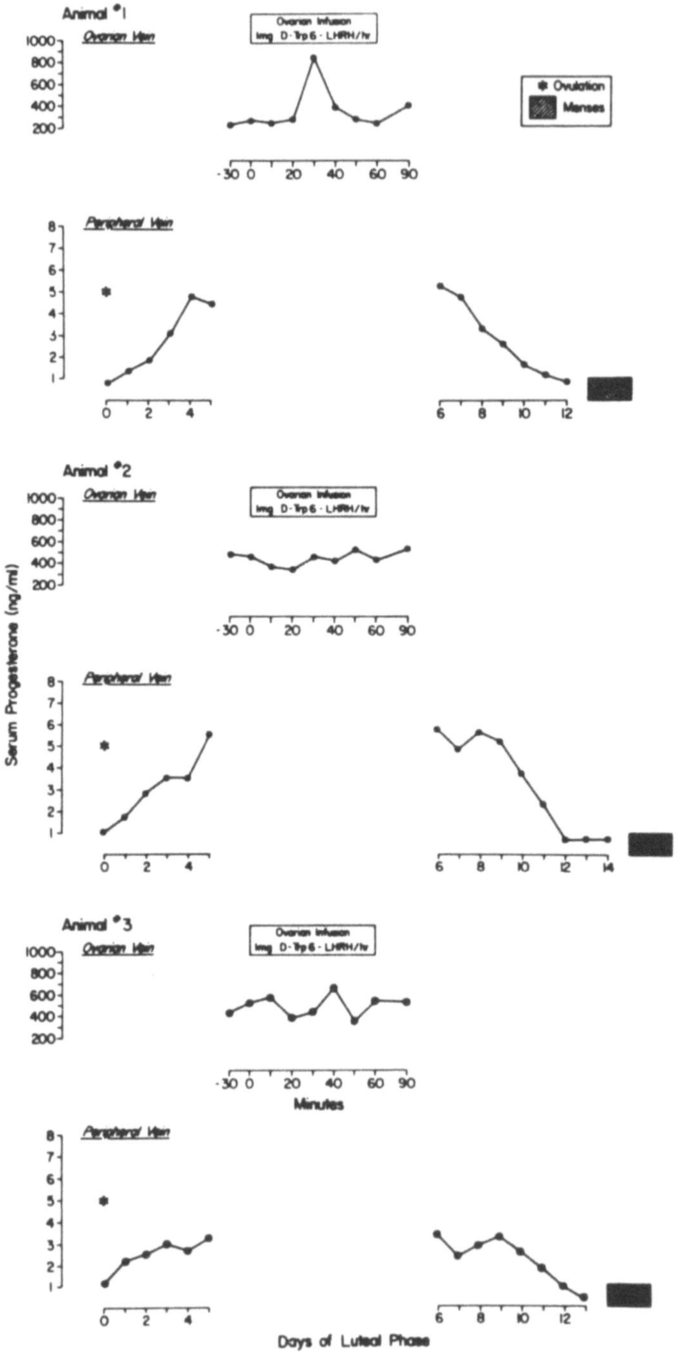

Fig. 2 Peripheral and ovarian vein progesterone (P) concentrations of induced ovulatory cycles in hypophysectomized rhesus monkeys that received an ovarian infusion of 1 mg [D-Trp^6]-LH-RH on day 5 post-ovulation [13].

Absence of LH-RH binding sites in corpora lutea of rhesus monkey

Extra pituitary binding sites for LH-RH have been described in several species. The experiment reported here was designed to determine if binding sites for the hypothalamic decapeptide were present in luteal cells of rhesus monkey [15].

Crude plasma membranes were prepared from adult male rat pituitary and rhesus monkey corpora lutea, lung, kidney, liver, and small bowel. Luteectomy was performed between days 5 and 8 after ovulation, using microsurgical techniques. The tissue obtained was used immediately for the study. The analog was radioiodinated according to the lactoperoxidase method initially described by Miyachi and coworkers [16] and modified by Marshall and Odell [17]. Bio Rad Enzymobeads® were the source of lactoperoxidase and glucose in the iodination reaction. Labeled and unlabeled analogs were separated using ion exchange chromatography on carboxymethylcellulose (fine mesh, Sigma, St. Louis, MO). Labeled analog was stored at 4° C, pH 7.5, in 0.05 M ammonium acetate. The specific activity of the ^{125}I-labeled LH-RH analog was measured by selfdisplacement in the radioreceptor assay (800–1000 μCi/ μg).

Luteectomy induced early onset of menses in all the animals. Ovarian vein concentrations of P dropped as early as 10 min after luteectomy. Peripheral concentrations of serum P were markedly diminished on the day following surgery.

Specific binding of ^{125}I D-Ala^6 LH-RH to plasma membranes of various tissues was tested. The protein concentration per tube used in binding studies was as follows: 150 μg pituitary, 90.4 μg lung, 114.2 μg kidney, 165,6 μg liver, and 97.2 μg small bowel. For rhesus monkey corpora lutea were 122.8 μg, 128,8 μg, 132 μg, and 138.5 μg, respectively.

Nonspecific binding was determined in the presence of 1000-fold excess of unlabeled analog. Rat pituitary plasma membranes specifically bound 27% of the radioiodinated analog (fig. 3). However, no specific binding of the LH-RH analog for lung, kidney, liver, small bowel, or corpora lutea from rhesus monkeys was observed.

Evidence concerning the presence or absence of LH-RH binding sites in human gonadal tissue is contradictory. Clayton and Huhtaniemi [18], utilizing a method identical to those described for rodents, did not find specific receptors for LH-RH in human corpora lutea or testis. However, Popkin et al. [19] described specific binding sites of very low affinity in human luteal cells for both native LH-RH and agonistic analogs. The differences observed in the literature may be due, in part, to methodology, and further research in this area is needed to elucidate whether LH-RH or its analogs can play any direct role in ovarian physiology.

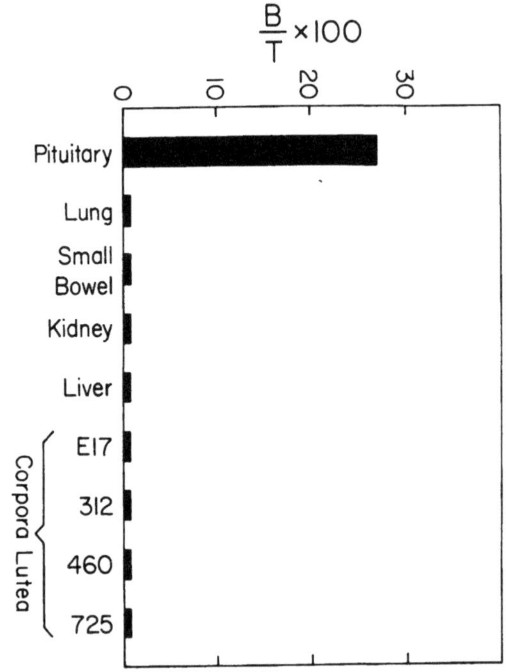

Fig. 3 Specific binding of ^{125}I D-Ala^{6}-analog to rat pituitary and corpora lutea, lung, kidney, liver, and small bowel from regularly cycling rhesus monkeys. (R. H. Asch et al.: Absence of LH-RH binding sites in corpora lutea from rhesus monkeys (*Macaca mulatta*) [15].)

5-LH-RH inhibitory analogs and luteal function

As we stated in the introduction of this chapter, the relative importance of post-ovulatory gonadotropin levels upon corpus luteum function is not entirely clear. If luteal function depends mainly on gonadotropin support, effective suppression of FSH and LH should alter progesterone production and shorten corpus luteum life span.

The following protocol was designed to study the effect of [N-Ac-D-Trp^{1,3}, D-pCl-Phe^{2},D-Phe^{6},D-Ala^{10}]-LH-RH, a potent inhibitory analog of LH-RH, administered after ovulation [20].

We used 20 regularly cycling female rhesus monkeys in this study. The protocol included two consecutive cycles. The first cycle was used for control. During the second cycle, the animals were divided into four groups for two separate experiments.

In the first experiment, group 2 (5 animals) received 1 mg of the antagonist daily by subcutaneous injection from the first day after ovulation until the onset of menses. Group 1 was the control and received daily injections of vehicle, following the same schedule. Cycle and luteal phase lengths for both groups are presented in table 2. No changes from the control to the treatment cycle were observed in any of the animals. Furthermore, no differences were detected between the animals treated with the antagonist and those treated with vehicle only. Figure 4 presents levels of LH, FSH, estradiol and P in peripheral blood. Although there was a significant decrease in circulating levels of both gonadotropins in the animals treated with the LH-RH antagonist, there was no difference in the estradiol or P levels of the two groups.

Table 2: Length of the cycle and of the luteal phase during the control and treatment cycles of the animals in experiment 1

	Animal	Length of Cycle Control	Length of Cycle Treated	Length of Luteal Phase Control	Length of Luteal Phase Treated
Group 1	1	28	29	14	15
	2	28	29	15	16
	3	31	29	15	14
	4	30	30	14	14
	5	26	27	13	15
Group 2	1	27	28	14	14
	2	28	28	14	15
	3	30	32	15	17
	4	31	30	15	16
	5	29	28	15	14

For the second experiment, the remaining two groups of animals were treated as described above. In addition, the animals received daily injections of hCG in increasing dosages from day 6 through 10 after ovulation. Again, the increase in progesterone secretion secondary to hCG stimulation was the same for both the treatment and the control group (fig. 5).

Although gonadotropin suppression was not complete, the results of these two experiments confirmed that a significant decrease of FSH and LH levels during the post-ovulation period does not affect the function of the corpus luteum. Also, animals treated with the antagonist at the dosage studied maintain intact the capacity to respond to hCG, suggesting no direct effect of the analog upon the corpus luteum.

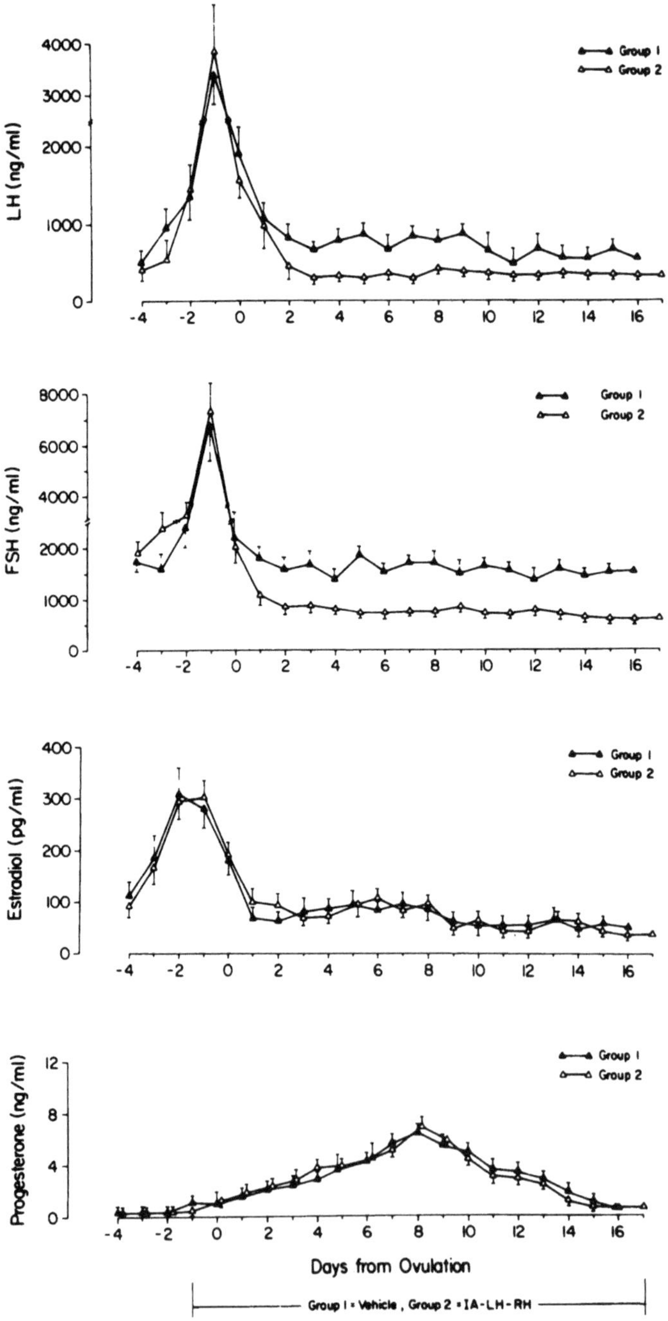

Fig. 4 Serum concentrations of luteinizing hormone (LH), follicle stimulating hormone (FSH), estradiol and progesterone (P) of animals treated with vehicle (Group 1) and and an LH-RH antagonist ([N-Ac-D-Trp$^{1/3}$,D-pCl-Phe^{2},D-Phe^{6},D-Ala^{10}]-LH-RH) (Group 2). Day 0 represents the date of ovulation (Experiment 1).

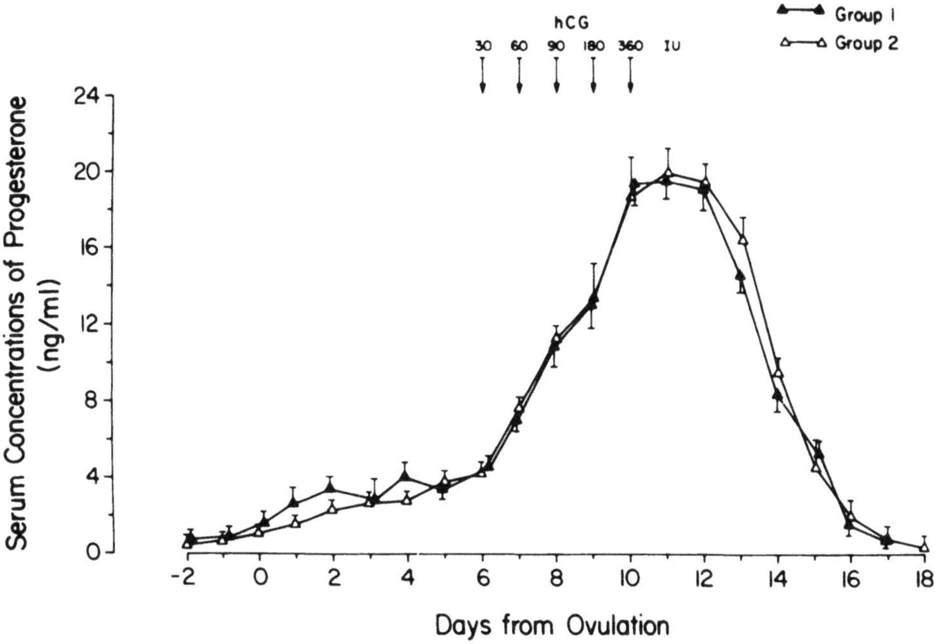

Fig. 5 Serum concentrations of progesterone (P) (1) of animals treated with vehicle (Group 1) and an LH-RH antagonist ([N-Ac-D-Trp$^{1/3}$,D-p-Cl-Phe^{2},D-Phe^{6},D-Ala^{10}]-LH-RH) (Group 2). hCG was given in increasing doses during the days 6 to 10 post-ovulation. Day 0 represents the date of ovulation (Experiment 2).

Acknowledgments

We are grateful to Drs. Andrew V. Schally and David Coy for their kind supply of different LH-RH antagonists and for their continuous intellectual motivation; to Organon, Oss, Holland for the recent supply of ORG30276B; and to Ms. Gretta Small for her excellent preparation of the manuscript. Support for this project was provided by the Ford Foundation (820-1073) and by the Program for Applied Research on Fertility Regulation (PARFR-347), Northwestern University, under a Cooperative Agreement with the United States Agency for International Development (AID) (DPE-0546-A-00-1003-00). The views expressed by the authors do not necessarily reflect the views of AID.

References

[1] Jones, G. S.: Fertil. Steril. 27 (1976) 351–356.
[2] Horta, J. L. H., J. G. Fernandez, L. B. DeSoto et al.: Obstet. Gynecol. **49** (1977) 705–708.
[3] Wilks, J. W., G. D. Hodgen, G. T. Ross: J. Clin Endocrinol. Metab. **43** (1976) 1261–1267.

[4] Ross, G. T., C. M. Cargille, M. B. Lipsett et al.: Recent Prog. Horm. Res. **26** (1970) 1–62.
[5] Stouffer, R. L., G. D. Hodgen: J. Clin. Endocrinol. Metab. **51** (1980) 669–671.
[6] Hanson, F. W., J. E. Powell, V. C. Stevens: J. Clin. Endocrinol. Metab. **32** (1971) 211–215.
[7] Moudgal, N. R., G. J. MacDonald, R. O. Greep: J. Clin. Endocrinol. Metab. **35** (1972) 113–116.
[8] Asch, R. H., M. AbouSarma, G. D. Braunstein et al.: J. Clin. Endocrinol. Metab. **55** (1982) 154–161.
[9] Karsch, F. J., L. C. Krey, R. F. Weick et al.: Endocrinology **92** (1973) 1148–1152.
[10] Balmaceda, J. P., G. Valenzuela, C. A. Eddy et al: Obstet. Gynecol. **57** (1981) 505–508.
[11] Asch, R. H., T. M. Siler-Khodr, C. G. Smith et al.: J. Clin. Endocrinol. Metab. **52** (1981) 565–571.
[12] Stouffer, R. L., W. E. Nixon, F. J. Gulyas: Steroids **27** (1976) 543–551.
[13] Asch, R. H., C. A. Eddy, A. V. Schally: Biol. Reprod. **29** (1981) 963–968.
[14] Wehrenberg, W. B., D. P. Chaichareon, D. J. Diersche et al.: Biol. Reprod. **17** (1977) 148–153.
[15] Asch, R. H., M. Van Sickle, V. Rettori et al.: J. Clin. Endocrinol. Metab. **53** (1981) 215–217.
[16] Miyachi, Y., J. Vaitukaitis, E. Neischlag et al.: J. Clin. Endocrinol. Metab. **34** (1972) 23–28.
[17] Marshall, J. C., R. A. Shakespear, W. D. Odell: Proc. Soc. Exp. Biol. Med. **149** (1975) 351–355.
[18] Clayton, R. N., I. T. Huhtaniemi: Nature **299** (1982) 56–59.
[19] Popkin, R., T. A. Bramley, A. Currie et al.: Biochem. Biophys. Res. Commun. **114** (1983) 750–756.
[20] Balmaceda, J. P., M. R. Borghi, D. H. Coy et al.: J. Clin. Endocrinol. Metab. **57** (1983) 866–868.

The effects of an LH-RH agonist on the premenstrual syndrome: a preliminary report

J. Bancroft, H. Boyle, D. W. Davidson, J. Gray, H. M. Fraser

Introduction

This paper reports preliminary work on the use of the LH-RH agonist, D-Ser $(Bu^t)^6$ LH-RH (1–9) nonapeptide-ethylamide (Buserelin) in the management of premenstrual syndrome, both as a method of treatment and as an experimental model for investigating its hormonal basis.

Many women experience cyclical changes in mood and physical well-being during their menstrual cycles, feeling best in the latter part of the follicular phase and worst in the late luteal or premenstrual phase. Common psychological symptoms in the premenstrual phase include irritability, tension, depression and tiredness; physical symptoms include breast tenderness, body swelling, urinary frequency and appetite changes. It is difficult to estimate the incidence of this so-called premenstrual syndrome as the intensity of these changes varies considerably from woman to woman as well as from cycle to cycle in the same woman. But probably the majority of women are aware of such a cyclical pattern and at least 2 to 3% are severely affected by it [1].

Very little is understood about the biological basis of this pattern. It is not yet clear whether those severely affected represent the extreme of a normal continuum or rather suffer from subtle abnormalities of their hormonal cycles. Women who suffer depressive illness are particularly prone to premenstrual syndrome which suggests that there may be some complex interaction between the mechanisms underlying depressive illness and the biological basis of the premenstrual cyclical pattern [2]. Obviously both personality and social circumstances influence the intensity of the syndrome and how well a woman copes with it. Typically the syndrome shows a close temporal relationship to the luteal phase of the cycle (fig. 1) [3], which has led some to assume that it is caused by some product or deficiency of the corpus luteum.

Many unseccessful attempts have been made to demonstrate differences between women with and without premenstrual syndrome by measuring circulating hormones during the luteal phase [4]. After participation in this type of research [3] we have come to the conclusion that this experimental model is unlikely to be helpful and we

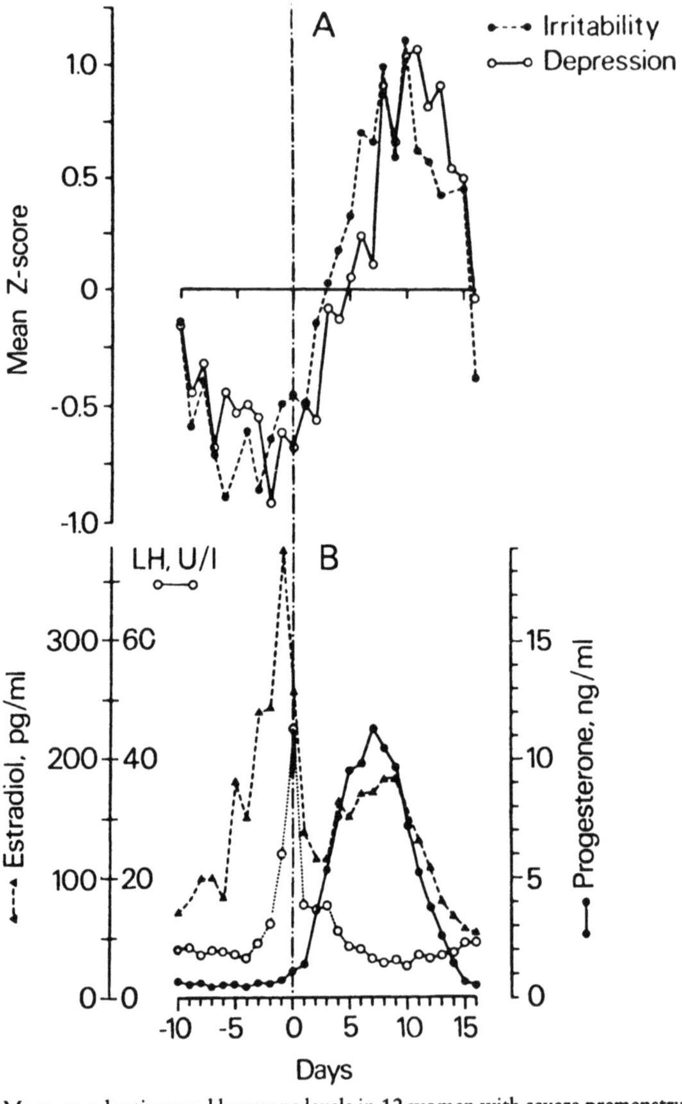

Fig. 1 Mean mood ratings and hormone levels in 12 women with severe premenstrual syndrome. Mood scores have been standardized and centerd around the day of the LH peak.

now favor a different research strategy which is to examine variations in hormonal cycles in the same woman and see how they relate to her cyclical symptoms. It is still not clear, for example, whether premenstrual syndrome can occur in anovular cycles.

The use of chronic treatment with LH-RH agonist to manipulate the ovarian cycle is one such model which has the added attraction of providing a possible form of treatment.

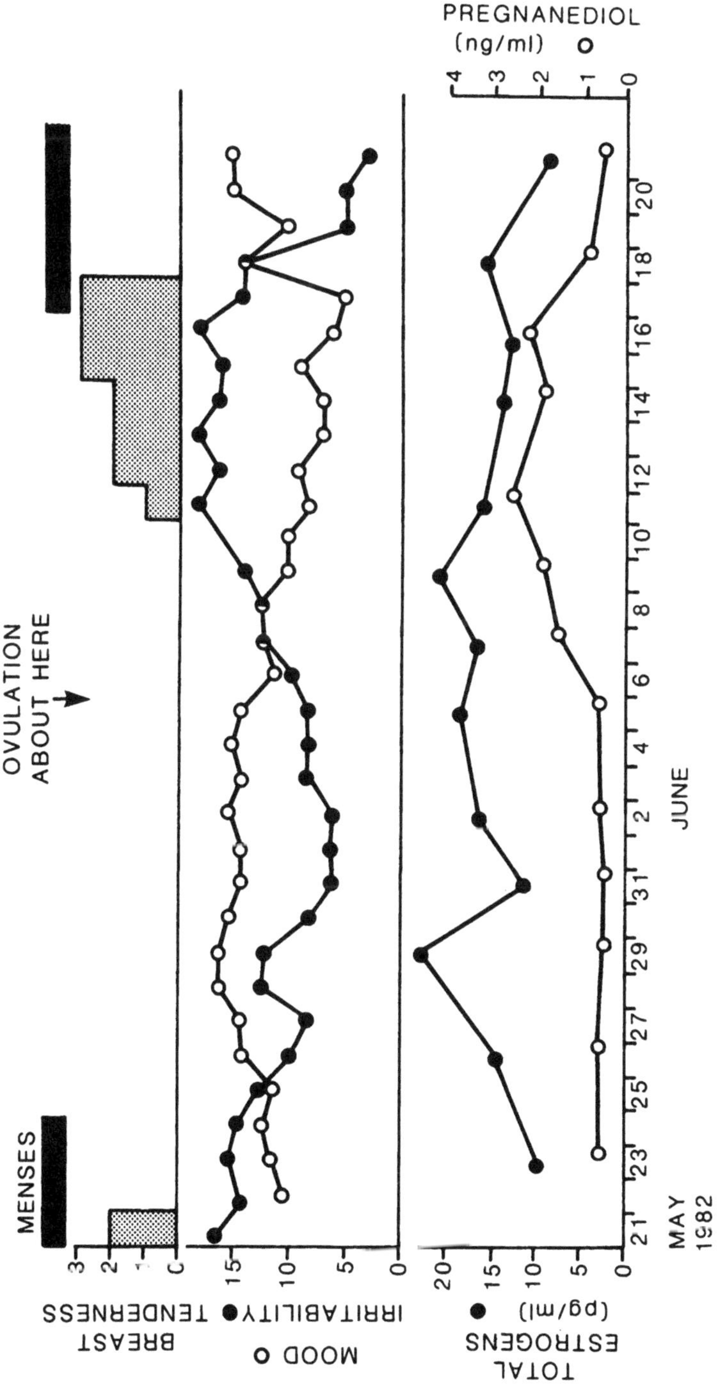

Fig. 2 A baseline month showing mood, irritability and breast symptom ratings together with urinary estrogen and pregnanediol. In the normal ovulatory cycle, irritability starts of increase and mood to deteriorate soon after ovulation. Breast symptoms follow in a few days (Case 4).

Method

Women complaining of premenstrual syndrome were asked to complete daily diaries, rating mood and physical symptoms [5] and to collect early morning urines 3 days a week for us to measure total estrogen and pregnanediol [6, 7] to assess follicular development and occurrence of ovulation respectively. An example of such data from one baseline month is shown in figure 2.

Before starting treatment a minimum of two baseline months showing a clear premenstrual pattern was required. The agonist, administered as a nasal spray, was given in the dosage of 200 μg twice daily in the early cases and 200 μg three times daily in the later cases, beginning on the first or second day of the next menstrual period. We have assessed 37 women with baseline data, selecting 14 as suitable for the agonist treatment. All these women had received at least one form of conventional treatment with either no or only transient benefit before starting on the agonist.

Therapeutic efficacy

It is not possible at this stage to assess the therapeutic value of the agonist. Controlled evaluation in larger numbers will be necessary for this purpose and the design of appropriate controlled studies will not be straightforward, for reasons that will become clear in this report. We can say simply, however, that in the 14 women, 8 were apparently helped and wished to continue on the spray for variable periods. In 6 women the treatment was stopped either because of unexpected side-effects or because of no worthwhile improvement. A brief description of the response to treatment will be given for each woman.

Response to treatment

The "Successes"

Case 1. A 36-year-old nurse with long history of severe premenstrual depression and breast tenderness. She has received two courses of agonist treatment for 12 and 10 months respectively. No evidence of ovulation was found during either course. In the first, involving the 200 μg twice daily dosage, she showed initial worsening of symptoms during the first two weeks. After the first month, however, she showed steady improvement month by month with moderately regular menstruation and some degree of follicular development. Further assessment was compliated by the development of spondylolisthesis which required hospitilisation and spinal surgery. Nine months after starting treatment both her premenstrual depression and follicular development were becoming more marked as though the spray was losing its effect.

Her breast symptoms however did not return. Treatment was stopped following which her severe premenstrual syndrome returned. She was re-started on a 200 μg three times daily dose 9 months later. Her reaction to the second course is presented in figure 3. This shows, once again, a marked aggravation of her premenstrual symptoms throughout the first month, with evidence of substantial follicular development (i.e. very high urinary total estrogens) but not apparent ovulation or corpus luteum development. This is therefore an example of severe premenstrual-type symptoms occurring during an anovular cycle. Later she shows a modest rise in urinary estrogen, accompanied by mild breast changes but no deterioration in mood. She then shows a stable pattern with no follicular development. In order to investigate the role of estrogen in causing these symptoms, a course of estradiol valerate, 2 mg

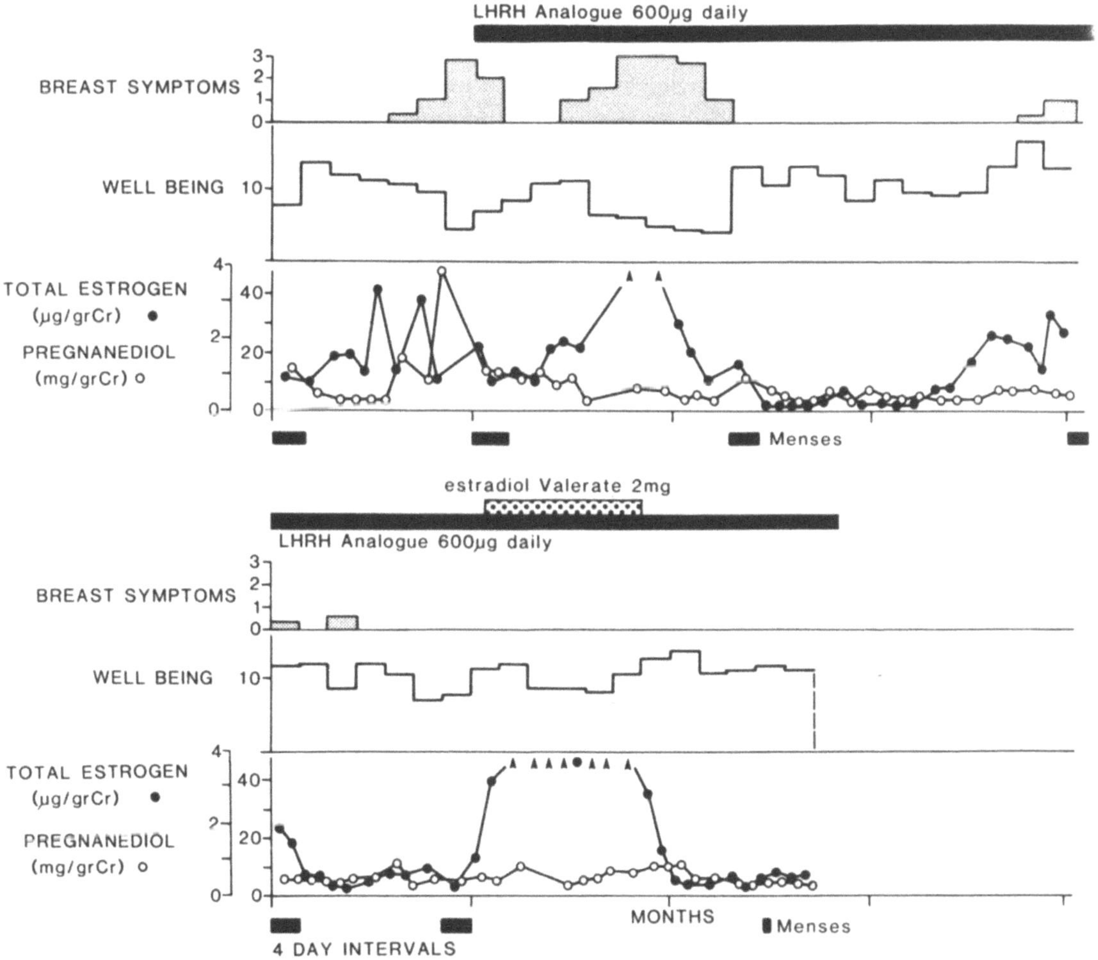

Fig. 3 The effects of Buserelin on premenstrual syndrome (Case 1). For description, see text.

daily, was given. This has no apparent effect, particularly on her breast symptoms. The very high urinary estrogens during the exogenous estrogen administration are presumably mainly the metabolite of estrone. But there is evidence that this dosage of estradiol valerate produces a five-fold increase in plasma estradiol in postmenopausal women [8]. This makes it less likely that her premenstrual syptoms result from the direct effects of estrogens.

Case 2. A 29-year-old teacher of maladjusted children. In addition to typical premenstrual symptoms she has severe bulimia nervosa with "binging" and self-induced vomiting which is much more frequent in the premenstrual phase of the cycle. She started treatment at 200 μg LH-RH agonist twice daily. Five days later she had a few days of severe symptoms followed by a further menstrual bleed. Following this she felt very much better and remained well with some follicular development but no further menstruation for 6 months. She was then sterilised at her request by tubal ligation and following this changed in a single blind fashion from active to placebo spray. Two weeks after starting on the placebo her psychological symptoms returned and her eating pattern deteriorated. After a month on placebo she returned to the active spray but it was thereafter impossible to regain the previous control of her cycle. Although she did not ovulate, she continued to have irregulare heavy bleeding preceded by her usual premenstrual symptoms. There was some improvement when the dose was increased to 200 μg three times daily but she was still troubled by periodic very heavy bleeding and developed fairly marked nasal congestion which required stopping the spray. The explanation for her altered response to the agonist after sterilisation and placebo treatment remains obscure.

Case 3. A 30-year-old social worker. Although she described typical premenstrual symptoms of tension and irritability her main complaint was a regular upper respiratory tract infection during the premenstrual week. Her initial reaction to treatment (200 μg three times daily) was good and during the first month her U.R.T.I. and premenstrual pattern were both modified. During the second month, she had a chronic "cold" for about a month but following this she remained very well and amenorrheic. During the first month and preceding the first and only menstruation after starting treatment she showed some rise in estrogens but thereafter her estrogen levels remained low. By the third month she was reporting hot flushes.

After 4 months on the spray and after two very good months when she felt better than she had for many years, she developed acute cholecystitis. She was told by the surgeon to stop the spray in case there was some link with her gall bladder disease.

Case 4. A 32-year-old health visitor. She started the spray on the 200 μg three times daily dosage. Her response to treatment is shown in figures 4 and 5. Initial reaction was severe PMS symptoms for two or three days and then an unstable month with

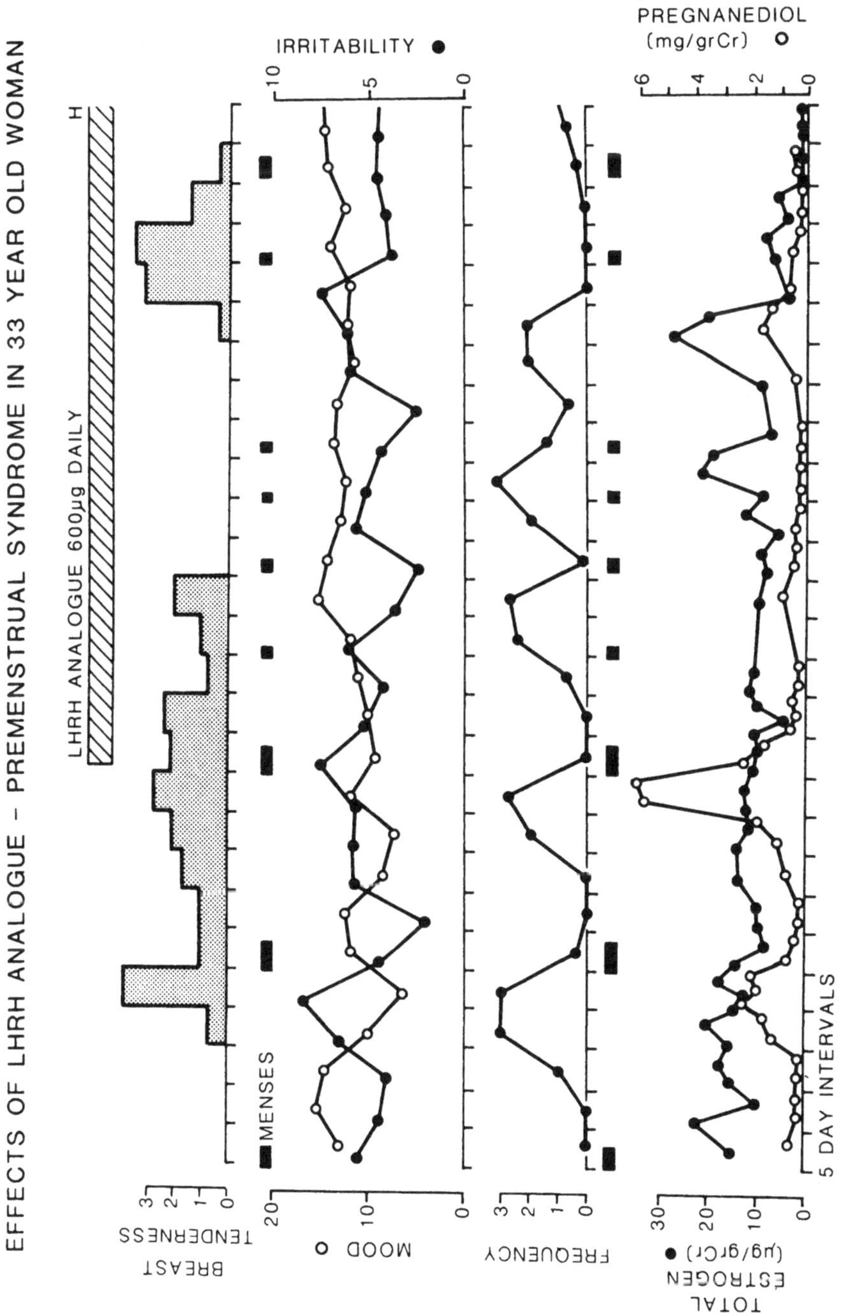

Fig. 4 Initial reaction to treatment with Buserelin in Case 4. Two pre-treatment cycles are shown. The first is typical, the second is less typical in terms of both symptoms and hormonal changes – menstruation starts when urinary pregnanediol is still high. Over the first 3 months of treatment with Buserelin there is irregular menstrual bleeding and follicular activity, with no evidence of ovulation. Psychological and physical symptoms (breast tenderness and urinary frequency) also occur irregularly and show no clear relationship with ovarian steroid changes or with each other. Response later in treatment is down in figure 5.

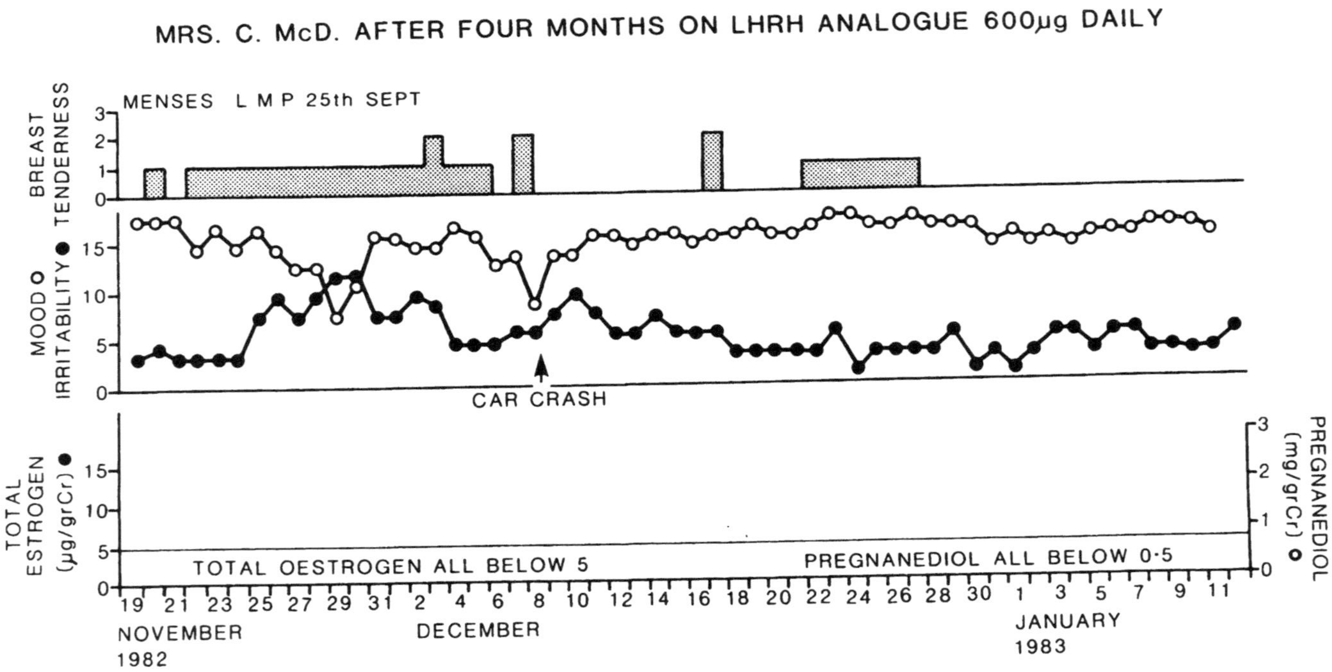

Fig. 5 Later stage of treatment in Case 4. (Fourth month onwards). By now ovarian activity is suppressed. There are still some variations in mood and occasional mild breast symptoms. By the 5th month the mood hat stabilized and the subject felt very well. Urinary frequency had ceased to be a problem by the 3rd month.

occasional spotting and a menstrual bleed 52 days later. There was no further bleeding after this. Estrogens were showing periodic rises for the first two months before settling at a low level. After two months her mood stabilized and she felt well but four months after starting treatment she was experiencing some hot flushes and slight vaginal dryness. The hot flushes became more frequent over the next months, occurring two or three times a day. The dose of spray was reduced to 500 µg and then 400 µg. The hot flushes stopped for a while and then returned at the previous frequency. In spite of lowering the dose her estrogens remained at the previously low level. Eight months ater starting treatment she was having problems with sinusitis and nasal congestion and in view of this, the hot flushes, and her wish to have a further pregnancy, the treatment was stopped. The hot flushes gradually reduced in frequency, stopping 30 days after the end of treatment when her estrogens were starting to rise.

Case 5. A 32-year-old housewife with a neurotic anxious personality. She started on 200 µg treatment three times daily and felt very well during the first month apart from a slight premenstrual drop. Thereafter she has been generally better, more stable and more self-confident. She has continued to menstruate on a regular basis with gradually lengthening intervals and showing fairly marked follicular development. After 2 months of treatment she reported some decline in her sexual response. This is difficult to assess because of problems in the marital relationship but it could be a side-effect of treatment.

Case 6. A 43-year-old housewife. She reported an improvement on the spray (200 µg twice daily) in spite of continuing to show ovulatory cycles throughout treatment. She was difficult to assess; she filled in the daily ratings in an inappropriate fashion and continued to report improvement when changed to a placebo spray. She is the only woman who has continued to ovulate on the spray and there must be some doubt as to whether she was using it properly.

Case 7. A 33-year-old housewife who started on 200 µg t.d.s. Her premenstrual pattern was not noticeable during the first month of treatment, but she was depressed for 3 weeks during the second month for no apparent reason. During the 3rd and 4th months she has felt well with no menstruation but continuing evidence of follicular development. She is continuing on treatment.

Case 8. A 39-year-old housewife who has been on treatment (200 µg three times a day) for 3 months. She ovulated during the first month and has continued to show follicular activity in the 2nd and 3rd months, with anovular menstruation. She has experienced a slight premenstrual decline before each menstrual bleed but with much reduced severity of symptoms and of shorter duration. She ist continuing on treatment.

"Treatment failures"

Case 9. This woman stopped treatment early in the second month as she felt no better. As we have more recently found that the benefits of treatment are often not evident until the second or third month, her trial of treatment cannot be considered conclusive.

Case 10. Aged 36. Housewife who had hysterectomy for endometriosis 2 years earlier, since when she has had fairly severe cyclical mood and breast changes and some degree of cyclical acne. Assessment showed her cyclical mood and breast changes to be related to her ovarian cycle. Within the first month on analogue (400 μg daily) she noticed aggravation of her acne and by the second month this was associated with some hirsutism of the legs and was severe enough for the treatment to be stopped in spite of some apparent improvement in her cyclical mood change. Assay of plasma showed slightly raised androgens prior to treatment with a further rise during LH-RH agonist treatment. She received thorough endocrine investigations and was found to have no evidence of polycystic ovaries. This woman was taking her 400 μg of agonist once daily rather than in divided doses.

The androgenizing effects of treatment in this case caused concern and androgen levels were checked in a number of other women on the spray for whom plasma samples were available. Results are shown in table I. Testosterone and androstenedione were assayed radioimmunologically after chromatography.

Case 11. A 35-year-old housewife with particular problems of premenstrual abdominal swelling and urinary frequency. She had shown herself to be very sensitive to hormone treatment and had remained amenorrheic and unwell for several months after an injection of medroxyprogesterone acetate.

She has had two courses of LH-RH agonist. In the first, using 200 μg twice daily for two months she showed an initial positive reaction for a few days, feeling unusually well and then her moods swung up and down with body swelling as a persistent problem. Some follicular development occurred during the first 4 weeks but during the second month her estrogen levels remained low. The second course was attempted about a year later using a higher dose of 200 μg three times daily and lasting two months. Basically her reaction was similar to the first occasion. Ovarian activity was suppressed earlier but her mood continued to fluctuate and there was more evidence of depression, particularly in the second month. Feelings of swelling persisted throughout the time on treatment.

Case 12. A 29-year-old housewife whose main complaint was tension and irritability premenstrually. She started on 200 μg three times daily and felt well during the first few days followed by a phase of unstable mood in spite of a flat hormonal profile. After 21 days body swelling became persistent and after 30 days there was a steady increase in irritability until she stopped taking her spray after 50 days. She had not

Table 1 Testosterone, androstenedione and SHBG levels in women before and during LHRH agonist treatment

Subject	Samples (n)	Testosterone nMol/L	Androstenedione nMol/L	SHBG nMol/L
Case 10		Mean (S.D.)	Mean (S.D.)	Mean (S.D.)
No treatment	(10)	1.92 (0.27)	3.47 (0.87)	34.3 (7.7)
Treatment – 1st month	(3)	1.86 (0.16)	3.11 (0.72)	25.8 (5.5)
2nd month	(7)	2.80 (0.57)***	4.53 (0.36)**	29.1 (5.2)
Case 1				
No treatment	(4)	1.33 (0.26)	–	–
No treatment	(3)	1.68 (0.21)	4.01 (0.15)	–
Treatment – 1st month	(10)	1.98 (0.69)	3.3 (1.36)	82.0 (15.6)
2nd month	(9)	1.52 (0.26)	2.89 (0.8)	83.0 (8.6)
3rd month	(7)	1.62 (0.31)	3.63 (0.96)	89.0 (6.4)
Case 2				
No treatment	(5)	1.49 (0.16)	4.31 (0.45)	51.0 (7.0)
Treatment – 1st month	(4)	1.23 (0.28)	4.36 (1.01)	46.0 (6.8)
2nd month	(4)	1.66 (0.58)	5.31 (0.85)	43.1 (5.6)
Case 9				
No treatment	(7)	2.86 (0.42)	6.27 (1.3)	55.3 (7.3)
Treatment – 1st month	(5)	3.19 (0.63)	5.61 (1.3)	62.5 (7.1)
Case 11				
No treatment	(14)	1.86 (0.5)	3.07 (0.75)	50.9 (12.6)
Treatment – 1st month	(4)	2.36 (0.3)	4.20* (1.21)	42.9 (5.1)

Comparison with no treatment – t-test *p = < 0.05 **p = < 0.01 ***p = < 0.001

menstruated during this time. She had had a number of quite severe headaches during treatment.

Case 13. A 26-year-old nurse who had a longstanding psychiatric history of suicidal behavior since her menarche. Only in the past 2 years had she shown regular menstrual cycles and these had been associated with marked premenstrual depression and suicidal ideas. Within a week of starting the spray she showed a marked mood change, first becoming hypomanic and then after 3 or 4 days swinging into a profound depression. She stopped the spray at this stage and admission to a psychiatric hospital was arranged. The spray was re-started after a 3-day gap but stopped quickly as a further hypomanic change occurred and persisted as a moderately severe hypomanic illness for the next two months before eventually being controlled with psychotropic drugs and lithium. This case is of particular interest. The LH-RH agonist apparently triggered off the first hypomanic episode in this woman's life revealing a tendency for bipolar affective illness which had not hitherto been apparent. She had previously been daignosed as "a serious personality problem".

Case 14. A 31-year-old housewife who became chronically tired on treatment which was stopped after 2 months. She continued to show follicular development without ovulation for the two months.

Discussion

The control of ovarian cyclicity in these women has been variable, as reported in other clinical studies. With the exception of Case 6, which may be misleading, all other women showed suppression of ovulation though in two women (Cases 5 and 7) this did not occur until the second month of treatment. Follicular development either continued intermittently throughout treatment (Cases 1a, 2, 5, 7, & 8) or became suppressed after variable periods of time (Cases 3 and 4).

The most convincing therapeutic results were in those who showed follicular suppression (Cases 1b, 3 & 4) but it is important to note that suppression occurred early in two of the 'failures' (Cases 11 and 12). In one woman this was associated with very unstable mood; in the other with gradually increasing irritability and tension, and both women showed persistent feelings of body swelling.

As an experimental model for investigating the relationship between premenstrual symptoms and ovarian activity, this approach has considerable potential. We have already demonstrated how premenstrual symptoms can occur without ovulation or corpus luteum formation (Cases 1, 2, 8, 12). We have also seen how during the period of time when suppression of follicular activity is developing, irregular symptoms may occur. Also, as illustrated in figure 3, the state of ovarian suppression induced by the agonist allows the experimental evaluation of the effects of estrogen and progesterone administered exogenously. If it can be shown that in this ovarian suppressed state premenstrual symptoms cannot be provoked by administering ovarian steroids, this increases the likelihood that some central cycling mechanism, that normally accompanies the ovarian cycle, is responsible for the cyclical symptoms.

Some of the reactions of the 'failures' are also of interest. The stimulation of ovarian androgen in Case 10 may have been avoided with a larger dose, but the woman's response, together with a slight increase early in treatment in some of the other women assessed, warrants caution in women with acne or with initially raised androgen levels. The triggering of a hypomanic illness in Case 13 not only points to the possible link between hypothalamic pituitary mechanisms and the determinants of endogenous mood change but also reminds us that direct effects of the agonist on the brain cannot yet be excluded.

As a method of treatment, the agonist also holds promise though much more evidence will be required before its proper place will be established. The variable length of time to produce follicular suppression and the possibility of initial stimulatory effects will make double-blind placebo controlled studies difficult, but with further experience of various dosages, this may become less of a problem. While suppression of ovarian cyclicity may well afford substantial relief in some cases, the problems of hypo-estrogenization may pose difficulties for long-term use.

These difficulties may be resolved with the introduction of effective antagonists for human use with the much greater degree of control they would allow. Certainly, we believe that this experimental appraisal should continue and enter the next phase of more controlled systematic studies. There is a distinct possibility that apart from learning a great deal about the hormonal basis of the premenstrual syndrome, we will identify a form of treatment that will be attractive for some women with PMS; particularly when its contraceptive and menses-related effects can be combined with its alleviation of premenstrual symptoms.

Acknowledgements

We are grateful to Dr. P. J. Magill (Hoechst, U.K.) for the gift of Buserelin nasal spray used in this study.

References

[1] Andersch, B.: Thesis, University of Gottenburg, Sweden 1980.
[2] Clare, A. W.: Psychological Medicine. Monograph Supplement **4** (1983).
[3] Bäckström, T., D. Sanders, R. Leask, D. Davidson, P. Warner, J. Bancroft: Psychosomatic Medicine (1984), in press.
[4] Bäcström, T., D. T. Baird, J. Bancroft et al.: J. Psychosomatic Obstetrics & Gynaecology **21**, 8–19.
[5] Sanders, D., P. Warner, T. Bäckström et al.: Psychosomatic Medicine (1984), in press.
[6] Brown, J. B., S. L. Macleod, C. MacNaughton et al.: J. Endocrinology **42** (1968) 5–15.
[7] Chamberlain, J., S. F. Contractor: American J. Obstetrics & Gynecology **101** (1968) 649–657.
[8] Luotola, H., T. Pyorala, P. Lahteenmaki: Maturitas **1** (1979) 287–294.

Discontinous intranasal application of the LH-RH analogon Buserelin in combination with an oral progestin in healthy female volunteers

G. Hoffmann, H.-J. Grill, B. Manz, U. Wiesenecker, K. Pollow

Introduction

The model of pulsatile stimulation of the pituitary, originally established in primate models [1–3] is also in humans essential for a functioning menstrual cycle [4–6]. Long acting LH-RH- analoga lead to inhibition of ovulation in normally menstruating women by disturbing the secretion of gonadotropins from the pituitary [7–9]. Repeated application of an analogon reduces pituitary gonadotropin reaction also in amenorrheic [10–13] and postmenopausal women [14]. The contraceptive potency of Buserelin has already been prooven in several clinical trials [15–20]. Essential drawbacks of continous application are irregular bleedings up to amenorrhea [19, 21] and the occasional appearence of signs of early endometrial hyperplasia [19, 22]. With these results in mind a discontinous application scheme of the LH-RH analogon Buserelin (D-Ser(TBU)^{6}-EA^{10}-LH-RH) with additional oral application of a progestin (norethisterone acetate) was applied in order to prohibit these side effects of continous treatment.

Volunteers and methods

Volunteers: Twenty healthy female volunteers, 20–42 years of age (27±7 years), who showed regular biphasic basal body temperature (BBT) curves and had not used hormonal contraceptives during three preceeding months were taken up in this study. The cycle previous to treatment served as control cycle. BBT was measured daily and on days 19 and 23 of cycle serum progesterone was determined. 18/20 volunteers had biphasic BBT curves as well as progesterone levels above 8 ng/ml in this control cycle thus resembling normal ovulatory cycles. One volunteer showed a corpus luteum insufficiency (progesterone 4–5.5 ng/ml) and a second did not show progesterone levels above 1 ng/ml as a sign of anovulation.

Treatment schedule: After a control cycle all volunteers received from day 1–22 of the cycle daily 300 μg Buserelin by a nasal spray. Additionally from day 16–22.5 mg norethisterone acetate (total dosis 35 mg) were applied per os followed by 6 days without treatment. This therapy schedule was applied for a total of 6 months. Norethisterone acetate served for the induction of regular menstrual bleedings. Thereafter followed a cycle without treatment. No other contraceptive devices were used within the time of this study.

Diagnostic follow-up: During treatment blood samples were drawn weekly in cycle 1, 2, 4 and 6 for determination of LH, FSH, estradiol, prolactin, DHEA-S and testosterone. Ovarian function was monitored by daily measurement of BBT and weekly serum progesterone determinations. The thyreoidea function was checked by repeated TRH-tests. Before, during and at the end of treatment several metabolic parameters (blood picture, liver and kidney function, blood coagulation etc.) were controlled. In the last cycle of treatment endometrial biopsies were taken in order to investigate the stage of endometrial proliferation. In the cycle after treatment were the same hormonal parameters controlled again.

Hormone determinations: All blood samples were drawn between 10 and 12 a.m., followed immediately by determination of the metabolic parameters.

The serum hormones were determined using commercially available radioimmunoassay kits.

Results

Gonadotropin

The gonadotropin levels showed different secretion patterns for LH and FSH with a significantly increased LH/FSH ratio up to 3 and 4. Only during the 7-day-treatment' free intervals was this ratio reduced to an average of 2 (fig. 1).

FSH levels were throughout treatment with 4.1–8.9 mIU/ml in lower normal range (4–12 mIU/ml, fig. 1). No significant differences in FSH serum concentrations could be detected comparing weeks of cycle (fig. 2) or overall cycles (fig. 3). Only during the first weeks of therapy a few volunteers showed slightly elevated FSH secretion above 12 ng/ml resulting in a minor elevation of FSG levels to 10.0 ± 8.9 ng/ml for the whole collective.

On the other hand, the LH levels under Buserelin treatment were significantly elevated during the first two weeks (n = 40, LH = 32.0 ± 21 mIU/ml) and remained although lower (n = 280, LH 15 ± 11.3 mIU/ml), throughout the whole study above normal range which is 4–12 mIU/ml (figs. 1, 3), Only in the treatment-free intervals did they returned to normal range levels (n = 80, LH = 8.0 ± 5.3 mIU/ml). Analyzing the LH-levels of all cycles under treatment according to stage of cycle, in the first two weeks similarily elevated values (1. week n = 80, LH = 22.4 ± 16.8 mIU/ml;

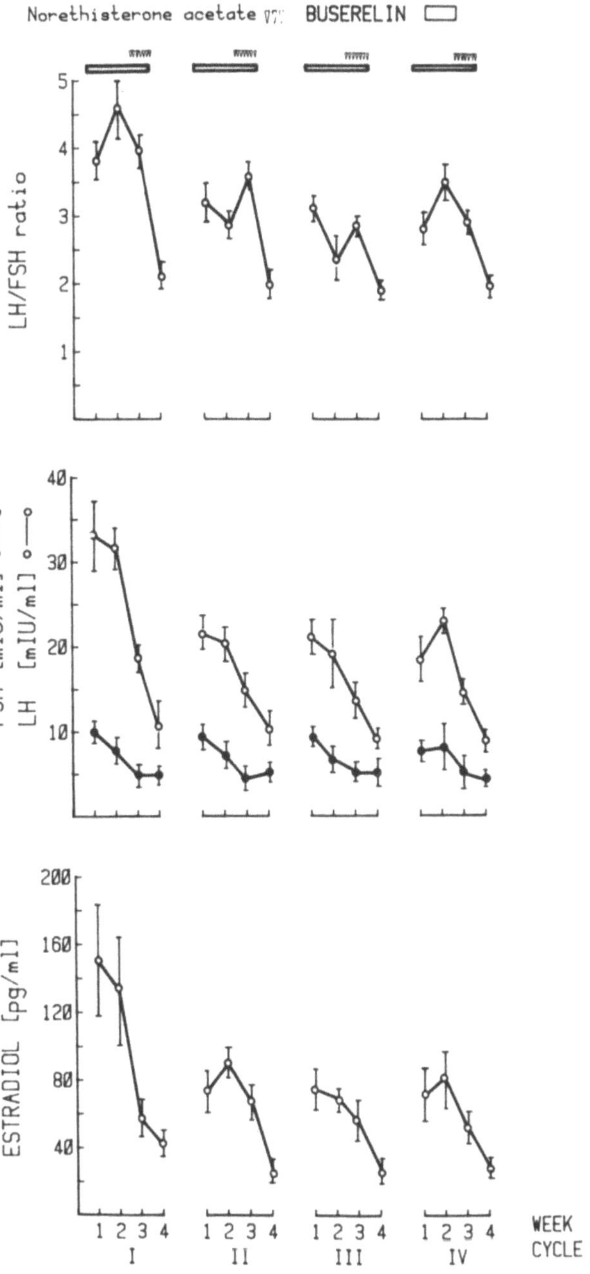

Fig. 1 Hormone profiles ($\bar{x} \pm$ SEM) of 20 volunteers under discontinous treatment with Buserelin and norethisterone acetate.

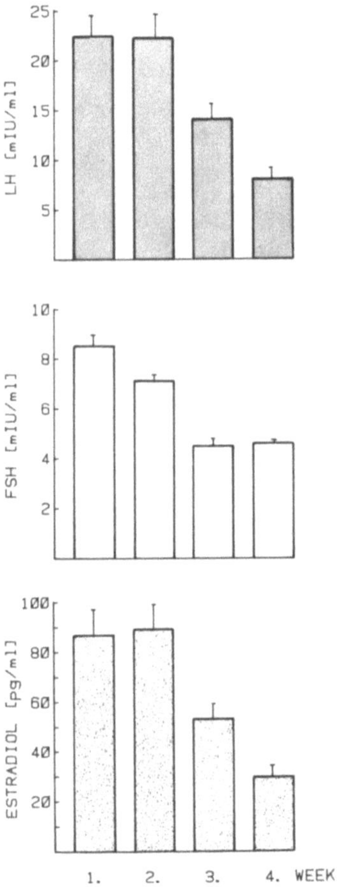

Fig. 2 Overall mean serum levels ($\bar{x} \pm$ SEM, n = 80 for each week) of the weeks of cycle under discontinous Buserelin/norethisterone acetate treatment: first and second week 300 µg Buserelin daily, third week: 300 µg Buserelin and 5 ng norethisterone acetate daily, fourth week: treatment free interval.

2. week n = 80, LH = 22.2±16.6 mIU/ml) could be found. In the third week with additional application of norethisterone acetate the LH levels decreased about 35% (n = 80, LH = 14.0±11.3 mIU/ml) and in the medication-free fourth week they returned to normal range (n = 80, LH = 8.0±5.3 mIU/ml) (fig. 2).

Estradiol

Estradiol serum levels increased at the beginning of treatment up to values similar to late follicular phase (first week n = 20, E_2 = 150.6±156 pg/ml); second week n = 20, E_2 = 136±128 pg/ml) but decreased drastically thereafter (third week

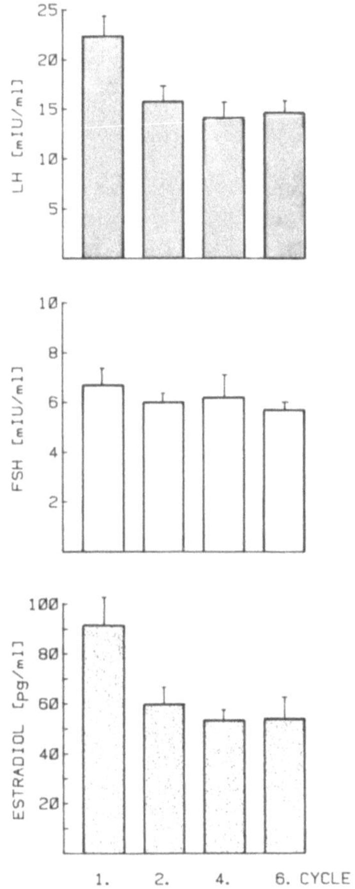

Fig. 3 Mean overall serum levels ($\bar{x} \pm$ SEM, n = 80 for each month) during 4 cycles under treatment.

n = 20, $E_2 = 58.6 \pm 31.4$ pg/ml; fourth week n = 20, $E_2 = 42.4 \pm 61.7$ pg/ml). A similar pattern could be seen in the following months of treatment, although the stimulation was less striking (fig. 1).

Taking all cycles into account E_2 levels were found to be 88.4 ± 94.3 pg/ml (n = 160) within the first two weeks, decreased to 53.1 ± 53.0 pg/ml (n = 80) in the third week and down to 29.6 ± 35.1 pg/ml (n = 80) in the fourth week (fig. 2).

Generally, the overall monthly E_2 secretion decreased especially in the first month until to the fourth month and then remained low. In the sixth month the overall monthly E_2 secretion remained around 55 pg/ml (fig. 3).

Due to the enormous range of the E_2 serum levels, the whole collective was split into 3 subgroups according to the E_2 secretion patterns (fig. 4). 6/20 volunteers (group I)

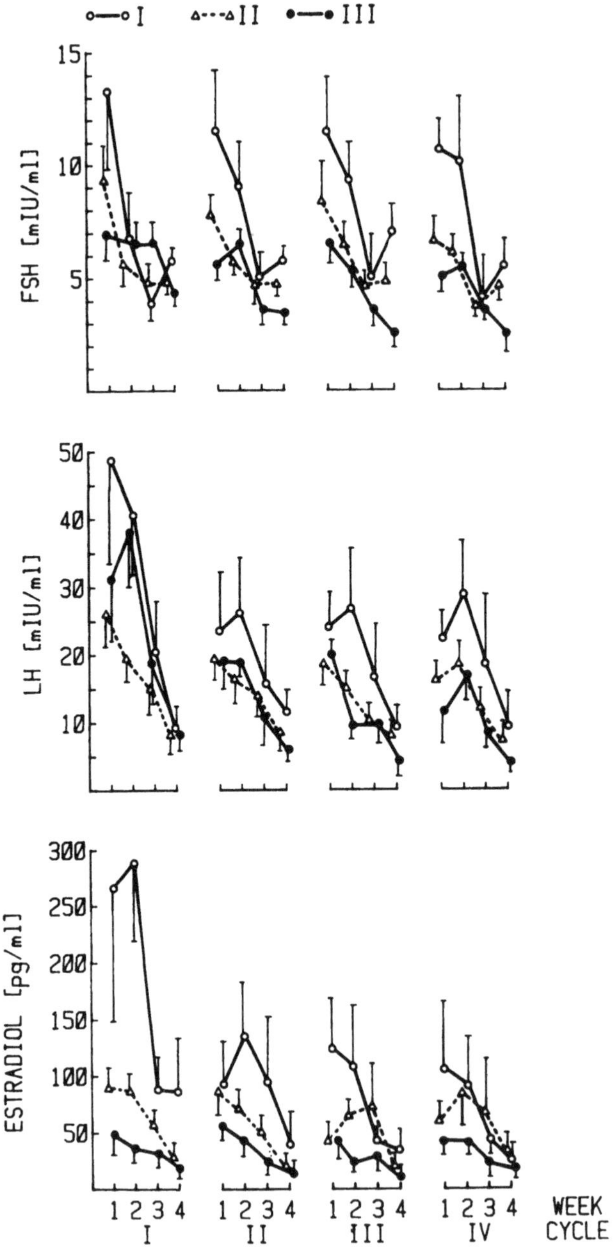

Fig. 4 Hormone profiles ($\bar{x} \pm$ SEM) of 3 subgroups depending on estradiol secretion pattern.
Group I (n - 6): marked estradiol suppression
Group II (n = 9): moderate estradiol suppression
Group III (n = 5): slight estradiol suppression

showed E_2 secretion up to preovulatory values (n = 12, E_2 = 277±217 pg/ml). Further treatment led to a reduction of the overall E_2 secretion in the first two weeks of each individual cycle where E_2 values similar to mid or late follicular phase were reached (100–150 pg/ml). 9/20 volunteers (group II) showed in the first two weeks of each cycle a stimulated E_2 secretion between 60.8–89.8 pg/ml, followed by a decrease. 5/20 volunteers (group III) had E_2 serum levels at any stage of the cycle below 50 pg/ml and ovarian function in this group was blocked from the first cycle under treatment. Also in this group could be found the two volunteers who had shown the above mentioned cycle abnormalities before the onset of treatment. Comparing the estradiol levels of the three groups to the corresponding gonadotropin levels, a similar behaviour resulted especially for FSH. It should be noted that the FSH levels of group I increased during the treatment-free interval, whereas in group III FSH further decreased.

Progesterone

In 105 of the 120 cycles under treatment the progesterone levels were below 1 ng/ml, indicating anovulatory cycles (tab. 1). In 8 cycles progesterone levels between 1–3 ng/ml were found once among the weekly spot checks. In another 5 cycles elevated progesterone levels up to 5 ng/ml of short duration appeared, which might have been due to premature follicle luteinisation or luteal insufficiency. One volunteer had in her first cycle under treatment progesterone levels of 5.6 ng/ml and in the middle of her sixth cycle lasting levels of 5.1–11 ng/ml (tab. 2, fig. 5).

Table 1 Serum progesterone levels under discontinous Buserelin/noresthisterone acetate treatment of 120 cycles

Progesterone (ng/ml)	20 volunteers 120 cycles
≦ 1	105/120 (87.5%)
> 1 ≦ 3	8/120 (6.7%)
> 3 ≦ 5	5/120 (4.1%)
> 5	2/120 (1.7%)

Table 2 Rate of ovulation under discontinous Buserelin/noresthisterone treatment in 120 cycles

Volunteer	Cycle/week	BBT elevation	Progesterone (ng/ml)
C.S.	*I/1.	4 days	5.0
C.R.	*I/1.	5 days	3.4
F.S.	*I/2.	6 days	5.6
	**VI/2.	9 days	5.7 and 11.0
Anovulatory cycles		116/120 (96.7%)	
* Corpus luteum insuff.		3/120 (2.5%)	
** Ovulatory cycle		1/120 (0.8%)	

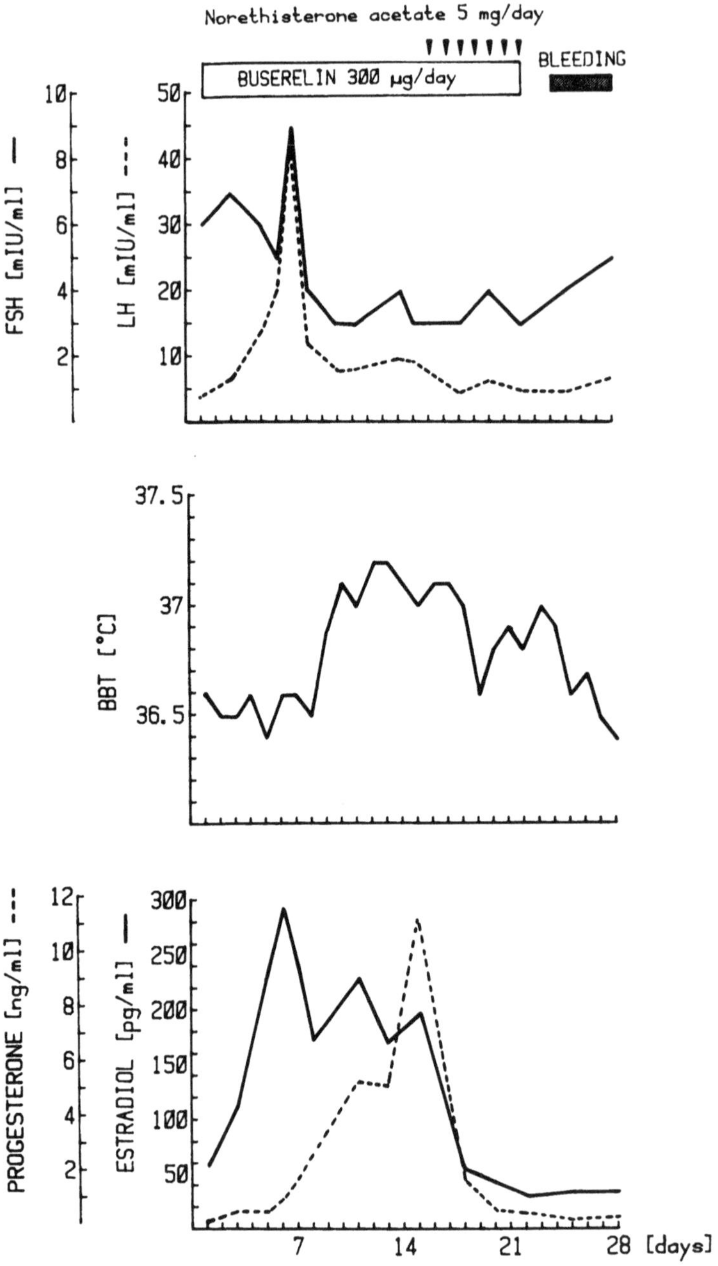

Fig. 5 Hormone profile of the only cycle (sixth cycle of volunteer F. S.) under Buserelin/norethisterone acetate treatment with possible ovulation.

Ovulation

Basal body temperature recordings were monophasic in 116/120 cycles. In synopsis with progesterone serum levels these cycles prooved to be anovulatory. In 96.7% was safe contraception therefore guaranteed. Three volunteers had brief elevated BBT during 6 days at the beginning of the first cycle under treatment together with increased serum progesterone values up to maximally 5.6 ng/ml, which can be interpreted as a corpus luteum insufficiency (tab. 2).

But also in these cases (2.5%) the cycles were disturbed in a way to provide safe contraception. One of these 3 volunteers had in her last cycle another BBT elevation for 9 days with luteal progesterone secretion. In this case ovulation cannot be excluded (fig. 5).

During application of norethisterone acetate there was always an increase of BBT measurable for 6–8 days due to the thermogenetic effects of this progestin. But ovulation within this time could be excluded because serum progesterone was below 1 ng/ml, as determined by RIA. Norethisterone acetate did not interfere with the progesterone RIA used.

Testosterone, DHEA-S and prolactin

The serum levels of testosterone and DHEA-S under Buserelin medication did not differ from the levels in the control cycles before and after treatment (tab. 3).

Table 3 Serum levels of testosterone, DHEA-sulfate and prolactin of 20 volunteers before, during and after discontinous Buserelin/norethisterone acetate treatment (n = number of samples)

Hormones (ng/ml)	Control cycle before treatment n = 40	Cycles under Buserelin and norethisterone acetate n = 320	Control cycles after treatment n = 40
Testosterone	0.7 ± 0.3	0.6 ± 0.3	0.6 ± 0.2
DHEA-sulfate	2.5 ± 1.7	2.6 ± 1.9	3.1 ± 2.0
Prolactin	12.4 ± 6.7	9.7 ± 4.2	9.2 ± 3.4

Only one volunteer, who showed previous to the onset of treatment signs of hyperandrogenaemia (testosterone 1.1 ng/ml, DHEA-S 4.8 μg/ml) as well as androgenic symptoms, had increased levels of testosterone (1.3 ng/ml) and DHEA-S (6.8 ng/ml) under treatment. After medication both hormones returned to starting levels (tab. 4).

Also, prolactin levels did not vary detectably under Buserelin (tab. 3). Only 4 volunteers revealed sporadically, levels between 25–59 ng/ml. These elevated concentrations were found independently of day of cycle or month of treatment.

Table 4 Serum levels of testosterone and DHEA-sulfate of 5 volunteers with androgenic side effects (acne, seborrhea, hirsutism) before, during and after discontinous Buserelin/norethisterone acetate treatment (n = number of samples)

Volunteer	Testosterone (ng/ml)			DHEA-S (µg/ml)		
	before	during treatment	after	before	during treatment	after
	n = 2	n = 16	n = 3	n = 2	n = 16	n = 3
A.B.	0.7 ∓ 0.2	0.8 ∓ 0.2	0.9 ∓ 0.2	7.1 ∓ 0.7	7.1 ∓ 1.6	7.8 ∓ 1.1
I.G.	1.1 ∓ 0.1	1.3 ∓ 0.3	1.1 ∓ 0.3	4.8 ∓ 1.5	6.8 ∓ 1.8	4.5 ∓ 0.7
P.H.	0.6 ∓ 0.1	0.6 ∓ 0.2	0.5 ∓ 0.1	2.5 ∓ 0.3	2.6 ∓ 0.5	2.4 ∓ 0.4
U.H.	0.6 ∓ 0.1	0.7 ∓ 0.3	0.6 ∓ 0.2	1.7 ∓ 0.1	1.7 ∓ 0.5	2.1 ∓ 0.5
S.P.	0.6 ∓ 0.2	0.6 ∓ 0.2	0.5 ∓ 0.2	1.8 ∓ 0.3	1.6 ∓ 0.3	1.6 ∓ 0.4

Thyreoidea function

The hormones of thyreoidea (total thyroxine, total triiodothyronine, free thyroxine) and thyroxine binding globuline (TBG) remained throughout treatment as well as in the cycles before and after medication within normal range. This was also found for basal thyreotropin (TSH) in serum. After i.v. injection of 200 µg TRH 17/20 volunteers showed a regular rise in thyreotropin (TSH_{30}) with a Δ TSH of 4.5–16.9 µU/ml during Buserelin treatment and afterwards. In two volunteers TSH could not be stimulated (Δ TSH < 1 µU/ml). A third volunteer developed under Buserelin treatment an enhancing latent hypothyreotic metabolic situation with Δ TSH of 14.6 µU/ml in the third, 21.4 µU/ml in the sixth and 24.1 µU/ml in the control cycle after treatment. This latent hypothyreotic situation does not seem to be associated with Buserelin treatment, as the total collective did not show any alterations.

Metabolic parameters

To ensure safety, the following metabolic parameters were determined: blood sedimentation rate, blood picture, differential blood picture, urea and creatinine, electrolytes, SGOT, SGPT, γ-GT, alkaline phosphatase, bilirubin, total protein, blood glucose, triglycerides, cholesterol, HDL-cholesterol, Quick's test and time. All determinations were carried out before as well as during the third and sixth month of treatment. No parameter revealed any statistically significant changes.

Bleeding patterns

The combined Buserelin/norethisterone acetate treatment led generally to reduced menstrual bleedings as well as duration for 1–2 days. In 102/120 cycles the withdrawal bleedings occured regularily. 8/20 volunteers reported short time intermediate bleedings (tab. 5) that appeared mostly in the first months of treatment. 2 vo-

Table 5 Side effects of discontinous Buserelin/norethisterone acetate treatment

Side effects of Buserelin treatment	Volunteers n = 20	Cycles n = 120
Hot flushes (strong)	6/20	17/120
Hot flushes (gentle)	7/20	23/120
Insomnia	2/20	4/120
Headache	2/20	5/120
Acne	5/20	22/120
Seborrhea	2/20	7/120
Hirsutism	1/20	3/120
Intermediate bleedings	8/20	18/120
Missing withdrawal bleedings	3/20	3/120

lunteers had had bleeding abnormalities before. Over all, in 18/120 cycles intermediate bleedings could be registered, and in 3/18 cycles a gestagen-induced-withdrawal bleeding was missing. In these cycles with intermediate bleedings and subsequent failure of withdrawal bleeding a corpus luteum deficiency could be demonstrated as already described above.

Endometrial biopsies

During the last cycle under treatment endometrial biopsies were performed on 4 volunteers 1–2 days before gestagen application and on 2 volunteers during gestagen treatment. Histological examination revealed in no case an exceeding proliferation or signs of hyperplasia. The samples before progestin treatment were of late proliferative stage, under progestin they showed an incomplet secretory transformation.

Side effects

13/20 volunteers suffered from hot flushes (tab. 5). These were hardly experienced by seven volunteers and were reported only after inquiry. 6 volunteers had distinct hot flushes, appearing in the second and third cycle under treatment and persistant in 5 volunteers even after treatment until the first spontaneous bleeding. The hot flushes may be a result of the partially marked decrease of estrogen levels. This assumption is supported by the fact that those volunteers suffered from hot flushes who showed a strong suppression of ovarian function (fig. 4, group III).

Under treatment, 5 volunteers developed signs of acne, often associated with seborrhea and 1 experienced additionally hirsutism, all of which are symptoms of hyperandrogenemia. Further more, 2 volunteers suffered from insomnia and headaches. The control cycle after treatment was generally 15 days extended compared to the control cycle before the onset of treatment (tab. 6). 12/20 control cycles were ovu-

Table 6 Length of cycle and rate of ovulations in the control cycles before and after Buserelin/norethisterone acetate treatment in 20 volunteers

Number	Cycles before treatment length (days)	Function	Cycles after treatment Length (days)	Function
12	28 ∓ 3	ovulatory	40 ∓ 13	ovulatory
4	27 ∓ 2	ovulatory	42 ∓ 10	CLI
2	29 and 30	ovulatory	29 and 78*	anovulatory
1	29	CLI	63*	anovulatory
1	34	anovulatory	59	anovulatory

CLI = corpus luteum insufficiency; * bleeding after induction with norethisterone acetate.

latory after treatment, while 4/20 showed had BBT and serum progesterone levels indicating a corpus luteum insufficiency. 4 cycles were anovulatory, and among these were the 2 volunteers with disturbed ovarian function.

Discussion

The pulsatile stimulation of the gonadotropic cells of the anterior pituitary via hypothalamic LH/RH is a prerequisite for the synthesis and secretion of gonadotropins, as well as for a functional physiological expression of the cycle [1–6, 23]. A permanent infusion of LH/RH leads via a so called "down-regulation" or "desensitation" of the LH-RH receptors to a complete inhibition of LH and FSH secretion [1, 24]. A change in the frequency or concentration of LH-RH results in a completely different secretion pattern for LH and FSH thus leads to different serum concentrations of these two hormones [25]. An increase in the frequency of LH-RH application leads to a suppression of serum levels for both gonadotropins. A decline in frequency on the other hand results in a decrease of LH and an increase in FSH-concentrations. A diminution in concentration leads to a decrease in the levels of both gonadotropins whereas an increased dosis results in unchanged LH but diminished FSH serum levels [26]. The synthetic LH-RH agonist Buserelin shows, compared to the genuine LH-RH, a higher affinity to the LH-RH-receptors and is less exposed to metabolic inactivation [27, 31].

The daily application of Buserelin led in our study to a marked decrease of FSH secretion while LH serum levels remained unchanged or slightly elevated. This was also expressed in the LH/FSH ratio of 3 to 4 under treatment, returning to a normal ratio of 2 in the treatment-free fourth week. Buserelin therefore does not inhibit gonadotropin secretion via a complete "down-regulation", as it can be observed under permanent infusion of genuine LH-RH, but induces – similar to a high dose administration of genuine LH-RH – a nearly complete inhibition of FSH and a slight elevation of serum LH levels. As the maturation of the follicle is almost entirely dependent on FSH, the discrepancy in secretion of the two gonadotropins but – not an exhaustion of the pituitary – is responsible for the anovulatory potency of this analogon.

The estradiol synthesis was influenced differently, resulting in marked intra- and interindividual fluctuations. Cyclic application of 300 μg Buserelin strongly suppressed estradiol synthesis in 5 volunteers. Among these were two women who suffered from disturbed ovarian function already in the control cycle before treatment. It can be assumed that these five volunteers had an unstable hypothalamic-pituitary-gonadal axis which reacted relatively independent of dosis with a prompt and long-lasting block of ovarian function [19]. In other cases a cyclic estradiol secretion pattern with a more or less marked but constant increase of estradiol serum levels at the begining of each cycle under treatment could be found. In relation to that, also the FSH levels reacted. Especially those volunteers with the least estradiol suppression (group I) revealed an increase in serum FSH levels during the 6-day medication-free interval. On the other hand, FSH concentration in women with blocked ovarian function (group II) dropped even further in the treatment-free interval. This stresses the above made assumption, that the disturbed ovarian function is not due to a complete exhaustion of the pituitary but depends on the isolated suppression of FSH-secretion.

According to serum progesterone levels and BBT in 96.7% of the investigated 120 cycles a clear inhibition of ovulation could be demonstrated. In 2.5% was the corpus luteum function disturbed; in one cycle (0.8%) an ovulation could not be excluded. Overall, 99.2% (120/120 cycles) obtained safe contraception, which is also confirmed by other investigators although in shorter observation periods [32, 33]. During the 6 months of treatment no volunteer became pregnant, and no other contraceptive devices were used. The anticontraceptive effectiveness of a discontinous Buserelin application with an additional progestin administration is therefore comparable to continous medication [15, 18–20, 22].

The incidence of intermediate bleedings was with 15% of all cycles under discontinous Buserelin/norethisterone acetate treatment significantly lower as compared to a continous medication [16, 19, 22]. Intermediate bleedings were reported mainly in the first two cycles under medication and were mostly of spotting nature. Two volunteers with repeated intermediate bleedings had been suffering from bleeding abnormalities already, before even using other hormonal contraceptives.

The 6 endometrial biopsy specimens obtained in the last cycle under treatment revealed in no case any sign of increased proliferation or even hyperplasia as observed under continous treatment [19, 22]. The discontinous Buserelin treatment with an additional progestin administration allows therefore a much better cycle control than the permanent treatment with the analogon only [16, 19, 21]. The induced withdrawal bleedings prevent the permanent stimulation of estrogens. Phases of longer lasting amenorrhea were not found in contrast to the continous treatment [15, 16, 19–22]. In 3 cycles with missing withdrawal bleedings were preceeding intermediate bleedings reported that can be traced back to a corpus luteum insufficiency.

No alterations in thyreoidea function were demonstrable in 19/20 volunteers except in one, who developed a latent hypothyreosis during treatment. In this case the functional impairment still persisted 5 months after treatment. It must not necessarily be connected with Buserelin treatment; above all, no alterations could be found in the remaining 19 volunteers. As found also in animal experiments [34], no alterations in blood picture, liver and kidney function, blood lipids and coagulation were demonstrable. The most prominent side effects were hot flushes in two thirds of volunteers, half of them experiencing them as bothersome. Mainly volunteers with markedly suppressed estrogen levels suffered from hot flushes which persisted after treatment in cases with estradiol levels below 40 pg/ml. The incidence of these side effects is in contrast to that found by other authors [32], who reported estrogen-induced side effects only under higher dosages and permanent treatment [19, 20]. Further side effects found in 25% were acne, partially connected with seborrhea and hirsutism, the typical symptoms of hyperandrogenemia. Preexisting androgen symptoms enhanced under treatment.

Several influences on androgen metabolism under discontinous Buserelin/norethisterone acetate treatment have to be discussed. The significant increase of the LH/FSH ratio might influence the androgen synthesis in theka cells [35, 36]. Except in one volunteer, who already had elevated testosterone and DHEA-S levels before treatment, both androgens remained unchanged during the study. As one of the main ovarian androgens, the Δ 4-androstene-dione [37, 38], was not determined, its influence cannot be excluded. An influence by elevated prolactin levels via a stimulation of adrenal androgen production [39–41] could be excluded because of unchanged prolactin serum levels.

On the other hand, a decrease in the concentration of sex hormone binding globulin [42], due to suppressed estradiol levels, could lead to an increase in the "free" (not protein bound), although overall constant, androgen fraction. This might induce or even enhance androgen symptoms, especially in borderline cases. Finally, the effects of norethisterone acetate have to be considered, which might induce such symptoms due to its androgenic side effects as a 19-nor-testosterone derivative [43]. Similar observations have not been made under continous Buserelin treatment. It seems therefore possible that the application of this progestin with a relatively high total dosis of 35 mg is responsible for the androgenic side effects.

In contrast to other reports [16, 19–21] disturbances persisted in parts of our collective in follicle maturation beyond treatment. Only 12/18 volunteers with regular ovulations in the first control cycle showed an ovulatory post treatment control cycle. However, these last control cycles were duration significantly prolonged with approximately 40 days. Another 6 volunteers showed in 4 cases a corpus luteum insufficiency with a 42-day cycle, while two cycles were anovulatory. The remaining two volunteers, who showed cycle abnormalities before treatment, had anovulatory cycles after treatment lasting more than 50 days. In two volunteers the bleeding had to be induced by gestagen application. In all cases, the additional influence of the gestagen in terms of delayed or missing follicle maturation after treatment should be discussed.

With respect to the better cycle control and the absence of long-lasting estrogen-dependent stimulation of the endometrium, the discontinous Buserelin treatment with a progestin-induced withdrawal bleeding is superior to the continous Buserelin medication for contraceptive treatment. Due to the side effects, but especially because of the more complicated mode of application, it is no alternative concept in comparison to the "pill". To what extent the side effects can be eliminated by choice of progestins with less androgenic potency, for example cyproterone acetate, has to be clarified by further investigations. This mode of contraception might still be of value for women, where other contraceptive devices are contra-indicant.

References

[1] Belchetz, P. E., T. M. Plant, Y. Nakai et al.: Science **202** (1978) 631.
[2] Knobil, E., T. M. Plant, L. Wildt et al.: Science **207** (1980) 1371.
[3] Knobil, E.: Biol. Reprod. **24** (1981) 44.
[4] Leyendecker G., Eur. J. Obstet. Gynecol. Reprod. Biol. 9 (1979) 175.
[5] Leyendecker, G. T. Struve, E. J. Plotz: Arch. Gynecol. **229** (1980) 177.
[6] Crowley, W. F., J. W. McArthur: J. Clin. Endocrinol. Metab. **51** (1980) 173.
[7] Dericks-Tan, J. S. E., E. Hammer, H. D. Toubert: J. Clin. Endocrinol. Metab. **45** (1977) 597.
[8] Nillius, S. J., C. Bergquist, L. Wide: Contraception **17** (1978) 537.
[9] Bergquist C., S. J. Nillius, L. Wide: Lancet **2** (1979) 215.
[10] Hanker, J. P., H. P. Bohnet, D. Mühlenstedt et al.: Acta Endocrinol. **89** (1978) 625.
[11] Schmidt-Gollwitzer, K., W. Hardt, G. Rebholz et al.: Acta Endocrinol. (Kbh.) Suppl. **225** (1979) 357.
[12] Hoffmann, G., R. H. Ackermann, K. Pollow: Arch. Gynecol. **232** (1981) 616.
[13] Friedrich, E., R. Baumann, H. Brandau et al.: Neuroendocrinol. Lett. **3** (1981) 53.
[14] Bergquist, C., S. J. Nillius, L. Wide: J. Clin. Endocrinol. Metab. **49** (1979) 472.
[15] Bergquist, C., S. J. Nillius, L. Wide: Contraception. **19** (1979) 497.
[16] Nillius, S. J., C. Bergquist, L. Wide: Int. J. Fertil. **25** (1980) 239.
[17] Baumann, R., H. Kuhl, H. D. Taubert et al.: Contraception **21** (1980) 191.
[18] Schmidt-Gollwitzer, M., W. Hardt, K. Schmidt-Gollwitzer et al.: Acta Eur. Fertil. **12** (1981) 275.
[19] Hardt, W., M. Schmidt-Gollwitzer, M. von der Ohe et al.: Geburtsh. Frauenheilk. **41** (1981) 791.
[20] Bergquist, C., S. J. Nillius, L. Wide: Fertil. Steril. **38** (1982) 190.
[21] Bergquist, C., S. J. Nillius, L. Wide et al.: Fertil. Steril. **36** (1981) 339.
[22] Schmidt-Gollwitzer, M., W. Hardt, K. Schmidt-Gollwitzer et al.: Contraception **23** (1981) 187.
[23] Skarin, G., S. J. Nillius, L. Wide: Acta Endocrinol. (Kbh.), 1983 (in press).
[24] Heber, D., R. S. Swerdloff: J. Clin. Endocrinol. Metab. **52** (1981) 171.

[25] Wildt, L., A. Häusler, G. Marshall et al.: Endocrinology **109** (1981) 376.
[26] Knobil, E.: Recent Prog. Horm. Res. **36** (1980) 53.
[27] Sandow, J., W. von Rechenberg, G. Jerzabek et al.: Fertil. Steril. **30** (1978) 205.
[28] Sandow, J., R. N. Clayton, H. Kuhl: In: Endocrinology of Human Infertility. New Aspects, p. 221. Academic Press, 1981.
[29] Sandow, J.: In: Neuroendocrine Perspectives (Eds. E. E. Müller, R. M. MacLeod), Vol. 1, p. 339. Elsevier Biomedical Press, 1982.
[30] Sandow, J., R. N. Clayton: In: Progress in Hormone Biochemistry and Pharmacology, vol. 2. Eden Press, 1982.
[31] Sandow, J., H. Kuhl, G. Jerzabek et al.: In: The Gonadotropins: Basic Science and Clinical Aspects in Females (Eds. C. Flamigini, J. R. Givens), p. 77. Academic Press, 1982.
[32] Hardt, W., K. Schmidt-Gollwitzer, J. Nevinny-Stickel et al.: Geburtsh. Frauenheilk. **42** (1982) 874.
[33] Lemay, A., N. Faure, F. Labrie: Acta Endocrinol. (Kbh.) **103**, Suppl. 256 (1983) 75.
[34] Sandow, J., G. Jerabek-Sandow, B. Krauss et al.: In: LH-RH Peptides as Female and Male Contraceptives (Eds. G. I. Zatuchni, J. D. Shelton, J. J. Sciarra, p. 338. Harper & Row, Philadelphia 1981.
[35] Erickson, G. F., K. J. Ryan: Endocrinology **99** (1976) 452.
[36] Tsang, B. K., Y. S. Moon, C. W. Simpson et al.: J. Clin. Endocrinol. Metab. **48** (1979) 153.
[37] McNatty, K. P., D. T. Baird, A. Bolton et al.: J. Endocr. **71** (1976) 77.
[38] Genazzani, A. R., G. Magrini, F. Facchinetti et al.: In: Androgens and Antiandrogens (Eds. L. Martini, M. Motta), p. 247, Raven Press, New York 1977.
[39] Carter, J. N., J. E. Tyson, G. L. Warner et al.: J. Clin. Endocrinol. Metab. **45** (1977) 973.
[40] Vermeulen, A., E. Suy, R. Rubens: J. Clin. Endocrinol. Metab. **44** (1977) 1222.
[41] Vermeulen, A., D. Ando: Clin. Endocrinol. (Oxf.) **8** (1978) 295.
[42] Anderson, D. C., C. David: Clin. Endocr. **3** (1974) 69.
[43] Elger, W., S. Beier: In: Aktuelle Aspekte der hormonalen Kontrazeption (Ed. J. Hammerstein), p. 9, Excerpta Medica, Amsterdam-Genf-Princeton-Tokio 1982.

Reversible down-regulation of pituitary-ovarian function induced by repetitive LH-RH agonist administration as a new approach for treatment and study of endometriosis in the human

A. Lemay, R. Maheux, N. Faure, C. Jean, A. T. A. Fazekas

Introduction

Endometriosis is a frequent disease during the reproductive years in women. It is frequently associated with abdominal pain and infertility. Persistance and spread of endometrial implants are related to ovarian function mainly to estrogen secretion.

Pharmacological doses of LH-RH agonist have been shown to cause paradoxical inhibition of ovarian function in various species. In normal women, once-daily intranasal insufflation of [D-Ser^6 (TBU)-des-Gly-$NH_2{}^{10}$] LH-RH ethylamide (Buserelin) inhibits follicular maturation and ovulation in a dose-dependent manner [1, 2]. A rapid return of normal ovulatory cycle has been demonstrated following prolonged periods of treatment [3]. The inhibitory effects of LH-RH agonists are also related to the frequency of drug administration leading to a rapid down-regulation of the pituitary-gonadal function [4, 5]. Repetitive subcutaneous or intranasal administration of higher doses of neuropeptides has been successful in suppressing gonadal function in prostate cancer [6, 7], premenopausal breast cancer [8] and precocious puberty [9].

We previously reported the beneficial effects of reversible pituitary-ovarian inhibition in an endometriosis patient treated with 300 μg of intranasal Buserelin every 12 hours during 173 days [10]. We have recently established a practical regimen for suppression of testicular steroidogenesis in prostate cancer patients administering the LH-RH sequentially by the subcutaneous and intranasal routes [5]. This paper reports data from a pilot study providing evidence for the clinical efficacy and safety of LH-RH agonist administration in endometriosis.

Material and methods

Endometriosis patients

Ten women, 17 to 34 years of age, were included in the study after signing informed consent. All women had a laparoscopy within 3 months of beginning the treatment showing various degrees of pelvic endometriosis according to the American Fertility Society classification [11] (tab. 1). Patients were in good general condition and had ovulatory menstrual cycles as evaluated by basal body temperature, except for patient no. 1, who had irregular menses.

Protocol

Prior to the treatment, baseline information included complete medical history, physical examination and laboratory investigation (complete hemogram, urine analysis, SMA-16, cholesterol, triglyceride, T_3, T_4, cortisol, prolactin, as well as LH, FSH, estradiol and progesterone). Treatment was started on day 3 to 6 of the cycle. During the first 5 days, 200 µg of [D-Ser^6(TBU)-des-Gly-NH_2^{10}] LH-RH ethylamide (Buserelin, Hoechst Canada Inc., Montréal, Canada) was injected subcutaneously every 12 hours. Thereafter 400 µg of the peptide solution was insufflated into the nose every 8 hours using a nasal spray (100 µg per spray applicated twice in each nostril). In order to properly evaluate the efficacy and safety of the treatment, patients were seen at the clinic every week during the first month, every two weeks during months 2 and 3 and monthly till the end of treatment at 6 to 7 months.

On the day of the visit at the clinic, blood sampling was obtained for hormone analysis and acute gonadotropin (LH, FSH), as well as estradiol responses to the ad-

Table 1 Age and laparoscopic staging of endometriosis patients according to the American Fertility Society classification

No	Initial	Age	Stage Clinical	Grade	Points
1	ML	22	Severe	III	21
2	DM	28	Mild	I	1
3	GF	33	Moderate	II	7
4	DN	32	Mild	I	2
5	GH	17	Mild	I	2
6	RL	31	Moderate	II	8
7	TY	32	Mild	I	5
8	FS	34	Extensive	IV	52
9	BL	24	Extensive	IV	35
10	MT	33	Moderate	II	11

ministration of the compound. Basal levels of progesterone were also measured at weekly and monthly visits. Basal body temperature was taken daily. Complete physical examination and biological tests were performed every two months. A control laparoscopy was carried out at the end of treatment including an endometrial biopsy or curettage.

Laboratory methods

Serum LH and FSH were measured by specific radioimmunoassays currently used in the laboratory [12]. Materials for LH and FSH were supplied through the courtesy of the National Pituitary Agency, National Institute of Health, Bethesda, Maryland. Results are expressed in ng/ml of LER-907. Estradiol and progesterone were measured by highly specific antibodies developed against 17-β estradiol-6(0-carboxymethyl) oxime and progesterone-3-(0-carboxyme-oxime) after extraction of duplicate aliquots in anhydrons ether, Radioimmonoassay data were analysed with a program derived from model II of Rodbard and Lewald [13].

Results

Serum gonadotropin and sex steroid levels and uterine bleeding

Gonadotropins and sex steroids profiles of patient no. 6 (RL) during the treatment period are illustrated in figure 1 and are representative of the general pattern observed in response to the treatment. Before beginning the treatment, basal levels of LH and FSH are, repsectively, 20 and 160 ng/ml. Four hours after the initial injecton of 200 µg of Buserelin serum gonadotropins are maximally stimulated, LH and FSH being 20 and 4-fold increased, respectively. Already at the second injection at 12 hours the LH response is blunted while the FSH response is completely prevented. FSH levels return to basal values on the second day of treatment and remain at that level for the entire period of treatment. A slower decrease of serum LH values is in the normal range although they remain 50–100% above pretreatment controls. For both gonadotropins, the acute response to LH-RH agonist administration was always abolished during the entired treatment period.

Following gonadotropin stimulation, serum estradiol rises from 28 pg/ml at time 0 to 157 pg/ml at 14 hours. At week 1 serum estradiol is 64 pg/ml and reaches a maximal value of 290 pg/ml at week 2. In the following 3 weeks the steroid level steadily decreases to stabilize around 20 pg/ml. Serum progesterone levels were measured at every weekly and monthly visit. There was no increase in this hormone at any time, levels always being below 0.5 ng/ml.

Following the fall of sex steroid, an estrogen withdrawal bleeding occurs as also shown in figure 1. Brownish spotting occurs on days 21 to 25 and on day 53. No other uterine bleeding occurred during the 6-month treatment period.

A similar gonadotropin response was obtained in all the patients. The stimulation of estradiol varied between individual women during the first month of treatment. After one week 5 patients had estradiol levels above 100 pg/ml, 3 in the early follicular range and in 2 below 25 pg/ml. At week 4 the mean level was 24±8 pg, which was 45% below starting levels of the early follicular phase and continued to decrease to 8±2 pg/ml at month 6 corresponding to an 81% inhibition. All the patients had spotting or light bleeding between weeks 1 and 4, depending on the level and dura-

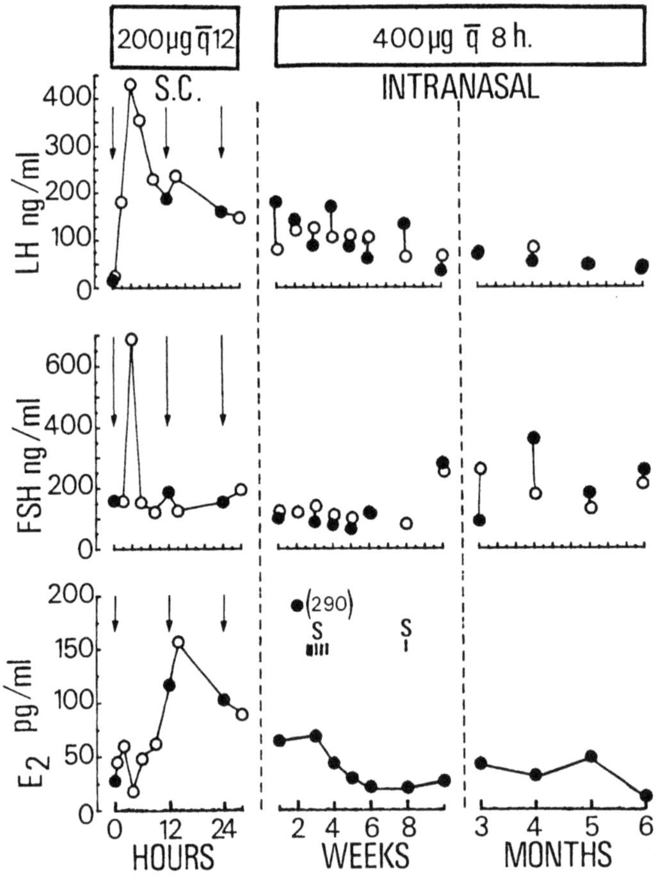

Fig. 1 Gonadotropins and sex steroid profiles during LH-RH agonist (Buserelin) treatment of patient GS. Buserelin was administered S. C. every 12h. for 5 days and then I. N. every 8 hours.
●: Hormone level at the time of drug administration
○: Hormone level at different times during the first day and 3 hours after treatment thereafter
S: Spotting

tion of estradiol stimulation. Two patients had an episode of light and moderate bleeding at weeks, 24 and 10 respectively while two others had occasional light bleeding or spotting and post-coital bleeding. The patient no. 10 (MT) having a uterine leiomyoma, had a prolonged episode of bleeding starting on week 5 although serum estradiol was suppressed; treatment was stopped at week 10.

Symptoms and signs of endometriosis

Five patients complained of moderate to severe intermenstrual abdominal pain before treatment. The pain was alleviated at months 2 to 4. There were no more complaints of profound dyspareunia, which was a significant problem in 4 patients.

Among the 9 patients who completed the treatment, 8 had abnormal findings at gynecological examination at the beginning of the treatment. At the end of the treatment, pain at the palpation of the uterus, ovaries and culs-de-sac was almost completely alleviated in 7 women. Nodules in the posterior cul-de-sac disappeared in one woman but one nodule was newly found in another woman at the end of treatment.

Laparoscopy and endometrial biopsy

At the second laparoscopy, performed at 6 months in the 9 patients who completed the treatment, there was an almost complete disappearance of small endometrial implants (tab. 2). When endometrial cysts were removed surgically no new implants could be seen. When adhesions were lysed, new filmy adhesions could occasionally be seen. According to the American Fertility Society, grading and/or scoring was objectively improved in all cases except in one patient (no. 8) who had a frozen pelvis

Table 2 Laparoscopy

		Before treatment				After treatment			
		Implants		Adhesions		Implants		Adhesions	
		<1 cm	>1 cm	Filmy	Dense	<1 cm	>1 cm	Filmy	Dense
1	ML	2	1	1	1	0	0	1	1
2	TM	n*				0			
3	GF	4		2		0		1	
4	AN	2		1		0		1	
5	GH	n				0		1	
6	RL	2		2	1	0		1	0
7	GY	2	1	1		2	0	0	
8	FS		2		n		0		n
9	BL	n	2		4	1	0		3
10	MT	n	0	1	1	–	–		–

* n: numerous

with multiple dense ahdesions. Excluding this last patient, there was a significant decrease of individual endometriosis score which decreased between 0 to 6% of initial values.

Endometrial biopsy was performed in 6 patients at the time of the second laparoscopy at the end of treatment. In 4 cases, atrophy was observed. A similiar histologic appearance of inactive endometrium was found in 3 specimens as illustrated in figure 2. A small number of thin endometrial glands are scattered in a dense cellular stroma. Trichrome staining revealed the presence of collagen fibers. In the 4th case showing atrophy, fibro-vascular tissue replaced normal stroma. The number and appearance of glands were relatively normal. In the fifth patient the histologic picture corresponded to an early follicular phase. In the sixth patient the specimen obtained at the curettage contained only blood without endometrial tissue.

Return of ovulation and fertility

Two patients had an anovulatory bleeding on day 34 and 38, after cessation of treatment. In the other 7 patients, the longest time interval before presumptive ovu-

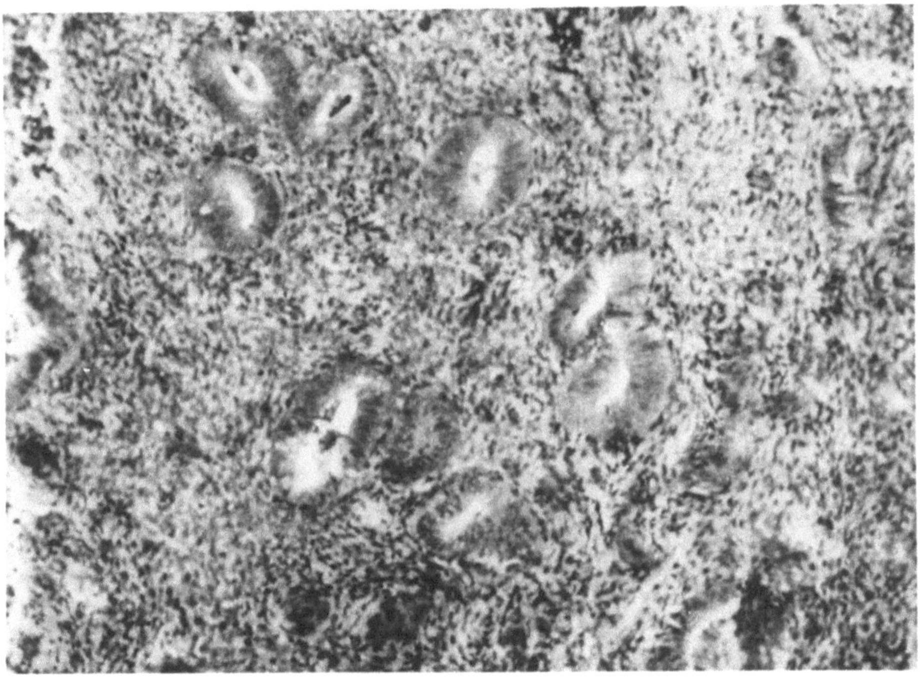

Fig. 2 Histology of endometrial biopsy in patient RL at the end of 6 months of treatment by LH-RH agonist (Buserelin) showing atrophy with cellular stroma similar to inactive endometrium of early menopause.

lation was 45 days. During the first recovery cycle 2 basal body temperature curves showed short luteal phases of 9 and 11 days. Subsequent cycles of a 6 month follow-up period were apparently normal as evaluated by basal body temperature and clinical history. The amount and duration of uterine bleeding was normal and no patient experienced significiant dysmenorrhea except patient no. 1, who complained of abdominal cramps similar to those before treatment. Patient no. 2, who had mild endometriosis but a 4, year unexplained infertility, conceived during the fifth post-treatment cycle (fig. 3). After an uneventful pregnancy she delivered a normal boy. Patient no. 3 (GF) became inadvertently pregnant on the third posttreatment cycle but an interruption of pregnancy was requested.

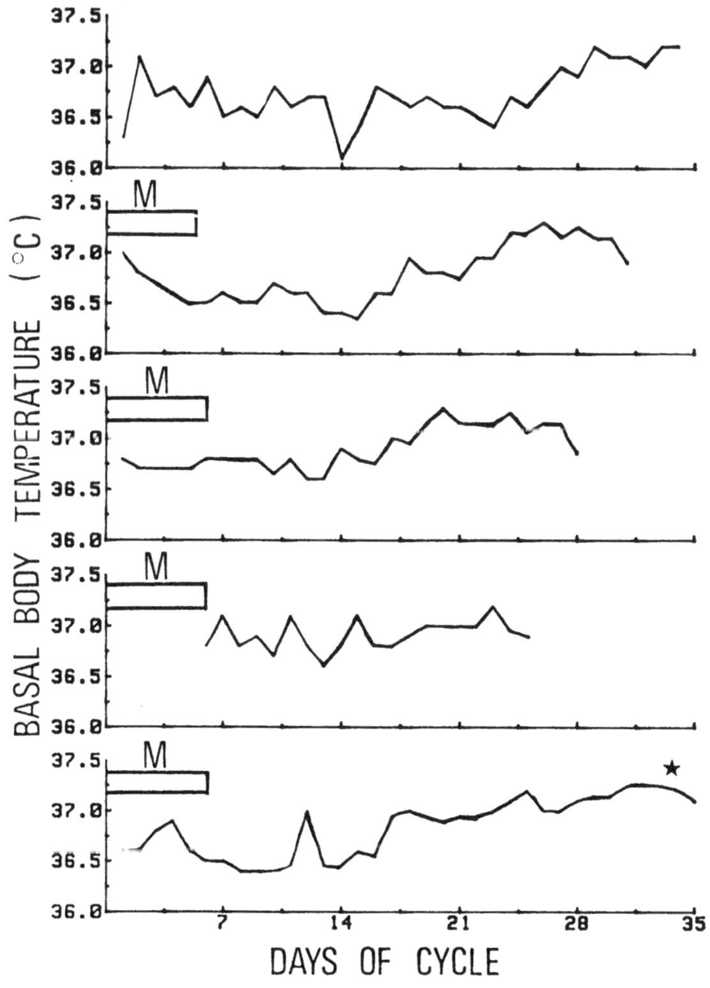

Fig. 3 Basal body temperature curves in patient DM following cessation of Buserelin treatment. Pregnancy occurred during the 5th cycle as detected by B-hCG determination (*).

Side-effects and laboratory safety data

A progressive number of women started to have hot flushes 4 weeks after beginning the treatment. At week 10 all the patients experienced significant or numerous hot flushes. In two patients hot flushes stopped at months 4 and 5.

Three women complained of vaginal dryness starting on weeks 6 to 8 and persisting until the end of treatment. In a fourth woman vaginal dryness was noted during months 5 and 6 whereas another patient was bothered by the absence of vaginal secretion during months 2 and 3.

Among 7 sexually active women, a constant decreased libido starting on month 3 was reported by 3 patients. One patient also reported discontinuous decreased libido on weeks 8, 10 and on months 5 and 6. Occasional but light breast swelling or tenderness was noted by 4 patients (nos. 6, 7, 9, 10).

There was no problem of local irritation during the subcutaneous injection period. No patient complained of nazal irritation. Overall the treatment was well accepted or tolerated by all the patients. All the inconveniences related to the state of hypoestrinism rapidly disappeared as ovarian function quickly returned after cessation of treatment.

Prior to the treatment, all biological parameters concerning hematology, urine analysis, serum biochemistry, lipids and complementary basal hormonal determinations, were within the normal range. There was no change in these clinical chemistry data as evaluated at months 2, 4 and 6 of the treatment period and at months 2 and 6 after cessation of therapy.

Discussion

Hormonal changes

The results obtained in this study show a biphasic effect of repetitive LH-RH agonist treatment. The stimulation of gonadotropin secretion was only transient. Already at 12 hours after the primary maximal increase of gonadotropin the LH and FSH responses to the agonist were almost completely prevented. We recently reported such a rapid refractoriness of the pituitary after the second intranasal administration of Buserelin in the luteal phase in normal women [14]. The transient stimulation of serum FSH was particularly short, with rapid return to basal levels on the second day of treatment. The decrease in elevated serum LH took a much longer time (4 weeks). A similar effect on serum LH and FSH has been documented recently, in normal women and polycystic ovarian disease after subcutaneous administration of 100 µg of an LH-RH agonist daily for 4 weeks [14].

A biphasic response was also observed at the ovarian level. Estradiol values already started to decrease on the second day of treatment. After 4 weeks of treatment the mean levels of estrogens were 45% below basal levels of the early follicular phase. Thereafter serum estradiol levels were further suppressed to reach menopausal levels. Such a profound inhibition of LH-RH treatment on serum estrogens also has been reported after 1 month of treatment with 100 μg of an LH-RH agonist administered daily by the subcutaneous route in 5 polycystic ovarian disease cases [14] and in 5 endometriosis patients [15].

The inhibitory effect of LH-RH agonist on follicular activity possibly could be explained by low gonadotropins levels and disruption of pulsatile secretion of gonadotropins. Frequency and amplitude of episodic gonadotropin secretion was markedly attenuated when frequent blood sampling was performed after down-regulation of gonadotropin following repetitive administration of LH-RH agonist [14, 16]. In LH-RH-treated prostate cancer patient, biological activity of serum LH was reported to be inhibited to a much lower level than the immunological activity [17].

Efficacy of treatment

The resorbtion of active endometrial implants would correlate with the profound inhibition of ovarian follicular activity. At the endometrial sampling at the time of the second laparoscopy, a limited amount of tissue could be recovered and atrophy similar to inactive endometrium of early menopause was demonstrated at histology in 4 out of 6 cases.

Improvement in abdominal pain, dyspareunia and dysmenorrhea corresponded to objective findings at gynecological examination and at the laparoscopy at the end of treatment. There was disappearance of previously identified small endometria implants. When adhesions had been previously lysed, less numerous filmy adhesions were noted. These observations provide evidence for the predominant role of serum estrogen levels in the pathogenesis of endometriosis and for the regression of implants following important inhibition of serum estradiol levels during long-term LH-RH agonist treatment.

Recently an intermittent regimen of LH-RH agonist treatment has been reported to suppress ovulation, menses and experimental endometriosis in monkeys without achieving maximal suppression of serum estradiol [18]. Preliminary observations on nuclear estrogen binding sites indicate a dissimilarity and asynchrony in human uterine endometrium versus intraovarian ectopic foci, the endometriotic foci appearing independent of the phase of the menstrual cycle [19].

Recovery of ovarian function and fertility

One important aspect of this therapeutic approach with LH-RH agonist is the rapid return of normal ovulatory cycles with normal uterine bleeding after cessation for therapy. In a 6 month follow-up period one of three patients consulting for unexplained primary infertility had a normal pregnancy. Another pregnancy occurred in a previously fertile patient wo requested an interruption.

Side effects and safety

Signs and symptoms of estrogen deprivation were the only side effects noted. Hot flushes were encountered in all the patients whereas vaginal dryness, penetration dyspareunia and decreased libido were reported in several patients but were not significant inconvenients to the treatment. No medication was given to alleviate these symptoms which rapidly disappear after cessation of treatment.

The LH-RH agonist buserelin appears to be safe since no changes in clinical chemistry data could be found during 6 months of treatment and 6 months of follow-up period. Similar safety data have been documented in prostate cancer patients in whom various amounts of neuropeptide have been administered for more than 3 years [20].

Because of its specificity and lack of side effects in tissues not under estrogenic control, this therapeutic approach appears as very interesting. Much larger studies with comparative aspects will have to be carried out to further demonstrate the efficacy of the LH-RH agonist in endometriosis. The use of very small amounts of a drug that specifically suppresses ovarian estrogen secretion in absence of other added steroids should open a new way to study the pathophysiology of endometriosis in the human.

References

[1] Bergquist, C., S. J. Nillius, L. Wide: Contraception **19** (1979) 497–506.
[2] Schmidt-Gollwitzer, M., W. Hardt. K. Schmidt-Gollwitzer: Contraception **23** (1981) 187–196.
[3] Bergquist, C., S. J. Nillius, L. Wide: Fertil. Steril. **38** (1982) 190–193.
[4] Lemay, A., N. Faure, F. Labrie et al.: Fertil. Steril. **39** (1938) 661–667.
[5] Hanker, J. P., J. Knippenberg, A. J. Kastin: Int. J. Fertil. **25** (1980) 7–17.
[6] Faure, N., F. Labrie, A. Lemay: Fertil. Steril. **37** (1982) 416–424.
[7] Tolis, G., D. Ackman, A. Stellos et al.: Proc. Natl. Acad. Sci. USA **79** (1982) 1658–1662.
[8] Klijn, J. G. M., F. H. De Jong: Lancet **I** (1982) 1213–1216.
[9] Crowley, W. F., F. Comite, W. Vale et al.: J. Clin. Endocrinol. Metab. **52** (1981) 370–372.
[10] Lemay, A., G. Quesnel: Fertil. Steril. **38** (1982) 376–379.
[11] American Fertility Society: Fertil. Steril. **32** (1979) 633–634.
[12] Lemay, A., N. Faure, F. Labrie: Fertil. Steril. **37** (1982) 193–200.

[13] Rodbard, D., J. E. Lewald: Second Karolinska Symposium on Research Methods in Reproductive Endocrinology (edited by E. Diczfalusy), pp. 79–103. Bogtryheiret Forum, Copenhagen 1970.
[14] Chang, R. J., L. R. Laufer, D. R. Meldrum et al.: J. Clin. Endocrinol. Metab. **56** (1983) 897–903.
[15] Meldrum, D. R., R. J. Chang, J. Lu et al.: J. Clin. Endocrinol. Metab. **54** (1982) 1081–1083.
[16] Doelle, G. C., R. M. Evans, A. N. Alexander et al.: Encyclopedia in Reproductive Health Care, in press.
[17] Kelly, S., F. Labrie, A. Dupont: Endocrinol. Soc. Meeting, Abst. 3, San Antonio, June (1983).
[18] Werlin, L. B., G. D. Hodgen: J. Clin. Endocrinol. Metab. **56** (1983) 844–848.
[19] Gould, S. F., J. M. Shannon, G. R. Cunha: Fertil. Steril. **39** (1983) 520–524.
[20] Faure, N., A. Lemay, G. Tolis et al.: Encyclopedia in Reproductive Health Care, MTP-Press, in press.

The treatment of endometriosis with LH-RH agonists

W. Hardt, T. Genz, M. Schmidt-Gollwitzer †

Introduction

Female sexual steroids can have an unfavorable effect on the course of hormonal-dependant disorders such as endometriosis or mammary carcinoma. Similar to the uterine mucous membranes, the ectopic endometrium is also subject to the influence of cyclic secretion of ovarian sexual steroids, particularily estradiol, which can lead to further spreading of the disorder [9]. Endometriosis in particular, with its many variations, although defined as a benign hormone-dependant condition, can lead to severe physical and psychological distress, ultimately resulting in invalidity. The characteristic and commonly extreme complaints such as dysmenorrhea, dyspareunia and chronic discomfort of the lower abdomen can often result in severe disturbance of intimacy even in non-extreme cases. Furthermore this obscure disease frequently occurs in the reproductive years and is commonly associated with female infertility.

Since endometriosis is a disease of hormonal-dependant tissue, causal therapy invariably involves disruption of the gonadal function. One therapeutic possibility is irreversible surgical castration, another is the reversible pharmacologic suppression of the gonadal function [5]. The choice of treatment depends on the extent of the disorder, age and, where relevant, the woman's desire to have children. The object of the treatment is invariably the suppression or reduction to an acceptable level of discomfort, inhibition or regression of tumor development, maintenance of the woman's fertility or a total cure. The latter can usually be achieved by drastic surgery, as a rule involving castration. Where conservative surgery is required, commonly in younger women, involving retention of the internal genital organs, particularily the ovaries, recurrence of the disorder is to be expected even when only remmnants of the endometriosis are left.

The value of medicational hormone therapy is readily appreaciated in terms of the time period required for suppression of the symptoms and possible regression of the tumor. Requirements of the medication are speed and efficiency, full reversibility, good tolerability and as few side effects as possible. None of the currently available drugs, such as the various gestagens or danazol meet all these requirements. Danazol, for example, although of proven efficiency in the treatment of endometriosis, commonly has such severe sideeffects that it only can be used in certain cases, i.e. long-term treatment with this substance at a therapeutic level is scarcely feasible [5]. Although the pituitary function is largely suppressed by this substance, estrogen secretion, with its not insignificant stimulatory effect on the ectopic endometrium, frequently remains to a certain extent.

Thus it seemed logical to use the paradoxical antifertility effect of the LH-RH agonists, such as Buserelin, in the medicational treatment of endometriosis. This peptide hormone, with its specific effect on the pituitary, simple degradation and metabolization and hence good tolerability, appeared predestined for use in the treatment of endometriosis [4, 6, 10].

Material and methods

The course of treatment was as follows: Buserelin was applied intranasally at a daily dose of 900 mcg over a period of six months. Along with clinical palpation, hormone determinations were carried out at frequent intervalls, accompanied where possible by endometrium biopsies and, on completion of the therapy, by second look laparoscopy or laparotomy, with subsequent histological examination.

Twenty-six female patients took part in the study, twenty-two of whom had severest endometriosis (stage III of the Acostaclassification [1]). Only 4 of the patients were afflicted with a mild or moderate endometriosis. Seventeen of the patients were primarily infertile. The age distribution lay between 20 and 44 years, with an average of 31.6 and mainly severe symptoms between 2 and 15 years. The diagnosis was confirmed in all cases by laparoscopy or laparotomy prior to the Buserelin treatment. Seventeen of the patients had undergone earlier surgery, most commonly involving partial or total unilateral ovarian resection. Particularily notable cases, involving for example extensive intenstinal resection or removal of a bladder tumor, will be considered in detail later.

Results

The most common symptoms were dysmenorrhea, chronic abdominal discomfort and dyspareunia. Defacational pain during he menstrual period, synchronal intestinal bleeding or cyclic vaginal bleeding following hysterctomy were less frequent (tab. 1). Endometrium tumors in the study group were located notably in the Douglas' pouch, in the parametrium, the lig. sacro-uterinum and the vagina. In 4 cases the intestine was involved to varying degrees and in 1 case the bladder was severely afflicted.

As far as size-description from palpation was possible, the ovarian endometriomas were described as of 3 cm diameter up to fist-size. In the Douglas pouch, the para-

Table 1 Main symptoms of endometriosis in 26 cases with severe endometriosis (multiple registration)

Dismenorrhea	18
Chronic pelvic pain	9
Dyspareunia	4
Defacation pain during menses	3
Bowel bleeding	1
Hamaturia	1
Vaginal bleeding after hysterectomy	1

metrium and rectovaginal findings were discussed as finger-thick, plum-, walnut- or tomato-size.

In a prior study on healthy fertile women, we were able to show that estrogen secretion could be suppressed by postmenopause values with a daily dose of 800 to 1200 mcg buserelin, although in a few cases, particularly in the first 2–3 months of treatment, a transitory estrogen increase could be detected (fig. 1). With the occurence of hot flushes, however, ovarian supression was constant in all cases (tab. 2).

Table 2 Side effects of the treatment with Buserelin

Appearance of hot flushes		
1– 4 weeks	15	21
5– 8 weeks	6	
8–16 weeks	2	
no	2	

As expected, the hormone profiles in the 26 patients with endoendometriosis followed a similar pattern. In 21 cases complete and constant pharmacological castration, with the accompagnying signs of estrogen depletion, was achieved within 2–4 weeks. In 3 cases the effect was delayed, i.e. within 3 months in 2 cases a more or less marked estrogen increase was noted before the end of the six month's observation period.

Hot flushes occured 2–4 weeks after the proven suppression of the gonad function, in 21 cases within the first two months.

In accordance with the initial short-term stimulation of estrogen-release, menstrual bleeding occured in 10 cases within the first 4–6 weeks. In two cases only accompanying pain was reported. Subsequently, particularily in the 3rd and 4th months, short-term painless bleeding occured in 6 cases. Only one patient complained of unchanged discomfort during the later bleeding. As previously mentioned, estrogen secretion could not be permanently suppressed in this patient. Earlier treatment of this patient with Lynestrenol and Danazol produced the same reaction. The endo-

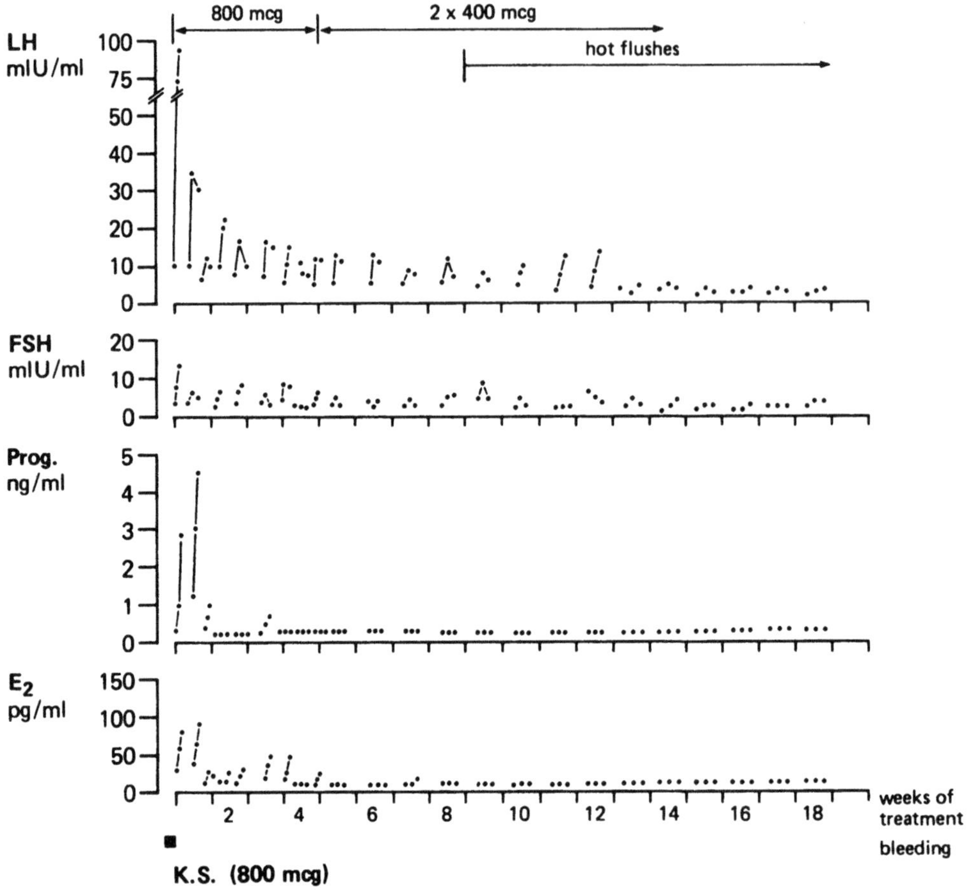

Fig. 1 Gonadotropin and sex steroid hormone levels during the treatment with 800 mcg Buserelin.

metrium biopsies carried out towards the end of treatment showed inactive endometrium in 11 cases (tab. 3). In 7 cases insufficient material was obtainable for assessment. Only one endometrium biopsy, performed in the 3rd month of therapy in one of the patients with persistant estrogen secretion, showed endometrium proliferation with transition to simple hyperlasia. Atrophic endometrium was found in 8 out of 9 endometriotic lesions obtained at laparotomy. Ovarian tissues showed only primordial follicels (tab. 4).

For the assessment of clinical applicability the decline of subjective discomfort or of the tumor itself is of greater significance than the effect of the drug on the endocrine functions (tab. 5). Twenty of the 26 women were completely without discomfort within 4–6 weeks. In 4 cases discomfort was reported to have decreased significantly, if not completely. In 2 cases pain remained unchanged up to the end of treatment.

Table 3 Results of endometrial biopsies taken during the treatment with Buserelin (n = 19)

Inactive endometrium	11
No material	7
Proliferation and hyperplasie (third month)	1

Table 4 Histological results of endometriotic lesions and ovaries after treatment with Buserelin

Endometriotic tissue (n = 9)

- 8 atrophy
- 1 mild-moderate proliferation

Ovarian tissue (n = 3)

- 3 quiescent ovary

Table 5 Clinical results of the treatment with Buserelin (n = 26)

Disappearance of pain	20
Relief of pain	4
No change	2

Table 6 Overall results of the treatment with Buserelin

- Relief of pain
- Tumour reduction
- Cessation of bowel bleeding or hamaturia
- No side effects
- High acceptability

In 10 out of 12 cases with readily palpable endometriose tumors mainly in the Douglas pouch or the rectovaginal area, a reduction in size of the tumor to a half or a third of its initial size was noted. Further, the tissue had generally softened and become less sensitive to palpation. In 2 cases the tumor remained unchanged both in size and sensitivity. A further ten cases with tumors which were difficult to define, the results could not easily be interpreted.

Hot flushes of varying intensity are not side-effects; they are the expected biological reactions to suppression of the gonadal function. Similarily subjective complaints such as insomnia and lack of concentration, as well as dry hair and skin, must seen as estrogen deficiency symptoms. In some cases slight loss in weight was recorded (2–4 kg) and in one case a gain of 2 kg. One patient reported increased activity of pre-existing acne, and another patient conspicuous muscular tension in arms and legs. All in all, side effects in the whole group over the 6-month observation period were very slight and particularily compared to Danazol, at no time gave grounds for discontinuing the therapy. The overall results are despicted in table 6.

Discussion

Although clinical studies with gestagens or Danazol are not available, it is clear, in view of the negligable side-effects and resulting tolerability of the LH-RH agonists that these would be the medication of choice at an equivalent level of effectiveness [2, 7, 8]. Since no serious side-effects occur it now remains to be investigated whether longer-term treatment with Buserelin can effect a cure in some patients. Our limited observations have shown that in advanced cases of endometriosis recurrence of the symptoms is to be expected within a few months. Even in so-called mild or moderate forms of endometriosis renewed ovarian function leads more commonly than postulated to recurrence of the disease. Reversible pharmacological castration is possible using the LH-RH agonist Buserelin in women as well as in men with advanced prostate cancer [3, 7, 8]. The advantages over the conventional medicational therapy are marked. Particularly where conservative surgery is to be attempted, treatment with LH-RH agonist should precede the operation.

In 10 out of 12 cases with readily palpable endometrium tumors, mainly in the Douglas pouch or the rectovaginal area, a reduction in size of the tumor was noted. Further, the tissue had generally softened and become less sensitive to palpation. In 2 cases the tumor remained unchanged both in size and sensitivity. In a further 10 cases with tumors which were difficult to define, the results could not be easily interpreted.

References

[1] Acosta, A. A., V. C. Buttram Jr., P. K. Besch et al.: Obstet. Gynecol. **42** (1973) 19.

[2] Bergquist, C., J. Nillius, L. Wide: Lancet II (1979) 215.

[3] Borgmann, V., W. Hardt, H. Adenauer et al.: Lancet **1083** (1982) 1097.

[4] Corbin, A., F. J. Bex: In: LH-RH Peptides as Female and Male Contraception (eds. G. I. Zatuchni, D. Shelton, J. J. Sciarra). Harper and Row, Philadelphia 1982.

[5] Dmowski, W. P., M. R. Cohen: Amer. J. Obstet. Gynecol. **130** (1978) 41.

[6] Fraser, H. M., N. C. Laird, D. M. Blakely: Endocrinology **106** (1980) 452.

[7] Hardt, W., M. Schmidt-Gollwitzer, M. von der Ohe et al.: J. Geburtsh. Frauenheilk. **41** (1981) 791.

[8] Hardt, W., M. Schmidt-Gollwitzer: Clin. Endocrinol. **19** (1983) 613.

[9] Kistner, R. W.: In: Gynecology and Obstetrics, Vol. II, Ch. 43. Harper and Row, Hagerstown 1968.

[10] Sandow, J.: In: Neuroendocrine Perspectives, Vol. 1 (eds. E. E. Müller, R. M. McLeod), pp. 339. Elsevier Biomedical Press, Amsterdam 1982.

Concluding remarks

We have now reached the end of this workshop. It has been shown during these three days that by the experimental work of Ernest Knobil and many others a wide and new field in basic and clinical research has been opened in which we are learning to better understand some of the basic physiological processes in reproduction.

In the list of new findings, new methods of therapy using LH-RH and its analogues are in their first stage of development.

The workshop has also shown quite clearly the areas of agreement in, and possibly even more important, the limits of our present knowledge. Braod areas of disagreement and controversy which will require elucidation in the future were recognized.

The extensive discussions following the contributions show that each individual paper has revealed new facts, ideas or opinions. Some of the papers were truly works of art in their clear presentation of data and their intellectual interpretation and evaluation. Highlights in the evaluation of facts against opinions – occasionally in the form of a "happening" – were also reached in the spontaneous discussions.

In trying to arrive at some general conclusions from a clinician's point of view, the following six items should be mentioned:

1. It has been established that the pulsatile administration of LH-RH with an infusion pump is a new method for the induction of ovulation of high practical value. Continuous pulsatile administration of LH-RH or substitution by HCG is necessary to maintain normal length and function of the corpus luteum.
2. Discovery of the LH-RH analogues, in form of agonists and antagonists, has opened up a new class of pharmaceuticals. We are still in the phase of pharmacological definition of many of these drugs, their actions and safety.
3. Safety and lack of severe side-effects would seem to be a clear advantage in using the pharmaceuticals in humans.
4. At the moment, the results of preliminary experiments in non-human primates and in humans allow cautious optimism that LH-RH analogues could gain some importance as an antifertility agent in women in the future. From the practical point of view, here again, the lack of side-effects should be an important factor.
5. Whether the new drugs will be of any importance for suppression of fertility in the male is still doubtful.

6. Many preliminary results on the positive reaction of different diseases in men and women to LH-RH analogues have been reported, including Carcinoma of the prostate and the breast, endometriosis, Pubertas praecox, premenstrual syndrome and others. More data and more time are necessary for final evaluation of the new drugs for these conditions.

In the name of all participants I would like to express our sincere gratitude to the Schering Company in Berlin for sponsoring this workshop. In particular I would like to thank Professor Gerhard, Professor Laudahn and Professor Neumann for their personal efforts and help in preparing this workshop. For more than half a century Schering has belonged to the pioneers of basic and clinical research in the endocrinology of reproductive processes. I would like to remind you of the early work of Dr. Hohlweg on the feed-back mechanisms which has been discussed many times in the course of this workshop. I remind you also of the early cooperation of Schering with Adolf Butenandt, at that time at the Kaiser-Wilhelm-Institut of Biochemistry, and with the gynecologist Carl Kaufmann working at the famous Charité in Berlin. This cooperation was of vital importance for the development of the clinical use of steroid hormones. It was introduced by Dr. Schöller from Schering. This gread tradition can be followed through up the present day. We are also happy that this extensive discussion of a new field in the physiology of reproduction has been possible in a city marked by many historical events in endocrine research.

The organization of any kind of a meeting was excellent, if everything went off smoothly, but nobody has the feeling it was organized. This has been the case during this meetint and we are obliged to Professor Schmidt-Gollwitzer as well as to Dr. Schreiber and Mrs. Schley. Final decisions for the invitations were made by Professor Schmidt-Gollwitzer. I think we all agree that he has been extremely successfull in calling together a group of experts tho were ready – as the discussions have shown – to learn from each other.

Thank you again Professor Schmidt-Gollwitzer, you have been a splendid host for these three days, thank you also Dr. Schreiber and Mrs. Schley for the invisible work you have done before and during these days. And last but not least, I would like to thank the organizers of the meeting for the warm and informal atmosphere we have enjoyed from the beginning.

J. Zander

List of First-mentioned Contributors

Asch, R., Health Science Center San Antonio, The University of Texas, San Antonio, Tx., USA
Balmaceda, J. C., Health Science Center San Antonio, The University of Texas, San Antonio, Tx., USA
Bancroft, J., Center for Reproductive Biology, MRC Reproductive Biology Unit, Edinburgh, UK
Berg, D., I. Universitäts-Frauenklnik, München FRG
Corbin, A., Wyeth Laboratories, Philadelphia, Pa., USA
Coy, D. H., School of Medicine, Tulane University, New Orleans, La., USA
Emons, G., Klinik für Frauenheilkunde und Geburtshilfe, Medizinische Hochschule Lübeck, Lübeck, FRG
Faure, N., National Institutes of Health Bethseda, Md., USA
Fraser, H. M., Center for Reproductive Biology, MRC Reproductive Biology Unit, Edinburgh, UK
Do Won Hahn, Ortho Pharmaceutical Corporation, Raritan, N. J., USA
Hardt, W., Universitäts-Klinikum Charlottenburg, Freie Universität Berlin, Berlin, FRG
Hodgen., G. D., Pregnancy Research Branch, NICHD, National Institutes of Health, Bethesda, Md., USA
Hoffmann, G., Abt. für Experimentelle Endokrinologie der Johannes-Gutenberg-Universität, Mainz, FRG
Labrie, F., Dept. of Molecular Endocrinology & Medicine, Université Laval, Quebec, Qu., Canada
Laudahn, G., Fachbereich Medizin, Schering Aktiengesellschaft, Berlin, FRG
Lemay, A., Endocrinologie de la Reproduction, Université Laval, Quebec, Qu., Canada
Merz, W. E., Institut für Biochemie, Universität Heidelberg, FRG
Nagel, R., Universitäts-Klinikum Charlottenburg, Freie Universität von Berlin, Berlin, FRG
Nillius, S. J., Dept. of Gynecology and Obstetrics, University Hospital, Uppsala, Sweden
Pescovitz, O. H., National Institutes of Health, Bethesda, Md., USA
Popkin, R., Center for Reproductive Biology, MRC Reproductive Biology Unit, Edinburgh, UK
Rivier, C., The Salk Institute, San Diego, Ca., USA
Sandow, J., Department für Pharmakologie, Hoechst AG, Frankfurt (Main), FRG
Schmidt-Gollwitzer, M. †
Swerdloff, R. S., Div. Endocrinology, Harbor UCLA, Med. Center, Torrance, Ca., USA
Vickery, B. H., Syntex Research, Division of Syntex (USA), Inc., Palo Alto, Ca., USA
Wildt, L., Universitäts-Frauenklinik, Bonn, FRG
Zander, J., I. Universitäts-Frauenklinik, München, FRG

Bei Fragen zur Produktsicherheit wenden Sie sich bitte an:
If you have any questions regarding product safety,
please contact:

Walter de Gruyter GmbH
Genthiner Straße 13
10785 Berlin
productsafety@degruyterbrill.com